W9-ANR-906

CRITICAL ACCLAIM FOR

Children and Teens Afraid to Eat

I CAN'T RECOMMEND THIS BOOK STRONGLY ENOUGH! Ms. Berg writes with compassion while exposing and dispelling many prejudicial beliefs. . . . One of the best messages that this book expresses is the basic human right to be treated as an individual.

— Journal of Family Life

BERG SERVES UP A FEAST of facts on dysfunctional eating, eating disorders, size prejudice and overweight. Condemning "diets," she instead proposes a wellness paradigm based on the Canadian "vitality" model.

The book contains advice for parents but emphasizes that social change is needed in schools, organized sports, and federal policies that focus too narrowly on antiobesity. The unique problems of boys and minority children are also explored. Berg's book is a valuable consciousness raiser.

Recommended for public libraries for both parents and concerned professionals.

— Library Journal

WHAT CAN WE DO to combat destructive influences and feelings about weight? . . . Setting a nutritionally-sound example, encouraging regular exercise, questioning advertising and role model images and focusing on accepting kids for who they are, rather than what they look like, Berg says.

— The New York Post

THE AUTHOR PRESENTS A COMPELLING CASE . . . the discussion on how to help overweight children and children with eating disorders is very well written, featuring excellent tables that highlight practical tips for parents and for nutrition educators.

Anyone who works in the area of weight control and disordered eating will want a copy of this book on his or her shelf.

— Journal of the American Dietetic Association

AS THE PARENT of a daughter who acquired a serious eating disorder in her teens, I can only wish that Frances Berg's book had come along sooner, and health and education professionals had heeded its advice years ago.

Thankfully we have it now. Berg provides badly needed ammunition to those who, like myself, have been groping for weapons in the battle to save kids, both thin and fat, from a lifetime of size oppression. . . . Long overdue.
— *William J. Fabrey*
Director, Council on Size & Weight Discrimination

FRANCES BERG POINTS OUT how the medical profession's insistence on ideal weight as a national health priority has reinforced and validated the obsession with body size and shape.

Instead of improved health, efforts that were supposed to help people manage their weight have backfired, contributing to an epidemic of body dissatisfaction, size discrimination, restrictive eating, bizarre eating disorders, poor nutrition, and increased depression, anxiety, frustration and low self-esteem among our nation's youth.
— *Joanne Ikeda, MA, RD, Extension Nutrition*
Specialist, University of California, Berkeley

BEST OF ALL, Berg provides many practical solutions to the problems she addresses. This is more than a penetrating analysis of a major public health problem; it is also a how-to book of solutions.
— *National Council Against Health Fraud Newsletter*

AN INDISPENSABLE RESOURCE . . . Her jewel of a book is a wake-up call to health education professionals to address all aspects of the problem. . . . This is not light reading. But it is extremely interesting.
— *BBW: Big Beautiful Woman*

TEACHERS WILL BENEFIT from the discussion of goals for elementary students, advice on how to spot weight problems in athletes and best address body image and self-esteem. If today's children are to grow up with normal eating habits, changes must come in attitudes, lifestyle, society and national health policy.

Berg states it is a major health crisis when more than two-thirds of high school girls are dieting, one-half are severely undernourished and one-third are occasionally smoking, mostly in an effort to be thinner. . . . Teenage boys mirror these same problems, but to a lesser extent.

Afraid to Eat promotes natural, wholesome eating patterns, healthy food relationships and regular physical activity — a new health paradigm for children.
— *Rochester Times Union, Rochester, N.Y.*

THERE'S A SILENT EPIDEMIC so large and extreme, it could only happen in this weight-obsessed culture: children's fear of eating. The good news is that *Healthy Weight Journal* editor Berg is out to change these attitudes. Her call to action is loud, clear, and above all, provides the framework for change. Anyone involved in shaping the eating habits of the young must read this book, especially parents and teachers.

— *CHOICE, American Library Association*

AS SCHOOL NURSES we regularly encounter students who may be struggling with negative body images and inappropriate eating attitudes and behaviors. *Afraid to Eat* provides insight into this nationwide weight-loss and thinness obsession, and offers assistance . . . Clear guidelines are presented.

— *School Nurse News*

CHILDREN AND TEENS AFRAID TO EAT **IS A MUST READ** for teachers. The pressures caused by the weight crisis are affecting academic achievement in our youth. It's time for school staff and students to become aware of the size bias pandemic and its consequences, and mobilize to liberate all students to achieve their fullest potential.

— *Linda L. Johnson, MS, Director of School Health Programs*
North Dakota Dept. of Public Instruction

A MUCH NEEDED BOOK . . . Berg dares to speak out on behalf of parents, educators, health professionals, and all members of society. The news (on nutrient deficiencies) should be alarming, but the media's attention is fixated on obesity fear rather than long-term health. . . . This is an issue that should touch our hearts deeply, make us angry, and give us motivation to bring about change. Inspires the reader to action.

— *EATING DISORDERS: Journal of Treatment & Prevention*

A GOOD BLEND OF FACT and research with personal experiences. . . . A resource for parents, teachers, coaches and health professionals.

— *Pediatric Nutrition*

AN EXTRAORDINARY contribution to both professionals and the public. *Children and Teens Afraid to Eat* identifies the cultural, social, physiological, emotional and spiritual issues facing kids today and how these issues collide, resulting in a generation of kids afraid to eat. Ms. Berg is an award winning writer and has a gift for gathering and clearly explaining how these forces influence our children relationally and developmentally.

A useful chart details dysfunctional eating from inconsistent eating to eating disorders. *Children and Teens Afraid to Eat* is also a storehouse of charts, graphs, lists, and short articles essential to nutrition professionals working with children and adolescents. Whether you are a workshop leader, counselor, author, educator, coach or in marketing and advertising, these resources will be valuable time after time.

Afraid to Eat demands that as a nation and as health care professionals we deal with these issues in healthier, more effective ways.

— *PULSE, Dietitians in Sports, Cardiovascular and Wellness*

A GROUND-BREAKING BOOK about an issue in our culture that is affecting almost every child in ways that range from detrimental to disastrous. . . . We need a national awareness of an intolerable situation that will not self-correct. *Afraid to Eat* needs to be read, discussed, argued about, and acted upon.

— *Academy for Eating Disorders Newsletter*

AFRAID TO EAT indicts society for this obsession with thinness and its impact on children's lives, which causes eating disorders, dysfunctional eating, size prejudice and overweight. The obsession and its consequences amount to perpetrating fraud on innocent children.

This insightful book shows how to challenge the status quo, and it's easy to read, too.

— *Kentucky Currents, Kentucky Dietetic Association*

ANYONE WHO HAS CHILDREN or works with children should read this book! *Afraid to Eat* charges parents, educators, and the medical field to wake up and take a stance to combat the prevalent thinking in our society — that the quest for thinness is healthy, when in reality, this quest has caused an epidemic of health problems for our children.

— *Wayne C. Miller, PhD, Exercise Science*
George Washington University Medical Center

Children and Teens Afraid to Eat

Helping Youth in Today's Weight-Obsessed World

■

Frances M. Berg

Edited by
Kendra Rosencrans

Published by
Healthy Weight Network

Acknowledgments

It's been my privilege and pleasure over the years to network with many outstanding leaders in the fields of nutrition, eating disorders, obesity, and size acceptance and I thank them for their contributions to this book. I'm especially grateful to Linda Johnson, Karen Petersmarck, Ellyn Satter, Linda Omichinski and Joanne Ikeda, and to Kendra Rosencrans for her superb editing, and to Ronda Irwin for her dedication and skill in production. Special thanks also to my family, my husband Bert, to Kathy and Dennis, Rick and Tracy, Cindy and Todd, Mike and Wendy, for their support and the many ways they inspire me.

Children and Teens Afraid to Eat:
Helping Youth in Today's Weight-Obsessed World
Copyright 2001 THIRD EDITION
Copyright 1997 SECOND EDITION
Copyright 1997 FIRST EDITION
by Frances M. Berg.
All rights reserved. Reproduction in whole or in part
prohibited without publisher's written permission.
ISBN: 0-918532-55-8 softcover
ISBN: 0-918532-56-6 hardcover

Afraid to Eat Series: *Women Afraid to Eat*
and *Children and Teens Afraid to Eat*
ISBN: 0-918532-70-1 hardcover
ISBN: 0-918532-69-8 softcover
Printed in USA

Edited by Kendra Rosencrans
Layout and production by Ronda Irwin
Published by
Healthy Weight Network
402 South 14th Street
Hettinger, ND 58639
Tel: 701-567-2646; Fax: 701-567-2602
hwj@healthyweight.net
www.healthyweight.net

Foreword

Children and Teens Afraid to Eat is one of the most important books of the decade. This isn't just a book about eating disorders or a book about the problems of children who are overweight. This is a ground-breaking book about an issue in our culture that is affecting almost every single child in ways that range
from detrimental to disastrous. Every adult who cares about children needs to understand the message that Frances Berg has
clearly articulated here.

The cultural obsession with slimness has reached a level which
is seriously hurting millions of our youth. Ms. Berg is one of the
few people in the country with a broad enough perspective to
piece together the destructive elements which contribute to a previ-
ously unrecognized national emergency — an emergency that will
get worse unless thoughtful and caring individuals from every quarter take positive action to change the situation.

Children today are flooded with messages telling them that they
are unacceptable and unlovable unless they somehow manage to
achieve a body size and shape which is biologically sustainable for
only a handful of human beings. Whereas natural diversity in other
physical characteristics is seen as normal (height, foot size, complexion, nose length), only individuals who fall within the lowest
range of weight for height are considered "normal." This message
is reinforced in hundreds of ways through the mass media, and it
is also unwittingly reinforced by well-meaning adults.

The result is that far too many children see themselves as defective simply because their weight is at a level that is genetically

and biologically appropriate for them.

The few children who happen to meet cultural standards for slimness are afraid to gain weight. Even the small weight increases which precede spurts in height in growing children are noted with alarm.

Fear of gaining weight and desperate desires to lose weight are daily realities for many, if not most, of our children.

The restrictions they make in quantity and variety of food are seriously threatening their long-term health, leading to epidemics of disordered eating. What is even more disastrous, however, is the pandemic of self-loathing based solely on body size which compromises the emotional development of the next generation.

Despite the dark picture painted in *Afraid to Eat*, the book is not depressing because Ms. Berg creates a clear vision of what is needed to change the status quo. By integrating the creative thinking of some of the finest minds in North America, she has formulated a set of reasonable, common-sense actions that can turn the situation around.

There will be some people who will consider this book controversial. That is good. We need controversy. We need debate. We need a national awareness of an intolerable situation that will not self-correct.

Children and Teens Afraid to Eat needs to be read, discussed, argued about, and acted upon.

KAREN PETERSMARCK, PhD, MPH, RD
Michigan Department of Community Health
Lansing, Michigan

HEALTH AT ANY SIZE
A new paradigm

Beauty, health and strength come in all sizes. This truth is affirmed by Health at Any Size, a health-centered approach that focuses on health and well-being, not weight.

It's about wellness and wholeness, eating in normal, healthy ways and living actively. It's about acceptance, self-respect and appreciation of diversity. It's health at any size.

Everyone qualifies!

— FRANCES M. BERG

Enjoy Health at Any Size

LIVE ACTIVELY

- Be active your way, every day
- Move for the sheer joy and power of it, for time spent with family, friends, nature
- Celebrate activity as a natural part of life — fitness feels good
- Pace yourself; choose fun activities
- Be creative — increase activity throughout the day
- Enjoy the benefits — meet new people, increase your energy, lower stress, sleep better, and improve health, bone strength, and resistance to illness. Take time to care for yourself
- Add years to your life, and life to your years
- Share the benefits with family and friends
- Have more fun!

EAT WELL

- Take pleasure in eating a variety of foods
- Think of food as a friend — celebrate, enjoy, taste, savor
- Meet your body's energy and nutrient needs
- Enjoy a nondiet lifestyle; keeping stable weight is worthwhile
- Listen to your body: eat when hungry, stop when full and satisfied
- Eat at regular times, typically three meals and one or two snacks
- Eat in a balanced way — enjoy all five food groups
- Trust your body to make up for mistakes
- All foods can fit; there are no good foods/bad foods
- To improve, make small changes over time
- Enjoy home cooking, eating with friends and family

RESPECT YOURSELF AND OTHERS

Beauty, health and strength come in all sizes ♡ Celebrate and enjoy your unique characteristics ♡ Like yourself and others in spite of imperfections ♡ Make peace with your genetic blueprint (avoid unrealistic goals, perfectionism, all or nothing) ♡ Wear clothes that fit comfortably and look good now ♡ Wear what you want, including shorts, swim suits or sleeveless tops no matter what your size or shape ♡ Think critically of media messages that portray unrealistic standards or suggest that happiness is based on appearance ♡ Accept, respect and celebrate diversity

Have confidence in your ability to make choices for better health ♡ Change your lifestyle gradually ♡ Nurture yourself ♡ Enjoy increased self-esteem ♡ Be flexible, go with the flow ♡ Keep in tune with your body ♡ Focus on quality of life, health and well-being ♡ Use positive language ♡ Embrace joy, pleasure, freedom, and self-discovery ♡ Nourish, listen, empower, explore, encourage, motivate, inspire, counsel, guide, validate, accept, respect, appreciate, self-care, heal, celebrate ♡

"I can if I choose"

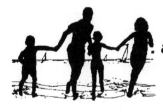 *a health centered approach*

for the 21st century

Developed by Frances M. Berg with adaptations from *Vitality*, Health Canada, and Linda Omichinski's HUGS programs, and credits to dietitians Ellyn Satter, Dayle Hayes, Nancy King, Karin Kratina and Gail Marchessault. Copyright 2001, 2000, by Frances M. Berg, *Women Afraid to Eat, Children and Teens Afraid to Eat*. All rights reserved. Healthy Weight Network, 402 South 14th Street, Hettinger, ND 58639 (701-567-2646; fax: 701-567-2602). Website: www.healthyweight.net

CONTENTS

Foreword

Enjoy Health at Any Size

PART I: CHILDREN AND TEENS IN WEIGHT CRISIS

PART II: HELPING YOUTH IN A
WEIGHT-OBSESSED WORLD

PART I

CHILDREN
AND TEENS
IN
WEIGHT
CRISIS

For the first time in the history of this country, young people are less healthy and less prepared to take their places in society than were their parents.

NATIONAL COMMISSION ON THE
ROLE OF SCHOOL AND COMMUNITY IN
IMPROVING ADOLESCENT HEALTH, CDC, 1990

CHAPTER 1

Growing up
afraid to eat

■

America's children are afraid to eat. It's a fear that consumes them, shatters lives, even kills. It's an obsession that dims their joy, their curiosity, their energy and their sense of what's normal. It's taking the fun from their teenage years.

Such a fear is irrational, but kids are succumbing to the same destructive cultural messages about body and weight that plague adults. To be overweight in American society today is to fail. Instead of growing up with secure and healthy attitudes about their bodies, eating and themselves, many kids fear food and fear being fat.

Some children can't eat normally. Others live with eating disorders. Still others fail to thrive because of the social shame they endure for being large. And we, as parents, educators, health professionals and members of society, have ignored them, punished them, and failed them.

Our daughters and sons are caught — and they need our help. They're not developing the eating habits, lifetime activities and self respect critical to becoming healthy adults with healthy weights.

It's a national public health crisis and we need to take action.

It should come as no surprise in a country where half of adults are dieting, that children see, hear and take to heart the cultural ideal that to be thin is to have the best of everything and to be fat is to fail.

These same pressures are growing globally, as attested to by our *Healthy Weight Journal* readers around the world, but they are especially acute in the United States, Canada and England, where they strongly affect kids of all ethnic and socioeconomic groups.

Weight issues have become an obsessive concern for American girls and boys of all ages, of every racial and ethnic heritage. Clearly it is a national crisis when harmful attempts at dieting are common in the third grade and even earlier. It is a crisis when more than two-thirds of high school girls are dieting and half are undernourished. One in five take diet pills, and many girls as well as boys are using laxatives, diuretics, fasting and vomiting in desperate attempts to slice their bodies as thin as they can.[1]

Crisis in eating and weight

Today's crisis consists of six major eating and weight problems:

1. Dysfunctional eating. Disturbed, chaotic, disordered eating has become the norm for kids. They are dieting, fasting, bingeing, skipping meals, undereating and overeating.

2. Undernourishment of teenage girls. Teen girls have the poorest nutrition of any group in America. Yet their widespread undernourishment and malnourishment go largely unnoticed, ignored by the policy makers who should care the most.

3. Hazardous weight loss. The methods kids use to lose weight can be very dangerous — vomiting, smoking, fasting, and taking laxatives, diuretics, diet pills. They can have lasting harmful effects, and can even kill.

4. Eating disorders. Extremely difficult to treat, eating disorders devastate families and claim many lives, a significant number from suicide. But their prevention and treatment is largely ignored in U.S. health policy. "The public is silent when young women die," charges Naomi Wolf, author of *The Beauty Myth*.[2]

5. Size prejudice. Large kids are easy targets for cruel and isolating taunts from their peers and others. Yet the harassment and stigma of size prejudice hurts youth of all sizes — in today's milieu no one is thin enough or perfectly shaped enough to feel safe. And some, especially boys, are stigmatized because of small stature or thinness.

6. Overweight. More kids are overweight today than ever before, yet we seemingly have no means to help them. Prevention efforts other than scare tactics have not moved forward, perhaps because most people still believe weight loss is fairly easy and safe. Research proves otherwise.

These six problems are interrelated and are intensifying. What affects one, affects others. For 16 years, I've been editing *Healthy Weight Journal* reviewing the latest worldwide research on these issues, and have seen all six problems growing worse year by year, yet little is being done to solve these problems in an integrated way.

Though no agency is keeping track, these problems are taking their toll of kids in injury and death. Every year young people die from eating disorders, hazardous weight loss, malnutrition, and suicides related to body image or size harassment.

When I first began looking at these issues, I was appalled at the disarray in the health field regarding weight and eating. Then I was hopeful, believing once the problems were better known they might be solved.

It hasn't happened. Instead, they have gotten worse.

I suppose I was naive, believing that once health policy makers understood the needs, they would be willing to make changes. But I underestimated the power of tradition, the marketplace, and the determination of those in power to hold onto it.

Yet, these are our children, our daughters and sons, who are growing up afraid to eat, afraid to gain weight, afraid to grow and mature in normal ways. They are desperate to have the right bodies, obsessed with the need to be thin, and fearful that they won't be loved unless they reach near perfection. This is the point to which our weight-obsessed culture has brought us. Our children are the innocent victims.

These are 21st century youth, the first to reach adulthood in the new millennium. How well prepared are they to meet the challenges of this new century?

Not well at all, according to the National Commission on the Role of School and Community in Improving Adolescent Health, at CDC in Atlanta. In 1990, the Commission warned, "For the first time in the history of this country, young people are less healthy and less prepared to take their places in society than were their parents."

When girls ages 11 to 17 were asked, "If you had three wishes, what would you wish for?" the top wish of nearly every girl was to lose weight. Not to cure cancer or save the rain forest or be a millionaire, but to be thin. In another survey young girls said they were more afraid of becoming fat than they were of cancer, nuclear war or losing their parents.[3]

A crisis in eating and weight

Possessed by this fear, many children don't eat normally. They shun certain foods, they diet, they fast, they binge. There's a new name for these eating patterns — dysfunctional. Instead of eating to satisfy hunger and nourish the body, dysfunctional eaters eat to be thin and binge to relieve stress.

Four-year-olds are asking, "Mommy, am I too fat?" Six-year-olds have full-blown eating disorders. As many as 81 percent of 10-year-old girls are eating in dysfunctional, disordered ways. And six out of 10 high school girls diet, as do one in four high school boys.

Almost every day, I hear new horror stories about how dysfunctional eating hurts children. Teachers tell me sad stories about the meager lettuce leaves girls put on their plates in the lunch line — and how they droop in class. They tell of the school's star wrestlers, thin-faced and gaunt, who shiver in winter jackets, light-headed, as they try to concentrate on writing a test.

A nutritionist tells of a four-year-old at Head Start who binges and purges. Caught in a three-way custody fight, the child is shuffled between parents and grandparents. Her art work reflects concern with the fat image. Is she trying to fix what's wrong through her eating, blaming herself for not being thin enough?[4]

Eating disorder specialists across the country are telling me about small girls and boys with fragile, stress-fractured bones, their growth stunted. Some children have been traumatized by radical animal rights groups that come into their schools and deliver graphic propaganda against eating animal-based foods. As a result, these kids won't eat eggs, meat, or milk — the building blocks of healthy growth and development which have for generations made America's youngsters among the strongest, tallest and healthiest in the world. A diet low in animal foods must be carefully planned, but these children don't have the skills for it.

I hear from parents that their college-age daughters are trying to eat zero fat. College girls who eat normally, or eat meat, are being harassed in their own sororities at Syracuse University in New York, says one of our subscribers, Cynthia DeTota, a registered dietitian and the campus nutritionist.

Young people who don't eat healthfully set themselves up for nutrient deficiencies and even malnutrition. Girls who are starving don't think straight. They don't feel well, or act normally. A recent national study revealed that at the median, girls age 11 to 19 are not getting the nutrition they need for healthy growth and development. The majority get less than two-thirds of the Recommended Daily Allowance for iron, calcium, vitamin A and other essential nutrients.[5]

One fourth — "the hungry one-fourth" — are drastically below these levels.[6]

Girls are also taking up smoking more and more as they grasp at every straw to lose weight. For the first time ever, in the 1995 U.S. Youth Risk Behavior survey girls surpassed boys in smoking rates. About 21 percent of white high school girls are regular smokers, compared with 18 percent of white boys.[7] This pattern is now being seen in advanced countries all around the world.

At least one teen in 10 struggles with the most serious kind of abnormal eating — potentially fatal eating disorders. Some are consumed by eating disorders through college and adulthood. Others die.

When Christy Heinrich died in 1994 of anorexia nervosa, she was 22 years old and weighed 60 pounds. The Kansas City gymnast had been weight-conscious as long as she'd been competing. But in 1988, a judge at an international competition told the then 16-year-old Heinrich that she needed to watch her weight if she wanted to continue winning. Her offending weight: 93 pounds.

At the same time as the country's obsession with thinness has soared, obesity among children and teens has skyrocketed. About 11 percent are overweight and obese, and the rates are much higher among ethnic and racial minorities and in lower income groups. Not only are more youngsters overweight, but they are more severely overweight than ever before. It's a complex problem with no surefire cure. Genetics, inactivity, poor nutrition, and the disruption of normal eating all play a role.

Meanwhile, large kids struggle with prejudice and stigmatization. A 16-year-old girl wrote to *Parade Magazine* of the anguish and humiliation she had suffered because of her weight and her efforts to reduce. "I can't speak for all fat people, but I do know that I am not lazy about losing weight. I'm always in the midst of planning a diet, in the middle of a diet or breaking a diet. I've tried sensible diets, liquid diets, crash diets . . . I've lived my entire life with people reminding me that it isn't okay to be fat. It isn't okay to be 16 years old, 5 feet 6 inches tall, have beautiful hair and eyes, and to be fat. It isn't okay, and it isn't fair."

No public outcry

Body image issues remain severe for young people — both girls and boys. Yet, except for overweight, there is almost no public recognition of the six eating and weight problems, and how closely entwined they are. The risks of overweight are often exaggerated, while the other problems are ignored or minimized, causing even more desperation to lose weight, and adversely affecting all problems.

I'm getting more letters and calls today from youngsters who seem suicidal. A 17-year-old boy from California wrote me a long and anguished letter about the bulimia that is taking over his life: "There is a war going on inside me . . . I don't know what to do. It is tearing apart our family . . . I sometimes feel that death would be better than being fat and having this destroy my family."

Joelyn M., 15, sent me an email message from Pennsylvania, "Can you help me? I'm a vegetarian, but mostly what I eat is lettuce. I'm afraid to get fat. I think a lot about doing away with myself."

So I was not surprised to see the suicide behavior statistics from the Youth Risk Behavior survey that show more than 30 percent of high school girls and 18 percent of high school boys seriously considered suicide during the year before the survey, and 21 percent of girls and 14 percent of boys went so far as to make a suicide plan.[8]

These numbers are self-reported and may even underestimate the despair our daughters and sons are feeling. How much does this desire for self-destruction have to do with body image issues, with not measuring up, with sexual violence, harassment, being stigmatized, and with depression related to malnutrition?

The shocking part of these latest reports on nutrient deficiencies, hazardous dieting and suicidal thinking is that there are no headlines, no public outcry, and no public health programs to deal with these problems. There is nothing but public apathy.

There is a better way

The good news is that there is a better way. In the midst of this crisis, a new paradigm or philosophy is emerging. It's called *Health at Any Size*.

Health at Any Size is an approach that focuses on health and well-being, not on weight. It reaffirms the truth that beauty, health and strength come in all sizes. It's about wellness and wholeness, eating in normal, healthy ways and living actively. It's about acceptance, self-respect, and appreciation of diversity. Everyone qualifies. And especially, every child qualifies!

By contrast, the current weight-centered paradigm holds that all bodies should be at a narrowly-defined weight and large people must lose weight to be healthy, even though they have tried many times and cannot do this in a healthy, lasting way.

Shifting to the health at any size approach helps focus on the goal of helping all children now at whatever size they are. The goal of healthy children at every size is practical and positive, whereas the goal to have all children at ideal size is impossible and causes endless problems.

In the model shown on the next page all children receive consistent messages that lead to this goal *(figure 1)*. If national health experts, health care providers, teachers, families, peers and the media — around the outside of the circle — consistently give messages that encourage eating well, living actively, and feeling good about oneself and others, then weight and eating problems will be diminished or prevented. This approach will have positive effects on the culture while strengthening children to withstand the negative messages they get.

Based on nondiet and size acceptance theories and the work of cutting-edge leaders in nutrition, psychology and public health, this philosophy encompasses living actively, eating well, emotional and spiritual health, positive family and social relationships, uniting mind, body and spiritual well-being.

It recognizes that we each have a natural weight at this time in our lives that our bodies *want* to weigh when we are well-nourished and living actively. For some of us, that weight will be higher, and for others, lower. And that's okay. It's wrong to say any child or adult should be a certain weight, just as it is wrong to say children of one age should be a certain height. We can respect size diversity just as we respect diversity in talent and experience.

It's not true that thinner is healthier. We have only to look at professional athletes for shining examples of "overweight or obese" individuals bursting with good health and exuberance. For example, during their heyday in the late 1990s, as perhaps the best basketball team ever, all the Chicago Bulls' team members reportedly weighed in at what is defined as overweight or obese (body mass index of 25 or more). So do most of the Los Angeles Lakers basketball players: Shaquille O'Neal has a BMI of 31.4; Rick Fox, 28.6.

The truth is that fit and well nourished people are healthier and live longer, regardless of weight, whether thin or heavy.

Within the health at any size approach we can help young people eat normally without fear, build self respect, learn assertiveness and healthy coping skills. Empowered to develop their unique potential as lovable, capable, valuable individuals, they can take pride in themselves and their bodies at any size, without being shamed or stigmatized. All children deserve this.

Health leaders using this new approach see weight and eating problems as interrelated. They understand that overweight cannot be resolved in a healthy way without attention to the potential disruption of normal eating, to size prejudice, hazardous weight loss, and mal-

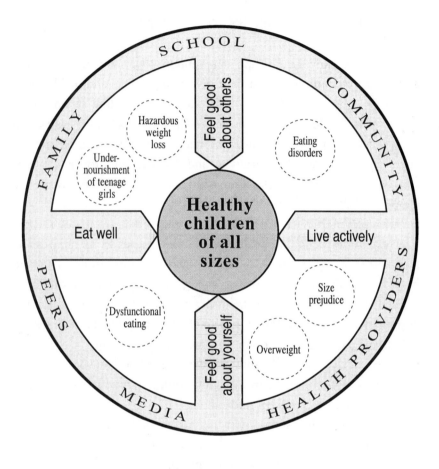

Figure 1

Health at Any Size

To achieve the goal of healthy children of all sizes, a health-centered approach is needed, whereby all children receive consistent messages that encourage normal eating, active living, self acceptance, respect and an appreciation of size diversity. If family, teachers, health professionals, peers and the media give these messages consistently to all children, then the six major eating and weight problems (dysfunctional eating, undernourishment of teenage girls, hazardous weight loss, eating disorders, size prejudice and overweight) will be diminished or prevented.

nutrition. How these issues interrelate is important in developing healthy treatment programs. We need to look at the big picture, ever wary of the harm so easily done to vulnerable youth by simplistic solutions.

Health at Any Size shapes prevention programs in new ways, empowering children to trust their own body signals and needs. They help kids understand they can be healthy and attractive at their natural weights, while growing normally. They can feel safe, assured of acceptance, liberated from false and narrow images based on appearance, and encouraged to evaluate and combat inappropriate media stereotypes. Programs with this new approach will empower and strengthen all youngsters.

The first step is to stop policies that may be harmful, such as the overwhelming focus on obesity, such as pressures to be abnormally thin, and to always be on low-fat, food-restricting programs. The next is to encourage healthy, normal eating, and to empower our half-starved daughters to nourish themselves. For many young girls, their current nutrition deficiencies are likely to have severe and lasting effects on their bones, growth and mental functioning.

Fortunately, what is healthy for the large child is also healthy for the thinnest — all benefit from eating well, living actively, and feeling good about themselves and others.

Canada has already adopted this health-centered approach, with a national campaign for active, holistic living that emphasizes health at every size, called the *Vitality* program.[9]

Current confusion

Today's policies are not working and they are hurting many children and adults.

What happens when we overemphasize the risks of obesity? How does this affect dysfunctional eating, eating disorders, undernutrition, size prejudice and the desperation to lose weight at any cost? I think they get worse. Unfortunately, our health bureaucrats in Washington have chosen to emphasize and, yes, exaggerate, the increases and risks of obesity — while ignoring the health hazards of their recommendations. Their policy is pushed by prominent obesity specialists who sometimes focus so narrowly on making weight loss happen that they seem unaware of the consequences of their actions. On the other hand, eating disorder specialists are keenly aware of dieting dangers, but may discount obesity problems. Few have seemed willing to stand back and view the whole picture. Few have examined the broad tragic network of weight issues that holds so many lives hostage. We need to do it now because the crisis continues to grow.

The diagram on the next page illustrates the current crisis, and the confusing ways that different groups are working to solve these problems (*figure 2*). Well-intended providers, specialists, parents and others work at cross-purposes depending on their area of concern, giving out conflicting messages, and allowing the negative aspects of culture to exert an even more powerful influence on children.

Health professionals, educators and parents need to work together, looking carefully at all six problems, closely aware of the harm that can be, and is being, done to vulnerable children and teens.

In particular, those who set national health policy need to take a broader view, since this sets the agenda for what happens throughout the country, and profoundly influences how the media and the medical community respond to these issues.

This nation has not dealt well with weight issues. Weight is a controversial issue, and differing viewpoints exist. The traditional view, which is official health policy today, is that fat is toxic and all large children and adults can and should lose weight. Americans are trying hard to comply.

Health and medical professionals who promote this view assume that any excess weight over a narrow range is unhealthy, dangerous and expensive to the U.S. health care system; that weight loss is always desirable and healthy for persons over this ideal, no matter how it is accomplished; and that all large persons can successfully lose at least 10 to 15 percent of their weight and maintain it.

They seem to believe that publicizing the risks of obesity and stressing the importance of thinness is helping people get thin, despite much evidence to the contrary. And there is fear that warning about eating disorders or the risks of weight loss may discourage people from trying to lose weight.

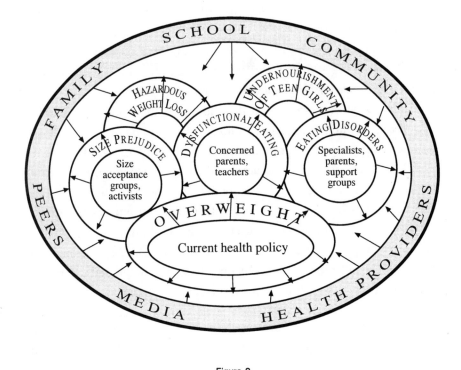

Figure 2

Today's weight and eating crisis

Children today are caught in a weight and eating crisis in which national health policy, health care providers, teachers, parents, peers and the media give out conflicting messages, working at cross-purposes, allowing the negative aspects of culture to exert a powerful influence that makes problems even worse.

CHILDREN AND TEENS AFRAID TO EAT 2001

In this official, traditional view, health professionals seem more concerned that people lose weight than that radical weight loss treatment methods are being prescribed for high risk patients and children, or that already underweight girls are severely restricting their nutritional intake to lose weight, or that more and more girls are smoking because of their fear of fat. Eating disorders are seen as unimportant, or at least irrelevant to public health's anti-obesity messages. This view ignores the possibility that national policy itself may be contributing to these problems.

It is clear that obesity is associated with health risks and that there are increases in obesity across the board. The question is, what should we do — and *not* do?

First, do no harm, warned the Greek healer Hippocrates. Canada puts it to health providers bluntly, "If you cannot help, at least do no harm." The cure for obesity may well be worse than the condition, and often it has been, causing swift death to many healthy young women. Why not admit this?

Industry exerts pressure

It's also true that many who set national health policy have vested interests in and may be unduly influenced by the powerful weight loss industry, which pulls in $30 to $50 billion annually in the U.S. alone.

For instance, the nine members of the federally-funded National Task Force on the Prevention and Treatment of Obesity, which sets our national health policy, finally disclosed their financial affiliations in the Dec. 18, 1996, issue of the *Journal of the American Medical Association*.

At *Healthy Weight Journal*, three times we had requested this information under the Freedom of Information Act, but were refused. No wonder. The list reads like a who's who of the diet industry. Of the nine members, eight are university-affiliated professors and researchers who have financial ties with at least two and up to *eight* commercial weight loss firms each. They serve as consultants, on advisory boards, conduct industry research, and reap honorariums and grants from diet drug and weight loss companies.[10]

The disclosure of vested interests in this field illustrates the charges Thomas J. Moore makes in his book, *Lifespan,* that it is "almost impossible to find any boundary between the government, the industry and the medical elite." He calls it "a closed circle of medical insiders operating without the normal checks and ethical barriers."

Since 1996, there have been no further disclosures of the vested interests in this field, to my knowledge — only that brief flash of truth, then again secrecy.

It's much like putting cigarette companies in charge of programs to stop teenage smoking. Wouldn't they keep self-interest uppermost, perhaps with programs that give short-term results, disguised as long-term? Putting diet companies in charge of America's weight plays to self-interest, too. Their results are also short-term, disguised as long-lasting. The difference is that the weight loss industry and its academic promoters would like lasting results — there'd be more profits — but diets and pills don't work. So they keep promising and pretending. Unfortunately, our government joins in the charade.

Few people fully believe the hype any more. They know diets don't work. Yet there's that blip of excitement with each new "discovery." Confusion reigns.

Many health officials and researchers do not share the traditional view of emphasizing weight loss, and refuse to support its policies; however, it is the one that currently determines U.S. health policy. It is a policy that powerfully emphasizes the risks of obesity and minimizes the risks of underweight, dieting, malnutrition, dysfunctional eating and eating disorders.

The heavy hand of the diet industry is evident in most federal reports on obesity. They emphasize obesity risks and the urgency of weight loss, and insist that current weight loss methods are safe and effective. Following are examples of this short-sighted bureaucratic policy and its pretense that all is well with obesity treatment:

■ The 1998 National Institutes of Health Guidelines on Overweight and Obesity tell doctors to urge weight loss for all large patients. *Motivate patients — by stressing obesity risks, and telling them new weight loss programs are different than any they've tried before* (though they are not), advise the guidelines. Thus, they urge doctors to manipulate their patients with scare tactics and false promises. Worse, the guidelines fail to advise screening for eating disorders or warn of hazardous weight loss.[11]

■ "Almost any of the commercial weight loss programs can work," declares the consumer bulletin *Choosing a Safe and Successful Weight-Loss Program*, by the Weight-Control Information Network (WIN) of the National Institute of Diabetes and Digestive and Kidney Disease (NIDDK). It gives no credible evidence at all for this astonishing statement.[12]

■ *Weighing the Options*, a federal review of weight loss programs, finds nearly all methods safe and effective. This 1995 book was published by the National Academy of Sciences, which is chartered by Congress to advise the nation on health policy.[13,14]

These reports claim that keeping excess pounds off for one year counts as long-term weight loss, despite all the evidence showing regain does not stop at one year, but almost inevitably continues until all lost weight is regained, whether one year or longer.

Federal leaders who author these kinds of policies are pressing hard to launch a major anti-obesity campaign in schools. They want to impress kids with the risks of obesity, to screen for overweight, to get large children on weight loss programs, and persuade insurance companies to pay for it all.

I'm concerned about the well-being of large children who would be further stigmatized, because no research indicates these programs would be successful or even safe. Insurance companies, too, often burned by overzealous claims for weight loss programs that didn't work and caused injury, for which they paid, are reluctant to back these efforts.

Certainly there is warranted concern among health leaders about the increases in obesity and potential health problems. Related to this is a fear that if obesity is not emphasized, or if officials openly discuss the undernourishment of teenage girls, eating disorders or dangerous weight loss methods, then this nation will be overwhelmed by a rising tide of excess weight.

Perhaps this is the fear of William Dietz, director of the Nutrition and Physical Activity Program at the Centers for Disease Control and

Prevention. Because he is influential in what happens to kids, I asked him why the Third Nutrition Monitoring report, which documents the severe undernutrition of teenage girls and which he helped write, does not mention a concern for these girls in its own summary. His comments are sobering. "Because obesity is more important. We need to focus on obesity."

"Yes, obesity is a concern," I agreed, "but what about teenage girls' undernutrition?"

"Later, perhaps, after we get obesity under control."

"And when do you expect to do that? Is it happening?"

"No, it's increasing."

So, when do we get around to the welfare of our hungry one-fourth of teenage girls? The implication that we have to fix obesity before considering related problems is absurd. In no other area of health would this be tolerated.

Healthy People 2010

It is this kind of thinking, and undeniable pressure from the diet industry, that has kept eating disorders off the nation's Healthy People 2010 health agenda. This huge, two-volume report claims to be "comprehensive" and to "reflect the very best in public health planning." It covers 467 objectives in 28 major focus areas, but appallingly, eating disorders is not among them.

The Healthy People steering committee was urged to add objectives aimed at reducing eating disorders, disturbed eating, hazardous weight loss efforts, the undernutrition of teenage girls, negative body image, and the stigma of obesity. But all were disallowed. Women nutritionists and eating disorder specialists struggled with an entrenched bureaucracy on this point, and lost.

Incredibly, the one crumb that was thrown — the only national health concern for eating disorders, apparently, to be considered for the next 10 years — is a need to prevent relapse in eating disorder treatment after hospitalization. It's true, *just that one!* And this brief two-paragraph mention appears in the mental health section, not nutrition, where obesity concerns dominate, to the distress of many nutritionists.

That eating disorders gained even this tiny toehold in the nation's health agenda, is due only to the dedicated efforts of many professional women. There is no doubt in my mind that women will persist until these critical issues are included, but the need is now.

Granted, weight is a controversial issue. But a balance is needed that will enable us all to work together. The current policy continues to jeopardize the health of America's children. Some children are dying because of their fear of fat.

These problems need to be addressed openly by leaders unswayed by vested interests. But at the many international and national obesity conferences I have attended, never has the tone been, "We have a problem with rising obesity rates, what can we do about it?" Instead, speakers invariably toe the commercial line: This works, and this works, and it's almost certain if *they* would just cooperate, this would work, too.

Yes, I am concerned about rising obesity rates, but I'm even more concerned about what health agencies might do about it, especially as it affects children. The truth is, we have no safe method of helping people lose weight in a lasting way, and our health and medical specialists should stop pretending that we do. It's all too clear that *everything* works short-term — and *nothing* works long-term. Health professionals need to reject those irrelevant short-term studies the diet industry keeps pushing. The scientific press needs to stop publishing them. And we all need to insist on proof of safety and effectiveness over two or three years, before we allow the promotion of new weight loss programs.

It's time to confess we don't know all the answers. Time to get serious about solving weight problems instead of letting uninformed or unethical leaders, the media, advertising, and the diet industry lead us into ever deeper trouble.

All this pretense and manipulation of reports and data gets in the way of solving urgent problems. As long as influential obesity experts insist that current diet drugs and treatments are safe and effective, we are prevented from moving ahead.

Why can't obesity be dealt with in the same way as other health problems, honestly, and in a straightforward manner? No one has pretended cancer is cured, then worked secretly backward to see what went wrong with the cure. We haven't burdened heart patients with the onus of curing themselves. But in the weight field, *it happens all the time.*

Miracle cures

Over the last 16 years of reviewing worldwide research, reporting, and attending national and international conferences, I've watched a steady stream of miracle cures come and go.

I was there when John Garren introduced the Garren-Edwards stomach balloon to an enthusiastic crowd of admiring physicians. I was there a couple of years later at a Harvard meeting as he stood alone by his posters, forlorn and rejected, his hastily-granted FDA approval withdrawn.

Already, enthusiasm had moved on to very low calorie liquid diets of 800 calories or fewer, with their "amazing, miracle" results. Large patients lost one-third of their size in months. Known as VLCDs, these were based, it was said, on safer formulas than the liquid diets that caused numerous deaths in the 1970s.

I knew Dr. Peter Lindner, one of the famed "diet doctors" of the 1980s, who co-authored with George Blackburn, MD, of Harvard, an early study that "proved" VLCD success. Theirs became a classic, oft-quoted study that launched liquid VLCD's soaring second wave of "miracles," which again ended disastrously.

Lindner was a magician and cheerleader, urging on his patients and colleagues alike with great enthusiasm. I feel sure his motivation was to help his many grateful patients. Was this why he grew increasingly despondent? His good friend told me it was because, as he confessed before he died, he made a five-year check of his former patients, and not one of them — *not one* — had kept off for five years any of the weight they had lost so successfully for him.

But by then the Lindner-Blackburn study had taken on a life of its own. So popular was the VLCD in the late 1980s and early 1990s that it is hardly an exaggeration to say that medical and scientific journals published thousands of nearly identical short-term studies, all lauding its success. None suggested there would be rapid regain and sometimes terrible side effects. Doctors and patients had to discover this for themselves.

Then came Slim Fast and its imitators in huge stacks blocking grocery aisles for a couple of years. Next, thigh cream. And after that, the fen-phen/Redux tragedy. Now again, new prescription diet drugs are being highly touted, again on the basis of irrelevant short-term studies. One cult after another, as one scientist complained. And these are just the legal, medically-sanctioned cures.

As editor of *Healthy Weight Journal* it has been my mission for 16 years to investigate and report the truth about these "miracle" cures. I've reported, as well, on more than 200 questionable and fraudulent products: acupressure earrings, appetite patches, hypnosis seminars, body wraps, vacuum pants, battery-operated belts, slimming insoles, herbal teas, Chinese soap, cookies, mushroom tea, starch blockers, fat blockers, herbals, bee pollen, cure-all pills and drinks to detoxify the body. Many have died from these so-called treatments. I get heartbreaking calls and letters from victims' families.

The one method that can work and does no harm — gradually changing activity and eating habits and relieving stress — is steadfastly ignored. There's no profit in it.

Current health policy has lost much support among doctors and educators because it runs counter to their experience. Time and again they have seen the failure of their best efforts to help. They are reluctant to put more pressure on large individuals and cause them more harm.

What is needed is a shift in how we deal with these issues. It is heartening that the National Center for Health Statistics and a few other agencies recognize this and warn that most people who lose weight by any method will regain it, and that adequate studies of safety and effectiveness are not available for any current methods.[15]

It's time to shift priorities and most experts know it.

It is my hope that this book will help them see these issues in clearer perspective, will help them recognize why a shift is needed, and will help them see how it can be done. Traditional ways of dealing with weight need to be replaced by a new way of living that helps children and does not harm them.

Part I documents the six major eating and weight problems (dysfunctional eating, undernourishment of teenage girls, hazardous weight loss, eating disorders, size prejudice and overweight), the social forces that have shaped them, the interplay of family, athletics, school, health care and peer pressure, and the profound effects of the thinness obsession on vulnerable youth. It explains why today's policies are not working.

Part II gives clear guidelines for dealing with these issues in healthier ways, using the health at any size approach. It gives practical steps that parents, teachers and health leaders can take now to help young people break free from weight obsession, overcome their fears, and fulfill their rich potential.

We must allow our children to eat without fear.

CHAPTER 2

Our culture fails
to nurture its youth

■

Modern culture is youth-centered, yet in many ways it does not
provide an environment that is nurturing or supportive for the healthy
growth and development of our children. In fact, it nurtures serious
problems.

This is especially true for girls, probably the reason their suicidal
thinking and attempt rates are double those of boys in nearly every
category.

"A girl-poisoning culture . . . a girl-destroying place," psychologist Mary Pipher brands our society in her book, *Reviving Ophelia*.[1]
Pipher says that in early adolescence girls are expected to sacrifice
the parts of themselves that our culture considers masculine on the
altar of social acceptability. They have to shrink their souls down to
petite size.

Appearance and, above all, thinness are the criteria by which
girls are being judged. Magazines for teenage girls give training in
lookism where the emphasis is on makeup, fashion, weight and how
to attract boys, with almost no space given to sports, hobbies, careers
or healthy body image attitudes. Young readers are being sold to
advertisers through articles and editorial copy linked to the ads. Boys,
too, are being taught body dissatisfaction through advertising and the
many new "muscle" magazines.

Boys are bewildered by their perceptions of what our culture expects of them. They live in a culture that showcases men as "macho," yet demands equality; that flaunts sexuality, but fears to discuss it. Young men are goaded by friends to select only girlfriends with thin "perfect" bodies, and to harass and exploit girls. And many of the girls and young women they know feed into this; obsessed with their bodies, eating and weight, they speak of little else.

And in their hidden lives, many boys, like their sisters, are emerging with shame and difficulty from childhood experiences of violence, trauma or sexual abuse that have damaged how they feel about and care for their bodies and for others.

The world has changed drastically for children in recent years. In 1960, less than 1 percent were children of divorce, 90 percent lived with both parents, and less than 20 percent of married women with children under six were in the work force. By 1990, nearly half of children had divorced parents, only 70 percent lived with two parents, and 60 percent of women with young children were working.[2]

Yet, what young people want most is to belong, to be accepted. They are ever searching, trying out and learning by trial and error. Culture, family, community and friends show them the way. But today family and community are losing out to the stronger influence of pop culture, the entertainment industries and peer group pressure. The messages kids get about how to belong are often confusing, conflicting and harmful to their well-being.

Pipher says there is a desperate need to build a culture for our children that is less complicated and more nurturing, less violent and sexualized and more growth-producing.

How thin is thin enough?

Television, movies and other social media probably have the strongest and most dangerous influence on children. At no time in history has the U.S. cultural obsession with thinness been more severe. What is it doing to children? Is it sabotaging their chances for healthy weight, healthy self respect and healthy, productive lives?

Both boys and girls are being taught that only thin people are worthy of love, attention and success. They turn that expectation on themselves and their friends, dieting to meet it, hating themselves when they don't.

Alicia Silverstone, a slim teenage movie star of *Batman* fame, was ridiculed in the press when she attended the Academy Awards, because she had gained five or 10 pounds since making her last movie (for which she had probably *lost* weight). Headlines read: "Batman and Fatgirl," and "Look out Batman, here comes Buttgirl." She was called "More Babe than Babe." Silverstone's director was outraged, "What did this child do? Have a couple of pizzas? The news coverage was outrageous, disgusting, judgmental and cruel!"

What message does her experience send to other young women? Will it keep them in line, dieting and starving? Will Silverstone be more careful next time about being seen in public between diets — at what may be her natural size?

With worldwide transmission of U.S. films and TV shows, the thinness obsession has gone global. Teenage girls in Moscow revealed that they shared the same thoughts on weight as girls who were surveyed in North Carolina. Girls in both places averaged 120 pounds but yearned to weigh 110 pounds. And they were dieting at the same high rates.[3]

Women on television and on film seem to get thinner each year. Their faces are gaunt and hollow-cheeked, sadly mirrored everywhere in real life. Often they show us their lean bodies from the side so we can get a good look at how hollow they really are, back to front.

We see this reflected in our own schools and communities. It breaks my heart to see a lineup of thin girls from the side — high school cheerleaders, for instance, their stomachs caved in, bony clavicles and hip bones protruding. Where are the bodies they have worked so hard to perfect? There's no body. Only bones, arms, legs, hair and that frighteningly skeletal face, screaming out cheers — or maybe, screaming for help from us adults who have abandoned them.

The cultural lesson: thin is in, fat is out. With most thinness messages aimed at girls and women, some feminists see links between the promotion of thinness and intentional oppression of women. The attack messages work best when the target is young. And young adolescent girls are most vulnerable.

"I am deeply concerned about what is happening to young girls in our society today," says Paula Levine, PhD, former president of Eating Disorders Awareness and Prevention. "Young girls up until the age of 11 are confident, unafraid of conflict, and willing to say exactly what is on their minds. As they enter puberty, however, they adjust to society's messages about what young women are 'supposed' to be — nice, kind, caring, self-sacrificing, agreeable and compliant."

In classrooms across the country, girls are encouraged to speak quietly, defer to boys, avoid math and science, value popularity and appearance over integrity and intelligence. I have clipped a set of Doonsbury cartoon strips in which a small girl keeps waving her hand in the classroom, eager to give the right answer, but is repeatedly overlooked by the teacher, in favor of boys. In the last frame, still ignored, she comes to the forlorn conclusion, "Maybe I should go on a diet."

Advocates for girls say our culture is splitting adolescent girls into true and false selves — one that is authentic and one that is culturally scripted. They can be authentic and honest, or they can be loved and admired, but seemingly, not both.

"If it is true that by the time young girls in this country reach puberty, they are voiceless, their self-esteem is at a low ebb, and they feel anxious, inferior and out of control, is there any more fertile ground for the development of an eating disorder? I think not," says Levine.

Researchers developing focus groups with teen girls were disconcerted to discover they often prefaced their remarks with, "I don't know." The girls used this qualifier before giving an opinion or fact, as in, "I don't know, I just love sports." In one group alone, girls repeated this phrase nearly 50 times in prefacing opinions. The researchers saw this as a way that girls protect themselves from criticism. More use seemed linked to lower self-esteem, less confidence and competence.

Girls fight to preserve their wholeness and authenticity, but most choose to be socially accepted, take up false selves, and abandon their true selves. In public, they become who they are supposed to be, she says. Thus, girls struggle with mixed messages, "Be beautiful, but beauty is only skin deep. Be sexy, but not sexual. Be honest, but don't hurt anyone's feelings. Be independent, but nice. Be smart, but not so smart that you threaten boys."

Today's co-educational liberal arts colleges promote these same stereotypical values, charges Sharlene Hesse-Biber, a Boston College teacher, in *Am I Thin Enough Yet?* She says colleges only encourage the most traditional roles for women and "serve more to preserve, rather than reduce stereotypic differences between men and women."[4]

Levine says teenage girls need to recapture the time in their lives when they were confident, courageous, and critical thinkers. "Only when they begin to value themselves as worthy human beings and not as objects of beauty will we begin to win the war on eating disorders."[5]

But the odds against that are incredibly high.

Molly Barker, who developed a running program designed to celebrate the gifts of girlhood, *Girls on the Run*, for ages 8 to 12, calls this trap the *Girl Box*. "Girls feel the push toward the Girl Box around the time they enter middle school. Reluctantly, we enter the Girl Box and leave behind our natural and uninhibited exploration of the world, our tomboyishness, and the spirited playfulness of girlhood, and step into the MTV images, the cultural and social expectations of an advertising industry gone haywire, and the '90s woman stereotype. Life becomes a series of performances as opposed to experiences."[6]

We can help to strengthen girls, encourage emotional toughness and self-protection, support and guide them, but Pipher says the important thing is to change our culture. "Our daughters deserve a society in which all their gifts can be developed and appreciated."

Advertising messages

Instead, advertising expertly conveys the message that "you're not okay — and here's what you need to buy to fix what's wrong." It sells body dissatisfaction a thousand times a day. The thinness craze is lucrative for the fashion and tobacco industry, for the makers of body products, weight loss services, diet drinks, and for every industry from cars to whiskey that advertises with striking models. Advertising is a $130 billion industry and the most powerful educational force in America. It has designed the cultural ideals for our time.

Here's how *Newsweek* recently described "the look" of the late 1990s: "It is a slimmer, more dissipated vision . . . reedy, women with hollow curves and sinewy lines . . . small, frail-looking . . . wan and disengaged . . . austere as the times . . . human coat hangers . . . Clothes fall off them." These images have toppled the "curvaceous supermodels" of the past decade. It's a "return to reality . . . down to earth." Inexplicably, *Newsweek* concludes this proves that "men and their appetites" don't rule the world.[7]

"Each era has exacted its own price for beauty, though our era is unique in producing a standard based exclusively on the bare bones of being, which can be disastrous for human health, happiness and productivity," says Roberta Seid, PhD, of the University of Southern California.[8]

Seid writes that in the past, excesses of fashion were severely criticized by social authorities, including doctors, teachers, clergy, parents and feminists. Moralists stressed that there were values more important than outward appearance. But no more. "In the late 20th century all these authorities, especially physicians, seemed to agree that one could never be too thin."

The *lookism* message is constantly sold through television and movies and magazines and billboards and novels and songs. To girls, the command is be thin, avoid fat and you deserve a wonderful life. To boys, the message becomes a command to build abdominals, sculpt, be the ultimate muscle man — or you won't be worthy.

And it's a success. Media pressure to be thin is stronger now than at any time in the last two decades, according to a recent study that compared numbers of TV commercials on diet foods, diet programs and reducing aids using advertising data from the *Network Television Books*.[9] Jean Kilbourne, EdD, author of *Still Killing Us Softly: Advertising and the Obsession with Thinness,* argues that advertising overpowers almost every other cultural message through sheer force. The average American sees 1,500 ads per day and spends a year and a half of a lifetime watching TV commercials.[10] Thus, "The tyranny of the ideal image makes almost all of us feel inferior," Kilbourne says. "We are taught to hate our bodies, and thus learn to hate ourselves. This self-hatred takes an enormous toll . . . (in) feelings of inferiority, anxiety, insecurity, and depression."

The ideal body, the ideal myth

The ideal female body type is now at the thinnest 5 percent of a normal weight distribution, say feminist writers. This excludes 95 percent of American girls and women. A statistical deviation has been made to seem the norm, with millions believing they are abnormal or "too fat." This mass delusion causes enormous suffering and becomes a prison for many — but it sells a lot of products.

"For women to stay at the official extreme of the weight spectrum requires 95 percent of us to infantilize or rigidify to some degree our mental lives," says Naomi Wolf, author of *The Beauty Myth*.[11]

The increasing pressures to be thin are vividly illustrated by a survey of Miss America winners from 1922 to 1999. These cultural icons dropped weight steadily from the 1920s when it was in the range considered normal — a body mass index between 20 and 25 — to as low as a BMI of 16.9. (Their height increased about 2 percent.) Nearly all winners since the mid 1960s have had BMIs below 18.5, defined as undernutrition by the World Health Organization. Worse, it is likely that every local and state pageant up through the national contest promotes this same ideal of female gauntness and hunger.[12]

The typical beauty contestant and model weighs in at 13 to 19 percent below "expected weight." The clinical criteria for anorexia nervosa is 15 percent below this point. To drop weight any lower is to risk death by starvation, say researchers.[13,14,15]

Young Olympic gymnasts, the role models of many girls, are becoming younger, smaller and much thinner.[16] The champions are often 16 or younger, weigh less than 90 pounds and are 4 feet, 10 inches or shorter. Body fat may be under 10 percent.

I felt somewhat more hopeful watching the 1996 Olympic games in Atlanta. These gymnasts were older — almost the women athletes we've been hoping for. Then I heard the piping, child-like voice of the injured 17-year-old. Was she almost a woman? I don't think so.

"Pathologically underweight women are being held up as cultural ideals," says David Greenfeld, MD, medical director of the Yale-New Haven Hospital Adolescent and Young Adult Treatment Unit.[17]

The 1999 Miss America pageant had an audience of more than 10 million, 11th in prime-time programs. Our girls were watching and coveting these figures. The more thin role models they see, the more dissatisfied girls are with their own bodies, and the less attractive they feel. One study found after briefly viewing a set of pictures of thin female models from magazines marketed to women, college girls felt upset, nervous, tense and had a disturbed sense of self-awareness. This did not happen when they viewed pictures of babies, children and older men and women.

Other studies confirm that girls exposed to media images of thin women rate themselves and women of average attractiveness lower, have increased depression, stress, guilt, shame, insecurity and body dissatisfaction. Advertisers target women far more than men with ads that create body dissatisfaction.[18]

One eating disorder specialist says her young patients tell her that reading teen and women's magazines makes them feel bad about themselves and more determined to restrict to lose weight.[19]

Even children's books reflect and repeat the obsession with thinness. One study found that illustrations have portrayed young girls as progressively thinner over the past 80 years, while no such trend was found for boys.[20]

Thin lesson teaches self-hate

"Because our society is so focused on appearance, body image becomes central to our feelings of self-esteem and self-worth, overshadowing qualities and achievements in other aspects of our lives," says Merryl Bear, coordinator of the National Eating Disorder Information Centre in Toronto, Ontario.

"This cultural focus on looking a particular way is taught. Today, being slender has come to have other meanings attached, such as being seen to be in control of one's self and one's life, successful, self-disciplined and attractive."[21]

The media creates a distorted picture of reality in three ways that adversely affect girls and women, reports Karin Jasper, PhD, of the Women's Center, also in Toronto. It does this by (1) frequently propagating myths and falsehoods, (2) normalizing or even glamorizing what is abnormal or unhealthy, and (3) creating the false impression that all women are alike by failing to represent whole segments of the real world. These false messages contribute to the prevalence of eating disorders, she says.[22]

Girls and boys believe it, react to it.

High school girls say they are terrified of being overweight. In a study of New York high school girls, 72 percent said they had tried to diet. Twenty percent of the underweight girls, 32 percent of the normal weight girls, and 54 percent of the overweight girls were currently dieting.[23]

A 1989 *Seventeen* magazine article described how "weight hate" has become a part of the American female identity, an insidious form of self-loathing that is reinforced everywhere a girl goes.[24] The article explained that girls talk about how they look — and how much they hate how they look — on the bus to school, between math and history class, during lunch, after school, and when they shop on the weekend. They think about the "cellulite" on their legs, their fat thighs, their not-flat-enough stomach all day long — whether they're on a diet or not, whether they "need" to be on a diet or not. It's an unquestioned part of their life, and it dictates how they feel about themselves and colors how they feel about everything.

Kris Adler of Bala-Cynwyd, Pa., is a 15-year-old girl described as "pretty, smart, very perceptive," happy at home, with lots of friends. She is slim, but obsessed with perfecting her body. Adler tells her story: "Every day at school at least one freshman girl comes up to me and tells me I have a great body. But I weigh myself three times a day so the scale doesn't creep up. It should be creeping down. It's not so much that I think I'm fat, it's just that I'd like to take some flesh from one part of my body and put it in other places . . . If I weighed five pounds less I'd be closer to perfect. I'd respect myself more."

Boys are also affected by pressures to shape their bodies to match current perfectionist ideals. They are increasingly being targeted by fitness, muscle and body sculpting magazines that tell them how to fix what's "wrong" with their bodies. The value being taught to boys, as to girls is that: *Only physical perfection is acceptable — you must keep trying.*

New muscle-bound action toys targeted to boys reflect the images of male actors, models, professional wrestlers and comic strip characters, all linked to boys' striking increases in body dissatisfaction.

The 1998 GI Joe Extreme doll dwarfs all earlier lines of GI Joe dolls. With his huge chest, shoulder and arm muscles, his expression of rage contrasts sharply with the mildly pleasant expressions of pre-1980 figures. In 1964, he had no visible abdominal muscles, but by 1994 GI Joe boasted sharply rippled abs.

Luke Skywalker and Han Solo dolls have swelled from their 1978 normal builds to new bodybuilder physiques, with massive shoulders and chests, narrow waists, and muscular arms and legs. Other popular 1998 figures — Iron Man, Batman, Wolverine — boast physiques and a ferocity far beyond any seen on the largest wrestlers or bodybuilders. Extrapolating the size of these figures to real life would give a 5-foot-10 man a 62-inch chest and 32-inch biceps.[25]

As boys take in this message, they're responding, also. Eating disorder specialists tell me they are seeing far more boys with eating disorders than ever before. Several community studies report an alarmingly high prevalence of severe weight concerns and unhealthy eating habits among boys and young men.

One study of students, age 12 to 19, found 2.4 percent of boys and 15 percent of girls had eating disorder-like symptoms. These boys were at the lower end of normal weight range.[26] Boys who think they don't measure up or are unhappy with their shape often struggle with dieting and weight loss in much the same way as girls, which can lead to extreme forms of exercise and body building. Some specialists view the drive for body shaping, often at puberty, as acting out a defense against conflict-laden concerns related to an overwhelming sense of insecurity, separation fears and uncertainties, and sexual identity fears. Emotional issues are expressed as body dissatisfaction and an intense desire to reshape that body.[27]

Still, weight obsession and dieting is far less prevalent for young men than women. Studies suggest that body concerns for boys usually focus on building and sculpting their muscles, rather than dieting and losing weight.

"How easily weight obsession is dismissed as an inevitable phase of female development," charges Susan Wooley, PhD, professor of psychology at the University of Cincinnati. "Would things be different if our hospitals and clinics were filled with young men whose educations and careers were arrested by the onset of anorexia nervosa, bulimia, or the need to make dieting and body shaping a full-time pursuit?"

We may yet get the chance to find out.

Socializing young girls

Where does it all begin? By age two, girls are watching television and starting their daily exposure to messages showing that women who are loved and successful are thin. They are hearing their mothers, sisters and other women objectify, distrust and battle their bodies to make them acceptably thin. They are hearing their fathers, brothers and other important males in their lives judge women's bodies, and talk about women as objects.

As pre-schoolers, they learn that certain bad foods will make them fat, and that people who are fat should diet and exercise until they get thin. Many girls in primary grades are so concerned about their bodies they have already tried to lose weight. By fourth grade, 40 percent or more of girls say they diet at least occasionally. Those who do not are gathering information and forming values and opinions about body shape and weight control.

Weight preoccupation and body dissatisfaction are occurring earlier and earlier. Forty percent of girls and 25 percent of boys in grades one through five in an Ohio study reported trying to lose weight. About a quarter of girls said they were restricting or altering their food intake. These are young children — six to 10 years old! In this study, girls who were trying to lose weight seemed more distressed about their shape than nondieting girls, as were dieting boys compared with nondieting boys.[28]

By fourth or fifth grade these concerns are strong. One-third of girls in a rural Iowa survey of over 400 fourth graders said they "very often worried about being fat" and nearly half of the girls "very often wished they were thinner." About 40 percent of the children dieted "sometimes or very often." Twice as many girls as boys expressed concerns about their size or weight. Some may be laying the foundation for eating disorders, warns the report, but concern is warranted even when dieting and body dissatisfaction fall short of this.[29]

In a study of fifth graders, University of South Carolina researchers found more than 40 percent of the kids felt too fat or wanted to lose weight, even though 80 percent were not overweight. They identified children as young as 9 with severe eating disorders, including anorexia nervosa and bulimia nervosa. This bodes plenty of trouble ahead, warn the researchers.[30]

An Arizona study that compared ideals of beauty for 300 adolescent girls found that rigid and fixed images held by white girls contrasts sharply with the more flexible beauty images of African American girls. Most of the white girls were dissatisfied with their bodies and wanted to lose weight as a way to be popular and "perfect." Over 90 percent were dissatisfied with their weight even when it was normal. Almost as one they described their "perfect girl." She weighed 120 pounds, had very long legs and long blonde hair. Comparing themselves to this ideal, the girls were very dissatisfied with their own weight and appearance. Perversely, they did not support their peers who were closest to this ideal, but felt envious and competitive with them. The younger girls in early adolescence were most severely affected by these kinds of self-defeating images.

By comparison, the African American girls in the study held images of beauty that were fluid and unrelated to a particular size. They were based on each girl's sense of self, style, confidence, and "looking good." Looking good meant a girl was projecting her self-image, establishing a presence, creating and presenting a sense of style, and "making what you have work for you." Unlike the white girls, they said they were supported in their efforts to look good by other girls and by family, friends and community.[31]

With more wholesome attitudes like these, it is no coincidence that African American girls in the Youth Risk Behavior survey are dieting at only two-thirds the rate of white and Hispanic girls, or that their suicidal behavior is only two-thirds as high.

Nevertheless, it is clear that African American girls, who average somewhat heavier, and other girls of color do feel the intense pressures of our weight-obsessed culture to lose weight. Perhaps because they see more thin models of their racial and ethnic groups in the media, or because they are simply responding to the overwhelmingly white, thin images everywhere. Many feel not only deep body dissatisfaction, but desperation to get their bodies "right." Research suggests they are developing rates of eating disorders similar to those of white girls.

Other messages in the mix

When Coca Cola launched a marketing campaign for Diet Sprite, they chose a bony girl listlessly nursing her diet drink and boasted in the advertisement that her nickname was "Skeleton." Public protest forced the company to pull the ad. "There's something very sick going on here," complained the mother of an anorexic daughter in a Boston consumers group that boycotted Diet Sprite because of the ad.

She's right. There is a cultural sickness when emaciated, vulnerable, passive, childlike women are idealized as role models for our daughters.

These advertisements also send other potentially harmful messages to girls. Take the recent Calvin Klein ads that feature thin, vulnerable waifs in sexually provocative poses. Many ads show models as young, wistful and sexually alluring, doing nothing at all but displaying themselves while males reinforce ownership of them by towering over or grasping them, points out Esther Rothblum, PhD, professor of psychology at the University of Vermont.[32] These cultural messages seem to promote child sexual abuse, which is often linked to eating disorders.

Barbie — one of the most enduring cultural icons for girls — has body proportions that can hardly exist in reality: tiny waist, large breasts, long legs and long, stately neck. She has thighs that never rub together, "big" hair, feet deformed from constantly wearing high heeled shoes, and outfits and accessories that glorify and promote self-absorption, primping, exhibitionism and materialistic behavior. The recent reshaping of Barbie's figure as leaner and more boyish to bring it in line with current fashion only confirms the power of ideal bodies.

Young girls want to be like their glamorous dolls, reports a British study that found 9-year-old girls wanted to weigh an average of 11 percent less and were influenced in this by their dolls, as well as by dieting mothers and the thinnest girl in class.[33]

"What better way to ensure a constant supply of these decorative, nonactivist women than to train little girls to emulate this look and attitude at a very early age?" asks Lynn Meletiche, a size-activist. "How better, than by giving them a sample, in the form of a Barbie — and all her attendant accessories, to serve as a constant reminder of the look and attitude they are expected to achieve?"[34]

One result of the Barbie ideal is that more girls are going under the knife to shape their bodies more like their latest idols: rail-thin, without womanly hips, but with large breasts. Girls as young as 14 are getting liposuction and breast enhancement surgery. Some surgeons hesitate to make permanent alterations during these transitional teenage years, but others are more than willing. In 1999, cosmetic surgeons performed some 25,000 elective procedures on teens, according to the American Society of Plastic and Reconstructive Surgeons, nearly double the number in 1992. They did liposuction on 1,645 girls and placed breast implants in nearly 2,000.[35]

Setting the stage

"Why are so many girls in therapy in the 1990s?" asks Pipher. "They are coming of age in a more dangerous, sexualized and media-saturated culture. They face incredible pressure to be beautiful and sophisticated, which in junior high means using chemicals and being sexual. As they navigate a more dangerous world, girls are less protected."

Yet, this is happening at a time when women have more freedom and independence than ever before. They can command companies, lead hospitals, hold public office and make millions. Girls have never had more opportunities to develop their minds, yet they grow up feeling as though their bodies are constantly being watched. They learn to feel disconnected from their bodies, as if observing themselves from the outside, especially when they have been sexually abused or harassed, say these experts.

"Girls do not simply live in their bodies but become aware of how their bodies appear in the eyes of boys . . . By seeing their own bodies as images in boys' eyes, they begin to observe rather than to experience their own bodies; their bodies become 'Other' to themselves," say Deborah Tolman, EdD, and Elizabeth Debold, MEd, of Harvard University.[36]

Some are asking: What is normal and what is disordered, for girls growing up in a culture that forces them to live as if their bodies are being "watched, desired and judged?" Ours stands accused of being a culture that encourages girls to use "the power of weakness," that allows high rates of violence and sexual assault on women, and at the same time demands that the female body be highly attractive and sexual.

Some experts are calling these demands a crime against our children, a monster. "The public conscience is fast asleep," charges Naomi Wolf.

Is it about women's freedom?

Why is this gaunt stereotype so persistently promoted and the diversity of women so ignored? Who is pressuring women to be abnormally thin, and why?

For the most part, this travesty is not perpetuated on women by individual men, who after all have female friends, lovers, wives, sisters and daughters, but by the political power structure and multinational corporations bent on shaping women into ultimate consumers, perennially dissatisfied with their appearance.

In a searing account, Wolf charges that this power structure unites to force women into a competition of continual striving for thinness and beauty. It's a cruel struggle they can't win. As Wolf points out, the adverse effect of self starvation in the ceaseless quest for a thin body is an important factor in keeping women weak, preoccupied, passive, and off track from career ambitions. Dieting and thinness began to be female preoccupations when women got the right to vote around 1920. Never before had there been idealized "the look of sickness, the look of poverty, and the look of nervous exhaustion." The new, leaner form replaced the more curvaceous one with startling rapidity, Wolf says.

This alteration of the female form was a great weight shift that must be understood as one of the major historical developments of the century, she asserts: It was a direct solution to the threat posed by the women's movement and her newly-won economic and reproductive freedom.

"Prolonged and periodic caloric restriction is a means to take the teeth out of this revolution . . . so that women just reaching for power would become weak, preoccupied, and mentally ill in useful ways and in astonishing proportions." Wolf says the cultural fixation on female thinness is not about beauty, but female obedience. It's "about how much social freedom women are going to get away with." Girls are still being admonished to keep their place, to not compete too seriously.

The "good girl" today is a thin girl, one who keeps her appetite for food (and for power, sex and equality) under control, says Kilbourne.

Sexual harassment

Sexual harassment, in addition to pressures to be thin, is experienced by both boys and girls. In one survey 83 percent of girls and 60 percent of boys report having been sexually harassed at school, and 72 percent say they have harassed others.[37]

Three Canadian researchers believe sexual harassment may be one of the important ways in which young girls learn to feel shame, embarrassment, rejection and hatred toward their developing bodies. June Larkin, Carla Rice and Vanessa Russell, women's studies specialists at the University of Toronto, organized focus groups in schools in which girls recorded in their journals and shared incidents of sexual harassment.[38] They suggest that sexual harassment or teasing is a tool of oppression that can alienate girls from their developing bodies and give them a distorted sense of self.

"We have heard countless accounts of this contempt being expressed by their male peers: the girl who is afraid to walk home from school because she is forced to walk past a gang of adolescent boys who routinely call her a 'fat bitch' while they pelt her with stones; the girls who do not want to walk down a certain hallway in their high school because they are afraid of being publicly rated on a scale of one to 10 and coming out on the low end; the girls who are subjected to barking, grunting and mooing calls and labels of 'dogs,' 'cows,' or 'pigs' when they pass by groups of male students; those who are teased about not measuring up to the buxom, bikini-clad girls that drape the pages of various newspapers; and the girls who are grabbed, pinched, groped and fondled as they try to make their way through the school corridors."

Having to ward off comments about being "as flat as the walls," or "a carpenter's dream" created a growing uneasiness about their developing bodies for many of the girls they talked with. A young girl's body image is developed through the messages she receives about her body, her own perception of her body, and her resulting feelings about her body. As one girl summed it up, "I feel bad about my body and I wish I was a boy."

The Toronto researchers charge that harassing words thrown at girls do not slide harmlessly away as the taunting sounds dissipate. "They are slowly absorbed into the child's identity and developing sense of self, becoming an essential part of whom she sees herself to be. Harassment involves the use of words as weapons to inflict pain and assert power. Harassing words are meant to instill fear, heighten bodily discomfort, and diminish the sense of self."

Sexual harassment is so commonplace it is often perceived as normal, an integral part of female development, and gets largely ignored. Yet it is one of the more pervasive ways that teenage girls are reminded of the hazards of living in a woman's body. Larkin,

Rice and Russell see harassment as a pervasive form of violence that contributes to young women's uneasiness about their bodies and results in a disruption of healthy female development.

Sexual harassment may be one of the most important ways in which their "excitement about their developing bodies is crushed," according to these writers. It's a process that brands girls as defective, inferior, and inadequate.

Stigmatizing girls, and youth in general, who don't measure up is a way of marking them as different, defining that difference as inferior, and using it to justify oppression. The rejection is experienced by the entire peer group. All absorb the message, and pass it on to younger kids. Stigmatizing large girls and boys not only hurts them, it's also a way to keep thinner girls in line, continuing to focus on diet and weight.

Sexual abuse

The dark side of every culture is its sexual abuse and violence against women and children. How does our culture allow — and even promote — sexual harassment and sexual abuse of girls and women?

When girls and women are treated as objects, in advertsing, television, men's magazines and pornography, and at the same time are rendered weak, dependent and self-critical, they are especially vulnerable.

Sexual violence is the most graphic and oppressive tool for subordinating women, Larkin, Rice and Russell suggest. An eating disordered girl often says she uses bingeing and purging as a way of expelling the frightening feelings that come from being sexually traumatized. She can't control her surroundings, the perpetrator, or the people around her, but she can control what goes in her mouth. Abused girls may develop eating and weight struggles, cut or burn themselves, or disassociate from their bodies as a way of disconnecting from the source of their vulnerability. Rape, incest or sexual abuse in childhood is reported by 30 to 40 percent of women, but is much higher in eating disordered patients.

Until very recently, nearly into the 1990s, the field of eating disorders was dominated by patriarchal specialists who refused to take childhood sexual abuse seriously. Sexual abuse was discounted as a factor in eating disorders, in much the same way it was disavowed by Sigmund Freud during the 19th century, in his treatment of "hysterical" women who insisted they were victims of incest and sexual abuse. Now such abuse is accepted as a known risk.

It's about shame

The consequence of this abuse is shame, often felt as the result of humiliation and failure to measure up to high standards of appearance. Shame is the response to being violated, harassed and stigmatized, the overwhelming sense of being inadequate and wrong. Shame as a result of harassment and oppression can make girls want to disappear, become invisible, disconnect from their bodies while engaging in "relentless body criticism and improvement in an effort to bolster their shattered self-esteem," say the Toronto specialists.

Rice says this can make girls vulnerable to chronic dieting and eating disorders: "For someone faced with unrelenting discrimination in the form of blatant public hostility and disgust, demeaning and dehumanizing jokes, and unwanted advice . . . losing weight becomes an attractive means of attempting to retrieve lost self-esteem as well as gaining and achieving success."

Girls who stop eating when called "cow" or "pig" may actually be finding a way to gain approval — by creating a more acceptable body. In a sense, this is a reasoned solution, rather than pathological, explain feminists.

Girls shut down

As girls move into adolescence, their growing preoccupation with their bodies has been interpreted as expressing the need for male approval. But this may not be the case. Feminist writers suggest their concern may be more about the struggle to gain some power and self-protection.

The Toronto writers say ogling by males quickly teaches girls the risks inherent in their maturing bodies. They find leering can be a process used by males to select those females who will be the target of their future sexual and abusive comments and behavior. They quote Marian Botsford Fraser: "At some point in their physical development, all female children lose the protection of baby fat and barrettes and become prey in a game in which there are rules only if the laws are broken . . . The worst messages come from men. I have watched the way that [a grown men feels] free to look at young girls . . . lets his eyes slide all over the body of a pretty teenage girl walking by . . . grunts when he encounters two teenagers young enough to be his daughters . . . mutters, 'check out the hot blonde' to his buddy; the hot blonde is not yet 16."

Thus, some girls attempt to take control of their bodies by shrinking them until the self seems to disappear.

Prevention of eating disorders and dysfunctional eating needs to begin by dealing with the sexual harassment of young girls as their bodies begin developing.

"I think if the women's movement has failed young girls in this country, which it clearly has, then they need a girls' movement," Levine says.[39]

Women must speak out forcefully about the dangers of obsession with thinness, says Kilbourne. "This is not a trivial issue; it cuts to the very heart of women's energy, power and self-esteem. This is a major public health problem, one that endangers the lives of young girls and women."

CHAPTER 3

Dysfunctional eating disrupts normal life

■

We are seeing great changes in the way kids eat today, changes in what they eat, how they eat, and when they eat.

You may recognize the eating patterns. The fourth grader who eats only a small amount of each food on her plate, never feeling really satisfied, because she's afraid of getting fat. The 12-year-old who comes home to an empty house and eats continuously on snack foods, crackers, cookies and chips. The teenager who skips breakfast and lunch, grabs a candy bar and Diet Coke after school, finds a way to skip the evening meal with her family — and then goes on an eating binge in the evening. The wrestler who fasts and spits for two days before his match to make weight, then binges a day or two before restricting again.

Dysfunctional eating describes these types of disordered and disturbed eating behaviors which disrupt normal life, sometimes up to the level of clinical eating disorders. Dysfunctional eating hasn't been investigated in much detail. Today there's such concern, almost an obsession, with *what* to eat, that *how* and *when* to eat are being largely ignored. Yet, when kids eat in normal ways, good nutrition is likely to take care of itself.

Concerned leaders have been writing about various aspects of dysfunctional eating for more than a decade. Dieting is one form that starts in children as young as age 7 or 8, or even younger, and by age 11 is so common that some researchers are calling it the norm for girls in America today. Children are growing up with skewed attitudes toward food because of fear of fat. They are turning away from normal eating and mealtimes with family to a restricted and chaotic form of eating.

A growing number of studies document this disturbing trend. More than half of 14-year-old girls in a study of 1,000 suburban Chicago girls had already been on at least one weight loss diet.[1] Similarly, 30 to 46 percent of 9-year-old girls and 46 to 81 percent of 10-year-old girls in a California study had disordered eating, restricting their food because of body image fears.[2]

If dysfunctional, disordered eating patterns are so prevalent, why don't we know more about them? What are their effects? How can they be measured?

It's time to take a closer look.

Defining dysfunctional eating

Dysfunctional or *disordered eating* is chaotic eating that is separated from its normal function of satisfying hunger and nourishing the body. It is aimed at reshaping the body, relieving stress or bringing comfort. Dysfunctional eating may be a response to anxiety, pain, anger, or loneliness. Not regulated in normal ways, the dysfunctional eater relies on inappropriate internal and external controls, such as will power, or a planned diet or pre-determined number of calories or fat grams. The dysfunctional eating may be triggered by emotional or sensory cues, such as seeing or smelling food.

In contrast, *normal eating* is eating at regular times, typically three meals and one or two snacks to satisfy hunger. The normal eater trusts his or her internal signals of hunger and satiety — eating when hungry and stopping when full. Eating at regular meals means people will usually be hungry at those times, and eating to satisfaction tends to hold them over to the next meal.

Babies and toddlers eat this way, if allowed the freedom to do so. They eat when hungry and stop when full and satisfied. Normal eating nourishes the body for health, energy and strength, enhancing feelings of well-being. It promotes stable weight for adults and normal growth for children. But many children no longer eat this way, and their parents, too, may be eating in dysfunctional ways.

Instead of relieving stress, dysfunctional eating often makes the situation worse. After eating, it is common to feel guilty, ashamed, uncomfortably full, to regret or scold oneself or, if unsatisfied, to feel ravenously hungry and fear triggering a binge.

When a child or teenager binges, the amount of food he or she eats varies greatly. For some, it's really only a small amount; for others it may be 10,000 calories or more. But always there is the sense of being out of control and unable to stop. Often it follows a period of restraint and deprivation, when the diet is broken and the "floodgates" come down.

Dysfunctional eating can be located on a continuum between normal eating and eating disorders, and may be mild, moderate or severe *(see charts on pages 60-61).* The youngster may move back and forth across the continuum, returning to normal eating after bouts of dieting. Or she or he may restrict food so severely that she goes on to develop debilitating eating disorders from which she cannot recover alone.

Dysfunctional eating is also called *disordered eating,* but because this easily gets confused with clinical eating disorders in the

---

What is dysfunctional eating?

Dysfunctional or *disordered eating* is eating in chaotic and irregular ways — dieting, fasting, bingeing, skipping meals — or consistently eating much more or much less than the body wants or needs. Dysfunctional eating is separated from the normal function of satisfying hunger and providing energy for health, growth and well-being, and instead, seeks to reshape the body or relieve stress. It is not regulated by hunger and satiety, but by inappropriate internal and external controls, such as emotions or will power.

CHILDREN AND TEENS AFRAID TO EAT 2001

Dysfunctional eating

Compared with normal eating and eating disorders[1]

	Normal eating	Dysfunctional (disordered) eating *mild moderate severe*	Eating disorders
Eating pattern	Eating at regular times, usually three meals a day and one or two snacks to satisfy hunger.	Irregular, chaotic eating — skip meals, fast, binge, diet; or consistent pattern of eating much more or much less than the body wants or needs.	Eating typical of anorexia, bulimia, binge eating disorder, other eating disorders.
How eating is regulated	Eating regulated by internal signals of hunger, appetite and satiety; eat when hungry, stop when full and satisfied.	Eating often regulated by inappropriate internal and external controls such as dieting, counting calories, emotional events, sight or smell of food.	Eating regulated mainly by inappropriate internal and external controls.
Purpose of eating (function)	Eat to satisfy hunger, for health, growth, well-being (and at times for pleasure, social reasons). After eating, feel good.	Often eat (or restrain eating) for thinness; eat to relieve anxiety or stress; may feel too full after eating, or feel remorse, guilt, shame.	Eating almost entirely for purposes of body shaping and to relieve stress; eating may cause distress.
Preva-lence	Small children, persons who don't interfere with natural regulation; likely more males than females.	Large percentage of girls and women, perhaps at times as many as 50-81% age 10 and over (who report trying to lose weight); increasingly boys and men.	Estimated prevalence: 10% of high school and college age youth, 90-95% female.

Children and Teens Afraid to Eat, Women Afraid to Eat. Copyright 2001, 1997. All rights reserved. May not be reprinted without permisson from the publisher. Healthy Weight Network, 402 South 14th Street, Hettinger, ND 58639 (701-567-2646; Fax 701-567-2602) www.healthyweight.net.

Dysfunctional eating *(continued)*

	Normal eating	Dysfunctional (disordered) eating *mild moderate severe*	Eating disorders
Physical	Promotes health, energy; growth and development of children.	Often feel tired, dizzy, chilled; may have weak bones, delayed puberty, if undernourished; increased risk of eating disorders.	Severe physical effects; mortality high as 15-20% for anorexia, bulimia.
Weight	Normal, stable weight, expressing genetic and environmental factors.	Varies; eating pattern may cause weight to cycle up and down, decrease, remain stable, or increase.	Weight varies, depending on genetics, the disorder and its expression.
Mental	Promotes clear thinking, ability to concentrate.	Decreased mental alertness, concentration; narrowing of interests.	Diminished mental capacity, memory loss.
Thoughts of food, weight	Food thoughts low, usually at mealtime, about 15-20% of day; less if no food preparation.	Preoccupied with food; thoughts often focus on eating, planning to eat, counting calories or fat grams, body image; may occupy 30-65% of time awake.	Thoughts focused on food, weight; as much as 90-100% of time awake in anorexia, 70-90% in bulimia.
Emotional	Promotes mood stability.	Greater mood instability; easily upset, irritable, anxious, lower self-esteem; increasing concern with body image.	Mood instability, risk of functional depression.
Social	Promotes healthy relationships with family and friends.	Less social integration; may be withdrawn, self-absorbed, lonely; diminished capacity for affection, generosity.	Social withdrawal, alienation, often eat alone; worsening family relations.

Children and Teens Afraid to Eat, Women Afraid to Eat. Copyright 2001, 1997. All rights reserved. May not be reprinted without permisson from the publisher. Healthy Weight Network, 402 South 14th Street, Hettinger, ND 58639 (701-567-2646; Fax 701-567-2602) www.healthyweight.net.

public mind, the term *dysfunctional eating* may be preferred.

Studies suggest that dysfunctional eating is extremely prevalent, especially among girls and women. It appears to be increasing and striking at younger ages as the cultural drive for thinness continues to intensify. As many as 50 to 81 percent of girls and women in the United States, age 10 and up, say they're trying to lose weight. Increasingly, they are joined by boys and men who are responding to new pressures to have lean, muscular bodies.

A North Carolina college study found 23 percent of a large sample of women students, faculty and staff and 8 percent of men revealed disturbed eating patterns, testing high on the Eating Attitude Test. Of the women, 80 percent reported they were terrified of being overweight, 85 percent were preoccupied with the desire to be thinner, 84 percent dieted, and 83 percent used diet foods. About 15 to 27 percent of the men were in these same categories.[3]

Dysfunctional eating includes three general patterns:

• **Chaotic eating.** Chaotic and irregular eating — fasting, dieting, skipping meals, snacking, restricting, bingeing.

• **Consistent undereating.** Eating less food than the body wants or needs; ignoring and overriding hunger signals.

• **Consistent overeating.** Eating more food on a daily basis than the body wants or needs, above maintenance and growth needs; eating past satiety and overriding normal fullness signals. Reasons for overeating may be because of stress, to comfort oneself, to relieve anger or anxiety, or simply from habit, perhaps following family or cultural patterns, or because abundant and good-tasting food is there. However, needs differ, and body size does not identify overeating; it cannot be assumed that large youngsters consistently overeat, or eat past the point of satiety.

Chaotic eating affects emotions

Dysfunctional eating affects children mentally and physically. They may be moody and irritable when they go too long without eating, or lethargic if they are eating continually and not allowing themselves to feel hunger. If their eating involves undernutrition, the harmful effects, from fatigue and decreased mental alertness to delayed puberty, stunted growth and fragile bones, can be extensive. These effects of food deficiency are described more fully in the next chapter.

Food thoughts take up much of the time for kids who eat in dysfunctional ways. There is also increased preoccupation with forbidden foods, diet foods, delicious foods, good foods and bad foods. They are preoccupied with when to eat, and how to avoid or delay eating, and concerned with weight and their body image. Socially, kids preoccupied in this way may feel isolated and lonely. Shame and guilt may surface because of their eating or thoughts about eating. They might feel stigmatized because of real or imagined body imperfections.

Dysfunctional eating affects weight, yet in its various forms, it is associated with a wide range of weights as genetic potential interacts with lifestyle factors. Associated with chaotic eating, dieting, and bingeing, fluctuations in weight often cycle up and down in "yo-yo" fashion. Consistent undereating can be expected to result in a weight lower than normal for that child, while overeating may result in a higher weight than normal, adding excess fat to normal growth, year after year.

Dieting shrinks a child's world

For many children, a diet is where their chaotic, roller-coaster eating begins. Dieting may seem harmless, but few consider how disruptive it is. Even without nutrient deficiencies, dieting and fasting can affect development.

"Dieting is not just about eating, it is an entire way of life," warns JanetPolivy, PhD, a University of Toronto professor who has researched the detrimental effects of dieting for over 20 years. "Life has a different meaning for people when they become dieters. Their self-image and self-esteem is all tied up in this."

Polivy's research shows dieters respond differently than non-dieters in a range of situations. Chronic dieters are easily upset, emotional, moody, are more likely to eat when anxious, and have trouble concentrating on the task at hand if there is any kind of distraction. They are compliant, perfectionist, preoccupied with weight and body dissatisfaction, and have a diminished lifestyle.

They salivate more when faced with attractive food, and have higher levels of digestive hormones and elevated levels of free fatty acids in their blood. They can go longer without food and eat less under "ideal" circumstances than nondieters, but once started, they binge or eat more, then experience guilt.

The chronic dieter focuses on food, eating and weight, both for herself and in her awareness of others, has lower self respect, is eager to please and compliant with others' demands.[4]

Ellyn Satter, RD, MS, author of *Secrets of Feeding a Healthy Family,* and an internationally known specialist on feeding children, warns that dieting causes a child to cross the line to external restriction of food, leaving behind natural weight regulation and normal responses to internal cues of hunger and satiety. Satter says food restriction at an early age disrupts a child's ability to eat normally. It can lead to closet eating, hoarding food, and disturbed eating patterns. The child learns to distrust his or her own responses and relies instead on external factors such as calorie count, food selection patterns, lists of *do's* and *don'ts,* and body weight.

Yet the internal processes will not be ignored, Satter cautions. "You have to invest more and more time and effort in overcoming the physical and emotional symptoms of energy deficit: hunger, increased appetite, fatigue, lethargy, irritability and depression. And you become preoccupied with food and with yourself. In some cases, these negative feelings become very strong, perhaps because the person is depriving herself terribly . . . and she just keeps trying harder and harder."[5]

Eating disorder specialists Linda Smolak and Michael Levine agree: "Although weight/shape concerns and dieting behavior are common in elementary school children . . . they are not harmless. In the short run, caloric-restrictive diets generate irritability, distractibility, food preoccupation and fatigue. The long-term effects are more worrisome. Dieting children may be at special risk for developing severe eating disorders . . . Caloric restriction during childhood and adolescence can lead to stunted growth, menstrual dysfunction and decreased bone density."[6]

Top 10 reasons not to diet

1. Diets don't work. You lose weight and gain it right back (weight cycling), often regaining more than you lost.

2. Dieting is dangerous. It causes many deaths and injuries every year.

3. Diets are expensive and without value.

4. Dieting causes fatigue, lightheadedness, saps energy and strength.

5. Dieting disrupts normal eating, causes bingeing, overeating and chaotic feeding patterns.

6. Dieting increases food preoccupation, so half the day or more is spent thinking about food and weight.

7. Dieting diminishes women, subverting their dreams and ambitions, keeping them playing the anticipation game.

8. Dieting stunts the growth and development of children and youth, mentally and physically.

9. Dieting increases size prejudice, makes people more judgmental and critical of themselves and others.

10. Dieting decreases self-esteem and feelings of well-being. Instead, accepting and respecting yourself as you are brings confidence, health and a sense of wellness and wholeness.

WOMEN AFRAID TO EAT 2000

One chronic dieter says dieting made her less of a human being. "What I resent about dieting is that it makes one so terribly self-centered, so much aware of oneself and one's body, so preoccupied with things that apply to oneself only, that there is scarcely any energy left to be really spontaneous, relaxed and outgoing. It starts with thinking about what to eat and what not to eat, and gradually goes over to other fields, and it is this aspect that makes me resent dieting; it makes me less of a human being."[7]

"Dieting shrinks a woman's world," agrees Merryl Bear, coordinator of the National Eating Disorder Information Centre in Toronto.[8] Dieting shrinks a man's world, too.

Dieting is abnormal

The problem with dieting is that we are not able to integrate diet behavior into our normal lifestyle because it is abnormal, says Mary Evans Young, founder of No Diet Day and author of *Diet Breaking.*[9] "Dieting is based on deprivation, sacrifice and guilt, which are difficult to sustain. We lose touch with our natural hunger signals in responding to external cues which don't address underlying issues."

The diet industry has the perfect product, she observes. "It promises so much, and when it doesn't deliver the consumer blames herself and then goes on to the next diet." Dieting can make girls feel they are doing the right thing. They feel good just for having made the decision to go on a diet. Pursuing thinness is widely perceived to be the same as pursuing good health.

"That feeling of self-sacrifice can hook us into wonderful feelings of purity and goodness," notes Evans Young. "The diet becomes a kind of fanatical religion, requiring you to abide by a set of stringent rules or pay the penance of guilt. It's a guilt that starts by slowly nibbling and then steadily gnaws away at your body, spirit and confidence. Give yourself a break. You deserve much, much more."

Eating disorder risk

Many nutritionists and health professionals are concerned that the current high rate of dieting and dysfunctional eating is leading to increased rates of eating disorders as well as to obesity. This is a controversial issue, yet dieting is considered a step on the way to developing an eating disorder — a "necessary but not sufficient cause," as some explain it.

Clearly, many girls and young women who begin dieting and restricting food do go on to develop full clinical eating disorders. A recent review showed that up to 35 percent of normal dieters advance to pathological dieting. Of pathological dieters, 20 to 25 percent progress to partial or full syndrome eating disorders.[10]

Even the effects of one bout of dieting can perpetuate more disturbed eating, say Linda Smolak and Michael Levine, eating disorder specialists. "Children who are already dieting during elementary school may be at risk for developing eating disorders because of the physiological and psychological effects of caloric restriction and weight loss failures."[11]

How dysfunctional eating begins is not well understood. Disturbed eating patterns may start by following the example of parents and friends, or with their encouragement. When parents criticize their own or others' size or shape, it can teach the child to fear criticism of her own body, and launch her on an early diet.

Dysfunctional eating may not be so very different from clinical eating disorders. For some it's only a matter of degree. It is no longer possible to dismiss patients with severe eating disorders as uniquely pathological, as was often done in the past. They tend to have certain vulnerabilities, yet in many ways, they are expressing what most other girls and women are feeling.[12]

Culture promotes dysfunction

Modern culture encourages disturbed eating. Youngsters are being coaxed to overeat and at the same time, are urged to restrict eating. They are not being taught to trust their internal control systems of hunger and satiety.

Today, an abundance of inexpensive, good-tasting foods — tempting foods — is available, and a culture of eating for pleasure or recreation has developed, shaped by billions in advertising dollars. People eat out more and favor "all you can eat" restaurants, where they seem to get more for their money.

Advertisements for Pringles Right Crisps show people eating 10 or 20 chips at a time. Ritz Air Crisp ads implore kids to "inhale them." And Baked Lays Potato Chips challenges, "Betcha can't eat just one — bag."

Restaurants offer larger servings, larger meals, and more abundant buffets with many food choices. A study in *Restaurants USA* found customers expected larger quantities of food in 1993 than in 1991, and that people think of large servings as getting better value for their money.[13]

A *Healthy Weight Journal* subscriber in London recently sent me a news clipping titled: "Portions out of all proportion" that decried America's "elephantine cuisine." The writer compares national foods: hot dogs (350 calories in the U.S. versus 150 calories in Britain), cookies (493 vs 65), ice cream cone (625 vs 160), muffin (705 vs 158), nachos (1,650 vs 569), and a meal of steak and fries (2,060 vs 730). Until recently, our very large muffins were called "jumbo muffins," the article notes, now they are simply "muffins."

The Cheesecake Factory heaps food "practically a foot high on its plates and proudly serves up a 12-ounce burger." As for the cheesecake, each slice has about 700 calories. The Factory claims it tried to serve lower-calorie slices but "nobody wanted them."

We probably deserve the writer's final comment, "Europeans are a lot more quality conscious . . . Americans just want value for their money, and base value on size."

And it's true, when served larger portions, both children and adults eat more. Studies by Barbara Rolls, PhD, nutrition professor at Pennsylvania State University, show this happens by the time children are 5 years old. Children up to age 3 were not easily influenced, eating about the same amount no matter how much food was on the plate. However, when the 5-year-olds were served more, they ate portions half again as large as the amount that otherwise seemed to satisfy them. Whether the child was heavier or thinner made no difference in how much he or she ate.[14]

Studies show adults eat more when presented with many food choices, and whether they are lean or obese, they eat more when served larger than standard portions.

Nutritionists recommend that children serve themselves, or be served smaller portions and allowed to take more if they wish.

At the same time we are urged to overeat, dieting and thinness are held out as the ideal. Both extremes — undereating and overeating — ignore the fact that our bodies are wonderfully designed to maintain balance through internal regulating systems, if we let them.

Fear of eating so-called "bad foods" also comes into play. Parents are frightened and confused about the foods they eat today. It's no wonder, with the contradictory scare messages in the media. Kids listen to the food terrorist message of the day as they get ready for school.

Nutritionists deplore the damaging effects of the media's largely single-focused messages, especially messages urging restriction of food choices or based on fear of disease.

"I've never known so many people to be so worried about what they eat, or so many who think of the dinner table as a trap that's killing them," laments Julia Child, the noted chef and author.[15]

Family battlegrounds

Family attitudes can set the stage for disturbed eating early in life. Frequent family dieting, restricting food, compulsive eating, overeating to control anxiety, excessive exercising, disparaging comments, and obsession with appearance all play a part.

Parents feel confused and pressured about their own bodies and often feel more control is needed. Parents who are into control, not trust, may worry more about food than about the child, warns Satter.

They are the kind of parents who impose a feeding schedule on a baby, urge him to finish the bottle, disguise cereal with applesauce to get it down, hesitate to let a chubby toddler have seconds, make a pre-schooler stay at the table until she finishes her peas, insist the child eat "two bites of each food," or lecture a school-age child to get him to drink his milk. They reward, plead and force. All this is overmanaging, and it teaches children to ignore their natural signals of hunger and satiety.

In a recent study, 40 percent of parents believed that restricting or forbidding a certain food would cause their child to like it less. But they were wrong; instead, children's preference increased for that food. When foods were given in a limited way as rewards, they were liked even more. And the more control parents exerted over their children's eating, the less it appeared that children could naturally regulate their intake, and the less self-control they had. Forbidding or withholding candy is not the way to get kids to enjoy eating beans.[16]

Children most at risk for obesity are those whose parents fluctuate between being highly controlling in restricting food and impulsive eating or loss of control, according to a recent Boston University study. When parents fast and binge, cycling weight up and down, their children tend to reflect this chaotic eating pattern, perhaps leading to their own excessive weight gain.

Parents of the kids who gained the least weight in this study had more normal, consistent eating patterns. It's likely they kept a more stable weight.[17]

The uneasy relationships mothers have with food and their bodies are mirrored in their daughters at very young ages, too, warns Satter. She advises dieting parents to return to normal eating.

Eating disturbances may begin soon after birth, and may be modeled by parents, according to a study that followed 216 newborns in the San Francisco Bay area from birth to 5 years. The mother's body dissatisfaction, dieting, bulimic symptoms, and internalization of the thin ideal, were related to problem eating in the child. This included inhibitions, secretive eating, overeating and overeating-induced vomiting.[18]

Parents disrupt normal eating patterns in children when they insist on rigid rules and give frequent instructions, such as to eat more, eat less, clean the plate, or when they invest food with emotional value, giving food instead of affection. Parents need to remember the long-term goal is to help their child listen to and trust her inner signals, while learning to enjoy a variety of nutritious foods. It's not to get her to eat that broccoli tonight.

Satter says the parents' role is to select food, prepare it and get the family to the table. Then the child must be allowed to choose what and how much to eat. Unfortunately, this natural division of responsibility is often violated by parents with rigid or restricting eating styles, who try to take over their children's eating.

Making meals a family battleground can promote serious eating problems. In a healthy lifestyle program led by Christie Keating of Victoria, British Columbia, teenagers shared unfortunate family eating experiences, as quoted in the *HUGS Club News:*[19]

- "My mom knows I hate mushrooms and I told her I would throw up and she made me eat it and I threw up."
- "My grandmother serves me, so I can't pick."
- "Cooked peas and carrots make me gag and my parents wouldn't let me eat anything else until I was finished."
- "If we eat too much, we get this story about being greedy."
- "My mom won't give me any more, even if I'm hungry."

Are you a dysfunctional eater?

1. Do you usually restrict your food intake?
2. Do you often skip meals?
3. Do you fast or diet, and then binge?
4. Do you frequently eat too much, so your stomach feels overfull?
5. Do you count calories, fat grams, weigh or measure your food?
6. Are you afraid of certain foods?
7. Do you turn to food to relieve stress or anxiety?
8. Do you deny being hungry or claim to feel full after eating very little?
9. Do you avoid eating with others?
10. Do you feel worse (anxious, guilty, overfull) after eating?
11. Do you think about food, eating and weight more than seems reasonable?

If you answer *yes* to three or more of these questions, you may be a dysfunctional eater.

CHILDREN AND TEENS AFRAID TO EAT 2001

- "If you breathe through your mouth, you don't taste it."
- "We used to stuff our mouths with the foods we didn't like and then ask to go to the bathroom."
- "If I eat all my dinner, then I can have dessert."

Disruption of normal eating may also occur when parents fear a child is gaining too much weight and begin to restrict food. Feelings of deprivation can foster disordered eating and weight gain, warns Laurel Mellin, RD, MA, University of California, San Francisco. She reports that obese youngsters are at greater risk for developing disordered eating than normal-weight youth.[20]

The "fear-of-obesity syndrome" is a term health professionals use to describe the stunted, underfed babies they've been seeing in the last decade or so — children whose parents are so afraid they will get fat, that they keep them half-starved.[21]

"Even the fat child is entitled to regulate the amount of food he eats," Satter insists. This might be difficult for parents to accept, but they should never put a child on a diet, she advises. "Diets are not an option. Restricting food intake, even in indirect ways, profoundly distorts developmental needs of children and adolescents."

Satter says it's time to define problems of childhood obesity in ways they can be solved, rather than continuing to set kids up for failure by putting them on weight loss diets. "In my view, no person has the right to impose starvation on another, even if that other person is your child. Withholding food profoundly interferes with a child's autonomy, and you will both pay the price."

Distressing meal trends

Looking ahead, there are few signs our culture will be promoting normal eating any time soon. The opposite seems more likely. Meals are losing out, starting with breakfast. Many kids and their parents skip breakfast and thus miss out on a nutritious start for the day.

Recent reviews of the research confirm that starting the day without breakfast affects thinking, problem solving, verbal fluency, attention span, educational achievement, and ability to recall and use newly acquired information. Breakfast is especially needed by youngsters who are nutritionally at risk, or are dieting. Iron deficiencies, anemia, and other nutrition deficiencies found to be prevalent in these youth severely affect their thinking ability.

Children ages 9 to 11 who eat breakfast work faster and more accurately in school, and have better recall. Schools that provide breakfast find kids are more likely to come to school and they perform better in the classroom.[22]

Getting the family together for meals may not be easy for parents who have long workdays or long commutes and kids who are involved in sports and other activities, but it is critically important. American families eat together an average of only 4.8 times per week, according to a Food Marketing Institute survey. Less than half eat dinner together every night. Many families don't eat meals, but simply "graze" from the refrigerator and cupboard.

"You *have to* have meals," Satter insists. She says all kids need the structure of planned eating times, teenagers as much as toddlers. This structure helps them learn to like a variety of foods, consume a nutritionally adequate diet, and eat the right amount to grow well.[23]

Families who eat together value these times. Nearly all say they appreciate using mealtimes to talk over their day's events. One study found the number of family meals eaten together predicted whether a teenager was doing well or poorly in academic motivation, peer relationships, substance abuse and depression.[24] Eating regular meals also means kids are more likely to be following good nutrition principles of balance, variety and moderation.

Ominous road signs that suggest people are moving more toward eating fast and alone, and away from togetherness, says nutritionist Margaret Reinhardt of Minneapolis, include:

- Fewer family meals and foods eaten together
- More food sold in single serving packs means not sharing meals
- Fast, hot convenience foods sold in gas stations
- Over half of fast food is purchased from drive-through windows
- More all-you-can-eat and super-size servings at restaurants and take-out[25]

The will to change

All kids who eat chaotically will benefit greatly from a shift back to normal eating. Specialists consider this critically important if we are to prevent eating disorders, but we need the will to change.

We can get at the problems at an earlier stage than is being done today. Normalizing eating while a child is still at a mild or moderate level of dysfunctional eating is far more successful than waiting for her to develop a full-blown eating disorder, and then trying to treat that very difficult condition.

Numerous forces have contributed to the increases in dysfunctional eating, its engulfing of ever younger children, and increases in the adverse related effects over the past two decades. Reversing the trend cannot be easy. But perhaps bringing together this information on dysfunctional and disturbed eating will help.

If parents can understand how severely dieting disrupts their lives and their children's lives, perhaps they'll not be so quick to discard life's richness for the preoccupation of watching a few pounds come and go. Perhaps they'll restore normal eating in their homes, reach out with caring and concern, and become whole again with their children, in body, mind and spirit.

This is my hope.

CHAPTER 4

Undernourishment of teenage girls

■

Teenage girls have the poorest nutrition of any group in America. Taken as a whole, their diets are deficient in many important nutrients and in total calories. Yet this is a time in their lives when they have critical needs for growth and body development.

The appalling truth is that over half of teenage girls do not eat enough for health, energy and strength. They do not eat enough to feel or look their best. They do not eat enough for optimal bone growth, for energy, or even to warm themselves normally. They do not eat enough to be their best selves or to reach their greatest potential.

Instead, they are often weak and dizzy, light-headed, cold and anemic. Emotionally, they may feel anxious, irritable, moody, and depressed. And mentally these girls, all students of course, may have difficulty understanding and concentrating on their studies. Moreover, they feel so badly about themselves that one-third of high school girls report having seriously considered suicide in the past 12 months — double the rates of boys their age.[1]

What is the problem? Why are so many girls disheartened? Why are so many undernourished or even malnourished, starving in the midst of plenty? And why is this critical problem being ignored? The answers to these questions, I believe, are in a culture that pressures girls to restrict their eating in unhealthy ways.

Girls age 12 to 15 are at most risk from nutrient deficiencies. They have enormous growth needs. But a recent national study showed their median intake — what the girl in the middle is eating — provides only half to two-thirds of the recommended amounts of calcium, iron, vitamin A, magnesium, zinc, copper and other critical nutrients. She consumes about 79 percent of recommended calories. In the next age group, 16 to 19 years, girls fare little better.

The Recommended Dietary Allowance (RDA) provides an allowance over minimum, yet these discouraging statistics mean that half of all girls are eating much less than needed. Nutrients fuel growing brains and bones as well as strong bodies, but these girls aren't getting even the calories they need for healthy growth and development. They are severely undernourished or even malnourished.

This is a time when their bodies undergo major changes, when their childhood bodies mature. It's normal to put on some extra fat as the body develops curves and readies itself for healthy pregnancies. It's all part of normal female development — and it's going to add a few pounds. How sad that modern girls feel they must fight against the maturing of their own bodies with every weapon they can muster!

Will these girls develop into well-rounded, capable, healthy adults? Or will they face a lifetime of health problems, including osteoporosis, because they have kept vital nutrients from their bodies? Will they have financial and relationship troubles because they were too weak to learn in school or develop careers? Will their intelligence be affected? I think the odds for future problems are frightening.

The documentation for this appalling news comes from the Third Report on Nutrition Monitoring, published by the U.S. Department of Health and Human Services and the U.S. Department of Agriculture.[2] Unfortunately, even this extensive report is missing the needed analysis that nutritionists and policy makers need so they can see more than just medians and averages to evaluate what's really going on. What's happening to the "hungry one-fourth" of girls at the bottom? We don't know. What are they lacking, and how can they be helped? This is what health leaders need to know, but it's only available in a stack of unpublished pages or stored computer files at the National Center of Health Statistics.

Thus, their cry for help goes unheeded.

Lettuce and Diet Coke

Today these are frequent reports: 12-year-old girls who take only lettuce and non-caloric dressing in the lunch line; teenage girls who eat only a bagel and apple all day — after they break a two-day fast of Diet Coke and cigarettes; a female runner who exercises obsessively but refuses to eat a bite of strength-giving meat, eggs, milk or any foods she imagines might add a half-gram of fat; a college sorority in which members pay a penalty if they eat any fat at all; girls in a dancing troupe who eat fat, but don't swallow it. When these girls binge, their nutrition would be much improved if they would binge on a stick of beef jerky, a boiled egg or beef sandwich, but it doesn't happen. Their usual binge foods are cookies, cake, chips, snack crackers and candy.

It's such an unfortunate way to eat. Where are the protective fruits and vegetables? Where are the nutrient-dense meats and milk?

Half of girls are not eating well. And even the half with better intake levels often eat erratically, fasting, then bingeing on foods that fail to add up to a high quality diet, cutting out entire food groups. They are dissatisfied and discouraged with their bodies, and yearn to make them less.

But it is the lower 25 percent of girls — the *hungry one-fourth* — who are at most risk. Go to any high school basketball game or visit a classroom and you'll see them — the undernourished and malnourished girls. The bony girls, the half-starved girls with hungry eyes and hollow cheeks.

They make their first resolution on the scale in the morning: "Today I won't eat a single bite!" when they see it's a half pound over. Many avoid breakfast and lunch. They delay as long as possible for that first bite, judging this as a way to keep the appetite at bay. At 4 pm it's a candy bar and Diet Coke, maybe a cigarette. Not all thin girls are in this category, certainly: it's okay to be thin if well-nourished. But large girls are not exempt, either.

Is undernourishment a long-lasting problem for these girls? Or a temporary phase that soon passes? Maybe in the past it could have been called a phase, or a concern affecting only a few girls. But today, we can take no comfort in this. Undernutrition and malnutrition affect huge numbers of girls and they're not going away. Afflicted girls are younger than ever, and their hunger stretches far into the future. We see severe undernutrition among college-age girls with no end in sight.

The hungry one-fourth

Girls at the lower end of the nutrient intake levels are truly the hungry one-fourth. At the 25th percentile (the top point of the lower one-fourth) Mexican American girls are consuming only 1,300 calories, white girls, 1,358 and African American girls, 1,400 *(figure 1)*. None is even up to the lower range of needed calories (recommended daily intake is 2,200 calories, with a range of 1,500 to 3,000). At the

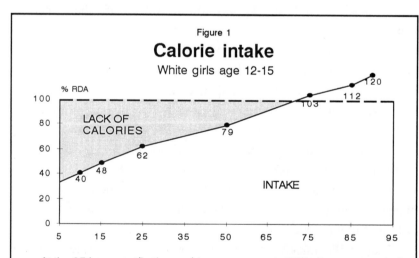

Figure 1
Calorie intake
White girls age 12-15

At the 25th percentile these girls consume only 62% of recommended daily calorie intake (2,200 calories). At the 15th they get 48% and at the 10th, 40%. Mexican American girls consume somewhat less, African American girls somewhat more. One day 24-hour recall.[1]

UNPUBLISHED DATA, NHANES III, 1988-91/
CHILDREN AND TEENS AFRAID TO EAT 2001

10th percentile, Mexican American girls get only 833 calories, white girls, 904 and African American girls, 1,064.

Looking at iron intake, girls at the 25th percentile get less than half the iron they need, and at the 10th only one-third *(figure 2)*. It's no surprise that iron deficiency and anemia are increasing among teen girls and now affect 11 percent of girls and women, including 19 percent of Mexican American and 15 percent of African American females, according to Healthy People 2010. This is even more severe for low-income pregnant girls; 29 percent of them suffer from anemia in their third trimester. Only one-fourth of females after puberty meet the RDA for iron.[3]

Warning bells go off when I see statistics like these on the limited food intake of Hispanic girls, added to studies that show their high suicidal behavior. What's going on with Mexican American girls? Who is standing up for these girls?

The calcium situation is even worse. Girls at the 25th percentile, are getting only about one-third of what they need, and at the 10th

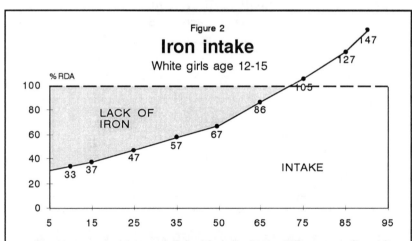

Figure 2
Iron intake
White girls age 12-15

Most teenage girls are deficient in iron. At the 50th percentile white girls this age are getting only 67% of recommended daily intake (RDA:15 mg); at the 25th percentile, 47%; at the 10th percentile, 33%. Mexican American girls get somewhat less iron, African American girls somewhat more. One day 24-hour recall.[2]

UNPUBLISHED DATA, NHANES III, 1988-91/
CHILDREN AND TEENS AFRAID TO EAT 2001

percentile only 20 percent *(figure 3)*. Only 19 percent of teenage girls meet their calcium requirements; 81 percent do not meet the RDA for calcium — the amount believed essential for building a strong skeletal structure for a lifetime. Even as calcium intake drops, the RDA has gone up. Recently, recommendations were raised to 1,300 mg for teenagers.[4]

Besides calories, iron and calcium, teen girls are deficient in many other nutrients. At the 10th percentile they are getting barely half the protein needed, one third the vitamin B12, one-fourth of the zinc, and 15 percent of the vitamin A. Median values for girls and women are shown in Table 1. It should be noted that percentiles are not averages, but the top intake at that point. If we figured the average intake for the bottom one-fourth of girls, these figures would be much lower.

Pre-teen girls from age six to 11 have more adequate nutrition,

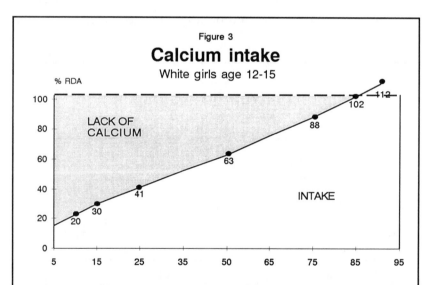

Figure 3
Calcium intake
White girls age 12-15

Teenage girls tend to be severely deficient in calcium. At the 50th percentile white girls are getting only 63% of recommended daily intake (RDA:1,200 mg); at the 25th percentile, 41%; at the 10th percentile, 20%. Mexican American and African American girls get less calcium than this at the 25th percentile, more at the 10th. One day 24-hour recall.[3]

UNPUBLISHED DATA, NHANES III, 1988-91/
CHILDREN AND TEENS AFRAID TO EAT 2001

overall. Their parents have more to say about what they are eating, and most are doing a good job of nourishing their children. Yet even in this younger group, many girls are dieting, skipping meals and restricting food. The hungry one-fourth of pre-teen white girls are getting only about one-half of the 2,400 calories recommended at this age. Their diets, too, are sadly deficient in many vitamins, minerals and protein essential for healthy growth. Our society's unfortunate overemphasis on reducing fat and increasing carbohydrates has meant that protein and animal product nutrients are being neglected by many girls and women.

The hungry one-fourth applies to college women, too. Ann Hertzler, PhD, professor of nutrition at Virginia Polytechnic Institute in Blacksburg, Va., cites three studies that indicate about 22 percent of women students daily consume less than 1,200 calories.[5]

Deficiencies in iron, zinc, calcium

Among the most critical nutrients for health and growth that American girls lack are iron, zinc and calcium. These deficiencies can cause long-term health problems, and most teenage girls consume less than two-thirds of what they need.

Teen girls are at more risk for iron deficiency than boys, yet many girls are so afraid of fat they won't eat even lean meat, its best source. Others see not eating meat as a way to avoid eating. For still others it is a guilt issue related to animal rights, for which girls seem especially susceptible. The trend is so strong that eating disorder specialists watch for the avoidance of meat as one of the steps along the way to an eating disorder.

Girls especially need the highly-absorbable heme iron from meat to make up for monthly blood losses, yet they usually consume less food and get less of all nutrients than boys.

Certainly a diet without meat can be healthy, especially for people who choose it for sound reasons and follow good nutrition practices. But unfortunately, as it is being practiced by many girls and young women in the United States today, vegetarianism is just one more self-abusing diet, unbalanced and sadly deficient in nutrients.

Iron carries energy-giving oxygen through the blood to cells. Girls

Table 1

Median daily intake — female

Percent of Recommended Dietary Allowances (RDA)

	12-15 years			16-19 years			20-59 years			≥60 years		
	NHW	NHB	MA	NHW	NHB	MA	NHW	NHB	MA	NHW	NHB	MA
Food energy	79	88	78	74	89	81	79	78	78	75	71	66
Protein	124	137	135	139	150	150	128	126	126	112	104	100
Vitamin A	63	64	59	73	60	54	75	52	66	104	63	60
Vitamin E	70	85	63	72	78	76	80	75	75	74	57	54
Vitamin C	106	180	144	102	140	127	110	97	110	143	135	102
Thiamin	108	120	107	105	118	107	112	111	112	121	106	95
Riboflavin	112	112	127	119	116	112	118	101	110	124	98	102
Niacin	97	115	100	100	112	96	118	111	103	129	109	90
Vitamin B_6	78	96	83	75	83	87	83	74	82	88	73	67
Folate	120	117	121	102	83	106	107	86	115	127	99	94
Vitamin B_{12}	169	145	170	170	154	148	156	146	150	140	116	114
Calcium	62	51	66	66	52	56	80	62	79	77	50	62
Phosphorus	87	81	94	88	87	90	130	113	134	116	96	102
Magnesium	64	70	74	62	58	66	85	66	85	83	67	65
Iron	67	65	68	63	69	68	74	66	72	103	96	84
Zinc	67	71	72	70	78	72	70	65	70	62	55	54
Copper	67	62	59	63	66	67	70	59	68	65	55	56
Sodium	108	124	106	103	129	106	110	111	106	96	83	76

NHW-nonHispanic white   NHB-nonHispanic black   MA-Mexican American

Shaded areas show median (middle) intake that are below recommended amounts (except for sodium, which is above) for females. Current public health issues considered to need attention for girls and women are the low intakes of food energy (calories), calcium, iron and zinc. Potential public health issues for which further study is needed are vitamin A, vitamin C, vitamin B_6 and folate. Low female intake of these nutrients is a serious health concern, especially for those below the median in each age and ethnic group. Values represent percentage of Recommended Dietary Allowances (RDA); for food energy, values represent percentage of the Recommended Energy Intake (NRC, 1989a). *See appendix for median intake of boys and men.*[4]

with low iron stores will likely feel fatigued, weak, listless, irritable and will be prone to headaches. And they'll have more difficulties in learning, and decreased verbal and memory scores.

In London, investigators recently found that one in four girls age 11 to 18 may be damaging their intelligence by dieting and depriving themselves of iron. "We were surprised that a very small drop in iron levels caused a fall in IQ," said Michael Nelson, PhD, study author and senior lecturer in nutrition at King's College, London. "We conclude that poor iron status is common among British adolescent girls and that diet and iron status play an important role in determining IQ." The researchers tested IQ and blood samples of 595 girls in three comprehensive schools in North London and, after controlling for social class, found a highly significant difference in intelligence scores between iron-deficient anemic girls, iron-deficient girls, and girls whose iron levels were normal.[6]

The damage young children suffer from lack of iron may be irreversible. Mental performance fails to improve in treatment for many anemic children, some studies show. Iron-deficient children commonly have shortened attention spans, lower intelligence scores, and reduced overall intellectual performance.[7] Other problems of anemia or iron deficiency include fatigue, palpitation, impaired work performance, temperature abnormalities, and a compromised immune system.

Worldwide, iron deficiency is one of the most common deficiencies for females. Fatigue and illness are typical, and anemia-related weakness may be a factor in women's treatment as second-class citizens in many parts of the world, especially where women eat last and get the poorest quality food.

Iron is not easily absorbed by the body. In fact, experts say 80 to 98 percent of iron may be wasted unless some heme iron from animal products is consumed. This has been called the meat factor — the substance in red meat that helps the body absorb iron. Hemoglobin tests find that on average the less meat a woman eats, the lower her iron levels, even when her total iron intake seems as if it would be adequate. Adding just a small amount of heme iron from meat, poultry, fish or eggs enables the body to absorb iron that is otherwise wasted. Vitamin C helps in absorption to some extent.

Girls with low iron stores usually have low zinc levels, as well, since zinc comes from similar animal sources. Zinc is need for optimal development and sexual maturation, and is of special concern in keeping the immune system healthy. Research shows all major branches of the immune system are compromised by even mild zinc deficiency. Other risks are retarded growth, birth defects and decreased short-term memory, problem-solving and attention.[8]

Calcium is also important for all youth to maximize bone development, but again is even more critical for girls because they have thinner bones and tend to be less active. Girls build bone mass until about age 25, but girls who don't drink enough milk, and especially if they are thin and often dieting (which can cause bone loss), may be setting themselves up for a lifetime of fragile bones, fractures and osteoporosis. Osteoporosis (literally, "porous bones") is painful, expensive, and lowers quality of life. It can rob women of their independent and active life. In severe cases, people with osteoporosis may break ribs by sneezing, or fracture a hip by standing the wrong way. Yet over 80 percent of girls today are *not* getting the calcium they need to build strong bones for a lifetime.

Experts fear an epidemic of osteoporosis when today's thin, dieting teenagers reach mid-life. Perhaps if these girls would help out in nursing homes, or visit the unfortunate women whose skeletons are giving way, maybe they'd value more highly the strong skeletal foundation they could be building now.

Why don't they drink milk? They fear it is fattening. Why don't they eat iron-rich meat or eggs? It's the same sad story — fear of fat, even though they could eat these foods with very little or no fat.

Fear of fat

Many teenage girls have taken their fear of fat to the extreme, cutting fat intake as close as possible to zero. This is painfully apparent in working with college students. Cynthia DeTota, MA, RD, university nutritionist at Syracuse University, New York, tells me their obsession with thinness is excruciating. Fat has become an evil.

During rush week at one sorority, girls who ate food containing any fat were required to pay into a penalty pot. In a drama group, students told her the newest trend is if a food has any fat, "You can eat, but don't swallow. Spit it out!"

DeTota says, "It's such a frustrating problem, because when I start talking about the dangers of over-restricting fat, these young women don't seem to value their health enough to make any changes. The value they place on physical appearance and body weight outweighs the value they place on their health."

"I have analyzed some students' fat intakes to be only four percent of their needs. When I give them the results, they are proud instead of concerned. They have an intense fear of fat. They really think if they increase their fat intake, they'll immediately gain weight. I encourage them to try a small change just for a week, anything else is overwhelming: 'If you could add one or two tablespoons of peanut butter on your bagels at breakfast. Just try it for a week and see if it makes a difference in how you feel.' Some will do it, and they say they feel so much better, are more alert, and don't fall asleep in class. But many are afraid to try."

Fat is important in the context of healthy eating, necessary for the absorption of fat-soluble vitamins, such as A, D, E and K. It also improves flavor, is more satisfying, helps delay hunger, and is important as an energy reserve. Girls who are eating in the range of about 2,000 calories, balanced with physical activity, can maintain their weight and meet the recommended 30 percent with about 67 grams of fat. This means a comfortable 22 grams of fat at each meal. It's a long way from zero fat.

Effects of undernutrition and malnutrition

What are the effects of long-term hunger, of undernutrition and malnutrition, of semi-starvation? If this is the norm for so many girls, can it be harmful? Unfortunately, yes. The effects can be physical, mental, emotional, social and spiritual. And they can be long-lasting.

Physically, the girl with inadequate nutrition may often feel tired, listless, light-headed, chilled. Bones may not develop normally, or demineralization may begin, leading to stress fractures. Puberty may be delayed and normal sexual development arrested. As weight drops, so do female hormones, sexual feelings, interest in the opposite sex.

Changes to personality can be dramatic. The undernourished girl easily turns moody and irritable, anxious or apathetic. She becomes intolerant, increasingly self-absorbed and focused on her appearance. As interest in food takes over and dominates her thoughts, she may withdraw from social activities and lose interest in school, career, family and friends. She feels lonely, alienated, disconnected from society. She may lose her sense of generosity, sharing and caring, stop volunteering and helping others.

These problems affect girls most acutely, but they also affect boys who are trying to lose weight. Boys who cut weight for sports such as wrestling often have these same effects. They feel weak, cold, light-headed, detached from reality, and have trouble concentrating on their studies.

Survival traits

Can some of these effects be explained as survival traits that kept our ancestors alive through periods of semi-starvation?

I believe they can. Closing down to preserve fuel during times of scarcity, the undernourished human body goes into a defensive or protective state. What happens to a person in this defensive mode — the many physical, mental, emotional, social and even spiritual effects — may be called the *starvation syndrome*. It's a closing down of the nonessential processes in the body, and focusing on survival.

Prehistoric humans lived through frequent feast and famine cycles, and even in Biblical times, famine could last those seven lean years. When this happened, human bodies shut down to conserve fuel, not just with lowered metabolism, heart rate and temperature, but in every process. Growth stopped or was severely stunted. Any fat eaten was routed to storage where possible, filling up empty fat cells instead of being burned. Sexual activity and fertility shut down; it was more important to survive than to conceive.

But our hungry ancestors did not simply lie listless in the cave awaiting death. There is no peace for starving people — they crave food, they think about food, they fantasize about food. Hunger drove them out to hunt food, despite the lurking saber-toothed tiger, howling blizzard, or fatigue. When food was again plentiful, they feasted. They binged and ate voraciously. And their bodies' natural efficiency likely increased to guard against the next famine.

Without this internal regulation, matching energy outgo with input, adjusting for fat loss, and increased hunger, the human race could hardly have survived. But it's an ancient legacy that haunts today's dieter. She cuts calories to lose weight, then burns fewer calories and craves more food. When she eats, her body rebounds quickly to its former weight, and may store extra fat against the next "famine."

The classic study of what it's like to live in a state of semi-starvation was done at the University of Minnesota in 1944 and 1945. In the *Minnesota Starvation* study, aimed at helping people in war-torn Europe after World War II, 32 male volunteers cut their daily food intake in half for six months and lost one-fourth of their weight.[9]

During this time, their metabolism dropped by almost 40 percent, heart work output per minute dropped by half, their pulses slowed, strength dropped by half, and body temperatures fell.

Mental and social effects were even more profound, and heart-breaking. The formerly idealistic, good-humored young men became argumentive, sarcastic, self-centered and intolerant of each other. They no longer enjoyed group activities, but became loners, complaining that dealing with others was too much trouble.

Even deeper social devastation than this was reported by anthropologist Colin Turnbull in his vivid account of the Ik, a starving tribe of east Africa in the 1960s. Turnbull relates in *The Mountain People* how ultimately, as starvation advanced, even children and the elderly were abandoned. The Ik came to fear and distrust each other. They seldom spoke. Cruelty took the place of love as their culture broke down. They lost their religion, spirituality, all sense of moral obligation. Men and women went out alone to forage for food, hiding any extra bits of food they found and returning empty-handed to avoid sharing with crying children, weakened parents or spouses.[10]

Today, U.N. relief teams working with starving people see this same sad desertion of family to save oneself. It seems that each person has a baseline of adequate nutrition, and when this is breached

Starvation syndrome
How the human body defends itself

Calorie restriction and weight loss cause the
body to close down into a defensive state

Metabolism, heart rate, body temperature and other processes
slow down, and the drive to eat increases
(after initial loss of appetite)

<u>Physical effects</u>
Weakness, fatigue, dizziness, headache, depression,
nausea, hair loss, anemia, chills, cold hands and feet,
diarrhea, constipation, muscle and abdominal pain,
reduced sexual function, amenorrhea, loss of bone mass,
irregular heartbeat, heart arrythmia,
risk of sudden death

<u>Mental, emotional, social effects</u>
Anxiety, irritability, intolerance,
distrust, moodiness, low self-esteem,
inability to concentrate or comprehend,
decrease in mental alertness and memory,
narrowed interests, reduced ambition,
decreased sexual interest,
intense food and weight preoccupation,
withdrawal from friends and family,
withdrawal from outside interests, loneliness,
self-centeredness, self-absorption,
diminished sense of generosity, spirituality,
love and compassion

In times of food scarcity or restriction, the human body strives to protect itself
against starvation by closing down into a defensive state that burns fewer
calories. The more severe the calorie restriction, the more severe and lasting
these effects. If food continues to be restricted, individuals may remain in this
defensive state, or they may return to it repeatedly during dieting and weight
loss cycles.

there is severe disruption of normal life and a diminishing of mind, body and spirit. These effects are well known to eating disorder specialists.

The chart on the facing page shows how the starvation syndrome defends the body against weight loss and death, as revealed in starvation and eating disorder studies. It shows the effects physically (weakness, fatigue, drop in metabolism and temperature, irregular heart beat), mentally (decrease in alertness and comprehension), emotionally (feeling anxious, irritable, moody), socially (withdrawal from friends and family, increasing self-absorption) and spiritually (loss of religion, moral values, generosity and love). In today's world, a person may maintain this reduced state indefinitely, perhaps as an eating disorder. Or the starvation syndrome may be part of a weight cycle in which the person repeatedly diets and loses weight, binges and regains weight, and begins the cycle all over again. (For more information on the starvation syndrome, see *Women Afraid to Eat,* Chapter 7.)

Food preoccupation

Even on half rations of about 1,570 calories, generous by today's dieting standards, men in the Minnesota Starvation study grew intensely preoccupied with food. They collected recipes, studied cookbooks and menus, toyed with and hoarded food. They took down photos of girlfriends and put up food pictures. Food was their central topic of conversation, and they talked of little else but hunger, food and their weight loss.

Similarly, food preoccupation is one of the most striking changes for the dieting or hungry teenager. Food craving drives her day, and she spends a major share of the day thinking about food, hunger and weight.

This food preoccupation has been studied by Dan and Kim Lampson Reiff, a husband-wife eating disorder team in Mercer Island, Wash. In their book, *Eating Disorders: Nutrition Therapy in the Recovery Process,* the Reiffs use a food preoccupation scale.[11] Patients are asked to write total conscious time spent thinking about food, weight and hunger at three periods in their lives (currently, at its highest, and at its lowest). Thinking time includes that spent in shopping, preparing food, eating, thinking about eating, food cravings, purging, weighing, reading diet books, suppressing feelings of hunger, using strategies such as smoking or chewing gum to distract from hunger, and thinking about or discussing weight.

The Reiffs have tested more than 600 eating disordered girls on this scale. Untreated anorexia nervosa patients report spending 90 to 110 percent of waking time thinking about food, weight and hunger (the extra 10 percent includes dreaming of food, or having sleep disturbed by hunger). Bulimic patients report about 70 to 90 percent.

Girls with restricted eating probably occupy 20 to 65 percent of their time this way, depending on how severe their restriction Those who eat normally think of food and eating only about 10 or 15 percent of their waking hours, usually around mealtime, suggest the Reiffs. In girls with eating disorders, they find that the intensity of food preoccupation is directly related to how much weight they have lost and the degree and duration of their semi-starvation.

Apathy in health policy and press

Apathy toward the plight of undernourished and malnourished teenage girls today, and increasingly, teenage boys, is truly appalling. Public health policy and the media take no notice. Even in the nutrition field, I find little concern.

As a licensed nutritionist who attends many international, national and state health and nutrition conferences, I scan the programs of many important meetings, and find concern for girls only in bits and pieces: iron deficiency problems, worse for adolescent females; calcium deficiencies, should be taken seriously in bone-building years; small birth-weight babies, worse with teenage mothers. No apparent concern for girls' problems as a whole.

The attitude seems to be that female dieting and weight loss is normal, so deficiencies are expected. Any blip in obesity merits headlines worldwide, but malnourished girls get only a shrug and silence.

Eating disorder specialists try to bring visibility to the effects of starvation. In their view, it seems obvious: If there weren't so many dieting, undernourished girls, there wouldn't be such high rates of eating disorders. Yet somehow their message is not being heard. In the U.S., eating disorder experts are rarely invited to serve on national advisory boards dealing with the very issues in which they specialize, as they are in Canada and other countries.

When I speak with policy makers, I urge them to take action to help undernourished and malnourished girls. But such requests are usually met with a stock answer, even by sympathetic officials who understand the problem: "The big national concern now is obesity. We have a Healthy People 2010 directive to reduce obesity — so that's our priority."

Hunger, yes, our officials can deal with that, but only if it is poverty related; then it fits a funding category. Obesity, yes, because it's on the national health agenda. But hungry girls don't fit anywhere.

It's true obesity is an urgent concern, and I'm concerned about it, too. But semi-starvation seems even more urgent. Girls are dying from heart irregularities, sudden imbalances, and other problems caused by self-induced malnutrition. Other girls and their families are scarred for life because of nutrition deficiencies which could easily have been avoided.

When the undernutrition of teenage girls and eating disorders become acknowledged as national problems, then obesity will have to be dealt with far differently than it is today, and that's a fear of some experts. But it can be done in ways that do no harm, and I believe this will happen — *must happen* — in the near future.

CHAPTER 5

Hazardous
weight loss

■

There are a hundred and more ways to lose weight. This alone should tell us something: *none work*. If even one method worked in a safe way, the others would speedily disappear.

Worse, many of today's quick fixes are outright dangerous, causing serious injury and sometimes death. Yet kids and adults are trying them all, often with a terrible sense of desperation that if they only try hard enough, they'll hit on the miracle cure. With all the glowing promises, it must be out there somewhere.

But wait a minute. Is the cure for obesity worse than the condition? This is the question asked by the distinguished editors of the *New England Journal of Medicine* in their 1998 New Year's Day editorial.[1] The editorial said flatly that weight loss is not effective, that it involves serious health risks, and that it is untrue that the risks of obesity are so high this kind of treatment is justified. It was a breath of fresh air, indeed.

The answer is, yes, in many cases the cure is worse.

Americans spend $30 to $50 billion annually on weight loss schemes. And this figure doesn't even include smoking for weight control, that unacknowledged and highly lucrative windfall for tobacco companies. The thinness culture has created a desperation in people from childhood to old age, and profiteers are quick to take advantage.

If this industry made cars, no one would buy them, and if they did, consumer groups would force a recall. If the diet industry promised any other health service, it would be required to prove safety and effectiveness. It would be held accountable for the harm it does.

But no agency even bothers to keep track of deaths or injuries resulting from weight loss treatment. Instead, the weight loss industry's unproven experiments are prescribed to millions of unsuspecting consumers — as were both the disastrous very low calorie diets and the fen-phen and dexfen diet pills in the last decade. Accountability, if any, seems to come only through hushed-up lawsuits and out-of-court settlements.

Failures of this industry comprise uncounted tragedies, emotional turmoil, death and injury. Worse, the industry exerts unprecedented control over our national health policy. Its agenda is literally being sold to long-suffering victims with their own tax money.

Failure of obesity treatment

Vast amounts of federal and private research money go into obesity treatment and its marketing. Yet, the fact remains: if even one of the many weight loss methods worked, would we have the others? I don't think so.

What happened with polio is an example: when polio was the scourge of summer swimming, it had many quack cures. But one success — an effective vaccine — ended them all. Now there's no quackery left in polio.

But the weight loss industry has little to fear, because no effective cure is in sight. The irony is that everything works short-term and nothing works long-term. This plays into the hands of promoters — they can boast of quick success and deftly shift blame for the inevitable failure to consumers.

C. Wayne Callaway, George Washington University endocrinologist and obesity expert, testifying at the 1990 congressional hearings for the American Board of Nutrition, said, "With rare exceptions, none of the popular commercially available programs for treating obesity is based on current scientific knowledge."[2]

When the National Institutes of Health and FDA asked the industry to verify their program effectiveness for the 1992 Technology Assessment Conference, only five companies sent research. Of these, only one provided adequate data, but that data — in 55 studies — failed to show any success at all in long-term weight loss.[3]

While promoters continue to claim dramatic results for obesity treatment, credible information that supports safety and effectiveness is simply not available. Some pediatric specialists say their children's results are better, but, again, their data is weak. They also likely benefit from the fact that most overweight kids will grow into their weight without intervention — 60 percent of overweight 7-year-olds achieve normal weight.

The lack of properly trained professionals working with children in the weight loss industry is another concern. "Supervision of such programs varies from none, to instantly created certified counselors, to physicians with little or no training in this area, to a few physicians and registered dietitians and behavioral psychologists who truly have the required expertise," Callaway reported.

Yet weight loss is a field in which anyone can claim expertise. Parents need to be wary, indeed, in their choice of health providers who will really help their child and do no harm.

Follow the money

The weight loss industry alone among health care sectors is allowed to parade pitifully weak studies, without challenge, at national and international obesity conferences. If we follow the money, we see why: obesity meetings are funded by the industry.

I've often been disappointed at the silence of knowledgeable scientists who guard their careers by saying nothing. Others try to bring balance, speaking out when they can, publishing articles that take a more objective view. But this is a protected industry. It is allowed to publish irrelevant research over and over again in the most respected medical and scientific journals of the day, as it did endlessly with the very low calorie diet and dexfenfluramine pills. Industry-paid scientists control editorial boards. They sit on tax-financed advisory groups and make federal policy decisions.

"Diet and pharmaceutical companies influence every step along the way of the scientific process. They pay for the ads that keep obesity journals publishing. They underwrite medical conferences. . . . Most obesity researchers would stand to lose a lot of money if they stopped telling Americans they had to lose a lot of weight," charges Laura Fraser, in *Losing it: America's Obsession with Weight and the Industry that Feeds on It.*[4]

Callaway agrees, "The so-called clinical research in this field has been largely paid for by the formula and drug companies."

Flawed guidelines

This compromised system, committed to propping up the failed weight loss industry, recently sent doctors a detailed set of "guidelines" on how to deal with obesity. The federal NIH report *Clinical Guidelines on the Identification, Evaluation, and Treatment of Overweight and Obesity* gives dire warnings about obesity risks and the necessity to lose weight, but fails to tell doctors how weight can be lost in a healthy way. Nor does it balance its warnings with others about the risks of weight loss or eating disorders.[5]

A low body mass index of 25 is set as the point where adult overweight begins. But far from finding health risks, the guidelines actually reveal a BMI of about 24 or 25 as the level of *least risk.* For African Americans, Native Americans, and older adults, especially women, the point of lowest mortality is even higher.

The guidelines recommend people lose one or two pounds a week for six months, then begin a weight maintenance program. However, there is no evidence this can work.

"No plan has demonstrated significant success in weight maintenance beyond six to 12 months," writes Ann Coulston, MS, RD, a senior research dietitian at Stanford University Medical Center.[6]

My concern is that these new federal guidelines can do a great deal of harm, especially to children, and there is no evidence they will benefit us in any lasting way. It seems unlikely that many experienced doctors will follow the guidelines advice. But if they do, and tell millions of already weight-obsessed Americans to lose weight, these are likely outcomes:

- More children will be harmed by their attempts to lose weight.
- More will begin smoking, and be less likely to quit.
- More teenage girls will be malnourished, and suffer stunted growth, arrested sexual development, and fragile bones.
- More kids will develop eating disorders and dysfunctional eating.
- Weight cycling will increase, along with its risks.
- The health community, the public and the media will intensify their focus on weight, rather than health.
- Media and advertising will increase the pressure on girls to be thin, and continue to emphasize weak, passive, vulnerable, self-absorbed role models.
- Large children will suffer even more from size prejudice, stigma and harassment.
- Health care costs will increase as more drugs are prescribed long term.
- Preventive efforts will remain stalled.

Kids are especially susceptible to advertising messages, the persuasive infomercial, the seductive voice of the quack.

Who's striving to lose weight?

About two-thirds of teenage girls are trying to lose weight, no matter what they weigh. So are one quarter of teenage boys. One of two adults diet, and children as young as six or seven are keying in to all this anxiety and following suit.[7] A nationwide study of 8th and 10th graders found 61 percent of girls and 28 percent of boys had been on a diet to lose weight during the previous year.[8]

These alarming statistics raise serious questions. What is happening to these kids as they restrict nutrients, pop pills with unknown ingredients, and yo-yo their weight up and down? What happens to their growth, their bones, their brain development, their lives? Is this supposed to be normal? Are we going to accept this?

Being overweight may have health risks, but this does not mean weight loss lessens the risks. It can do just the opposite. At the very least, the efforts kids make to reshape their bodies are diverting many from their important tasks of physical, emotional and intellectual growth and development.

A survey in Cleveland high schools found that 70 percent of white girls and 60 percent of African American girls had lost at least five pounds in a weight loss attempt, as had 40 percent of all boys. More than one third of these girls were currently dieting, including 40 percent of white girls and 38 percent of black girls. Many used dangerous methods, including semi-starvation, vomiting, diet pills, laxatives, diuretics and smoking. One-third of dieting girls and one-fourth of dieting boys said they fast for 24 hours at least once a week *(figure 1)*.[9]

"This is very disturbing," said Laurie Humphries, PhD, director of the Eating Disorders Clinic, at the University of Kentucky. "Frequently, we find these adolescents come in, 5-foot-1 and 100 pounds . . . and (say) they need to be 89 pounds."

"Our study confirms that high school students feel very pressured to shape their bodies into the popular mold, and that increasing percentages of both boys and girls are dieting and purging in an attempt to accomplish this," said Lillian Emmons, PhD, RD, the nutritional anthropologist who directed the Cleveland study. The high dieting rates she found among boys are much above earlier reports, and yet may be underreported, says Emmons. Of particular concern, she suggests, are the 10 percent of male dieters who lost 62 pounds or more through dieting, and lost 10 pounds twice as often as any other group.

Native American youth are using high risk weight loss methods at rates as high or higher than other kids, according to several recent studies. Up to 74 percent of girls and 38 percent of boys are trying to lose weight. A national survey of 13,454 American Indian students, grades 7 through 12, found 27 percent of girls reported self-induced vomiting, 11 percent used diet pills, and 7 percent dieted more than 10 times a year. Boys were using these behaviors less often, yet 12 percent of boys said they had vomited to lose weight.[10]

Emmons says meaningful education on the dangers of dieting and reasonable expectations for body size and shape need to be taught in schools before the pre-adolescent growth spurt. But it's certainly not happening, or if it is, "is not as powerful as other cultural pressures.

The amount of purging shown in this study is cause for concern because of the potentially damaging effects purging can have on health," she warns.

As noted earlier, not only are more kids dieting today, but they are starting younger.[11]

Young athletes in sports and performance arts that emphasize leanness are at special risk for harmful attempts to control the size and shape of their bodies. These activities include gymnastics, wrestling, judo, boxing, weight lifting, bodybuilding, figure skating, diving, ballet, dance, horse racing and distance running. Vomiting and laxatives are commonly used by female college athletes in several sports.[12] Many high school wrestlers use extreme fluid and food deprivation in their

---

Figure 1

Dieting and purging
Percent of high school students

	Girls		Boys	
	White	Black	White	Black
Dieting	77%	61%	42%	41%
Liquid diet	14	24	6	9
Diet pills	23	16	6	0
Laxatives	7	18	5	2
Diuretics	5	11	1	2
Vomiting	16	3	7	0
Monthly or more often	8	1	-	-
Fasting monthly or more often	35	40	29	25

Potentially harmful dieting behaviors are widely practiced by U.S. high school students. Total 1,269 students, Cleveland State University study.[1]

JADA 1992/ CHILDREN AND TEENS AFRAID TO EAT 2001, 1997

efforts to "make weight" for a match.

What methods are kids using?

Children fall victim to the many ways to lose weight, from fad diets, drugs, gadgets, smoking and purging, to surgery — methods which can damage the body, mind and pocketbook. None of them works in a safe and lasting way for very many, but each time kids are led on to a new miracle.

The trick is that they seem to work for a time. Since everything works short-term, and nothing works long-term, they keep looking, trying to discover their own "failure."

Even the Food and Drug Administration is vulnerable to pressure from this influencial industry. In April 1996, the FDA approved a diet drug, dexfenfluramine (Redux), which had only one-year safety and effectiveness data — even though to be effective, the drug had to be taken long term, perhaps for life. A year later, it was abruptly withdrawn, due to terrible complications and deaths.

While many children are taken from specialist to specialist for doctor-endorsed medical treatments, most are using do-it-yourself methods to lose weight. Here are some of their favorites — and most dangerous.

Diet pills

Kids don't need a prescription to buy diet pills off the shelf. Many teenage girls confess they shoplift and swallow the pills by the box.

Pills containing PPA (phenylpropanolamine) are readily available at grocery, drug, chain and convenience stores, under such names as Dexatrim, Accutrim and Dex-A-Diet. PPA is the only over-the-counter weight loss drug approved by the FDA, except for seldom-used benzocaine which is said to numb the tongue. (Both were approved back when FDA didn't know any better, and since then, industry pressure has kept them "on review" — a way to sidetrack action.) Over $40 million dollars is spent annually on advertising the profitable PPA diet products.

Parents and health professionals have pleaded with FDA and Congress to restrict PPA diet pills to prescription sales for adults. A bereaved father protested at the 1990 congressional hearings investigating the weight loss industry. "The lights went out in our lives on July 12, 1989, when our beautiful, fun-loving, and soon-to-be-married daughter, Noelle, died of cardiac arrest [after taking diet pills]. These stores have no more business selling these drugs to children than they do liquor to a minor."[13]

One in three teen girls has taken diet pills, according to some studies.[14] In a Michigan State University survey, nearly half of college women and 6 percent of men had taken a PPA diet drug. One in five said they'd started using these pills between age 12 and 16, reported L. R. Krupka, professor of natural science. About 27 percent of the women had taken it within the past 12 months and 3 percent in the past 24 hours.

None had ever consulted a physician, even though labels advise it under age 18. Many took more than the recommended daily limit of 75 mg of PPA. About one-fourth of the women students using diet pills had double-dosed, using other PPA-containing products at the same time. One young woman with a severe cold had taken a diet pill and four nonprescription decongestant cold medicines containing PPA within 24 hours of the interview — a total of 675 mg. Most users say PPA doesn't work in weight loss, and no data at all contradicts this.

Diet pills may cause fatigue, hyperphagia, insomnia, mood changes, irritability and, in large doses, psychosis, say Allan Kaplan and Paul Garfinkel in *Medical issues and the Eating Disorders*. Other documented side effects include fatal strokes, dangerously high blood pressure, heart rhythm abnormalities, heart and kidney damage, hallucinations, seizures, headaches, nervousness, cerebral hemorrhage, nausea, vomiting, anxiety, palpitations, renal failure, disorientation and death.

Even when used correctly, PPA can cause dangerous reactions. It leads all other major nonprescription drugs in the number of adverse drug reactions and in the number of contacts reported with Poison Control Centers, a total of nearly 47,000 in 1989.

Vivian Meehan, president of the National Association of Anorexia Nervosa and Associated Disorders, urged Congress to require that diet pills, laxatives, diuretics and emetics be sold only to adults from behind the counter, never from an open shelf, or near products identified as diet aids, and to minors only by prescription.

Herbal and quack pills

In addition to PPA, many herbal and quack pills, often illegally claim that they suppress appetite, speed up metabolism, block digestion of fat or calories, flush fat out of the cells, or otherwise alter body functions to bring about "safe, easy, fast" weight loss. Often sold as "natural" or "herbal," these products are usually labeled as food supplements to avoid being confiscated by FDA. However, the claims seen in the ad or infomercial usually are mysteriously absent from the label.

Pills like these are often spotlighted for the Slim Chance Awards we give each January from Healthy Weight Network and the National Council Against Health Fraud, for which I serve as national coordinator of the Task Force on Weight Loss Abuse. Awards go to the four "worst" weight loss products of the year. Always in hot contention are the latest versions of herbal pills.[15]

Ephedrine, often sold as the Chinese herb Ma huang, has proven one of the most deadly of these pills. In March 1994, 10 Texas teenagers were taken to emergency rooms after overdosing on ephedrine. After 37 hospitalizations and two suspected deaths, Texas Health Commissioner David Smith temporarily banned Formula One, a popular diet supplement containing ephedrine, and prohibited the sale of ephedrine products to young people under age 18.[16]

FDA warned consumers not to buy or ingest diet products that contain both Ma huang (ephedrine) and kola nut, because overdosing with ephedrine can start the heart racing, cause heart palpations and death. Yet overdosing is common with diet pills.

Since 1993, FDA's MEDWatch program has logged 38 deaths from ephedra products. But this is only the tip of the iceberg, warns the National Council Against Health Fraud. One company admitted receiving over 3,500 complaints about its ephedra-based diet program, and none of these complaints was passed on to FDA.[17] Life-threatening conditions include irregular heartbeat, heart attack, angina, stroke, seizures, hepatitis and psychosis. Temporary conditions such as dizziness, headache, memory loss, and gastrointestinal distress were also reported.[18]

Bee pollen, too, has caused fatal reactions. The FDA warns that bee pollen holds hazards for anyone with allergies, asthma or hay fever — although promoters claim it is "naturally safe" and "safe for any dieter."[19] Authorities in Australia recently linked royal bee jelly to a severe asthma attack that killed an 11-year-old girl.[20]

There's an endless supply of these "magical" quack pills, endlessly hyped. In the last 16 years, I've reported on over 200 questionable weight loss products in *Healthy Weight Journal* and our special report *Weight Loss Quackery and Fads*, and I have stacks of new ads on these kinds of products awaiting review. If these ads find me, they're finding the kids, too.[21]

Weight loss fraud works because kids and adults want to believe there are easy ways to lose weight. Con artists exploit this with a mixture of pseudoscience, mysticism and sensationalism, says Burton Love, FDA Midwest Regional Director. Authorities say there is more fraudulent and misleading information about nutrition and weight today than ever before, and it is being marketed more effectively in high-tech, highly targeted ways, with enormous profits.

Laxatives and diuretics

Taking laxatives or diuretics is a dangerous and ineffective way to lose weight. In the Cleveland study mentioned before, African American girls were most likely to use laxatives and diuretics to lose weight — 18 percent had used laxatives and 11 percent diuretics. About half of users took them at least every month.[22] In the Youth Risk Behavior Survey, laxatives and diuretics taken most often by Mexican American girls.[23]

Laxatives cause weight loss through dehydration due to a large volume of watery diarrhea. Calorie absorption is not really affected, but nutrients may be poorly absorbed.

Abuse of laxatives can cause both acute and chronic lower gastrointestinal complications, including abdominal cramping, bloating, pain, nausea, constipation and diarrhea.[24] They can cause loss of electrolytes, including potassium, essential for heart function.[25] Nerve damage may result in a sluggish bowel that can get so severe it requires removal of the colon.

Tolerance develops to laxatives over time, so abusers may increase to 60 or more tablets daily. Laxatives are probably the most common type of drug abused by bulimic patients.[26]

Diuretics or "water pills" are used less by youngsters, but their abuse is extremely dangerous. Using several purging techniques together intensifies the effects. The big concern is potassium loss leading to heart arrhythmias and kidney damage. A physician should be consulted immediately on signs of potassium loss, such as muscle weakness, fatigue and chest pain.

Vomiting

One in six white girls in the Cleveland study vomited in a desperate effort to avoid digesting the food they ate.[27]

Vomiting can cause sore throat, difficulty in swallowing, heartburn-like pain, esophageal rupture, tooth decay, loss of potassium, dehydration, cardiac arrhythmias, and sudden death.[28] Forceful vomiting may tear the mucosa of the gastrointestinal tract, revealed as blood in the vomitus.

Occasionally, the force of vomiting can break small blood vessels in the eyes and injure the esophageal sphincter, allowing stomach contents into the lower esophagus. The esophagus can rupture after ingestion of a large meal and subsequent forceful vomiting. This creates a medical emergency with severe upper abdominal pain, worsened by swallowing and breathing. It has high death rate if left untreated; surgery is usually required. Low levels of potassium, essential for muscle and heart functioning, can trigger cardiac arrhythmias, from prolonged vomiting.

Some kids use Ipecac syrup to induce vomiting, a practice that is especially dangerous and can cause cardiovascular, gastrointestinal and neuromuscular toxicity.[29]

Those who vomit three times a week or more will eventually cause erosion of their tooth enamel from acid vomitus in the mouth. Experts say this erosion can take as little as six months, or several years. Teeth become sensitive to heat and cold, open up spaces, lose fillings, and eventually deteriorate down to painful cores. Vomiting also causes "chipmunk" cheeks, probably from repeated gland stimulation by the acid contents of the stomach.

Smoking to lose weight

Nicotine is the most popular weight loss drug used today. Smoking rates are up for young Americans, especially girls, after a decline in the 1970s and 1980s.

For the first time ever in 1995, white high school girls were smoking more than boys, as indicated in the Youth Risk Behavior survey. Forty percent of white girls smoked, at least occasionally, compared with 37 percent of white boys. Twenty-one percent were regular smokers (20 or more cigarettes a month), compared with 18 percent of white boys *(figure 2)*. This percentage is highest for white

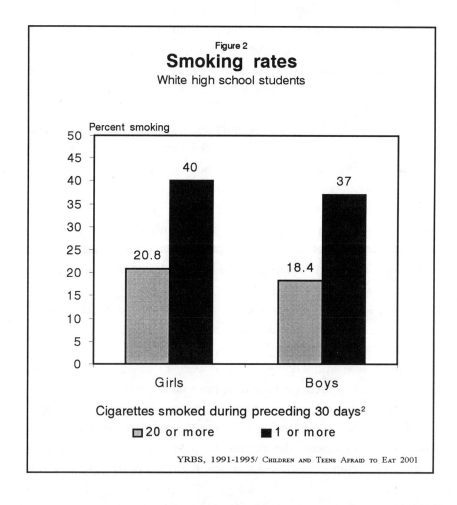

Figure 2
Smoking rates
White high school students

Percent smoking

Cigarettes smoked during preceding 30 days[2]

□ 20 or more   ■ 1 or more

YRBS, 1991-1995/ Children and Teens Afraid to Eat 2001

students, lowest for African American students. Only 12 percent of African American girls smoked occasionally in 1995, a figure that had increased to 17 percent by 1997.[30]

The pattern of girls smoking more than boys now exists in advanced countries around the world. In Canada in 1996-97, 31 percent of girls and 27 percent of boys age 15 to 19 were current smokers (smoked daily or occasionally), according to Health Canada's National Population Health Survey. There's one compelling reason: girls are desperate to control their weight.

And smoking among girls continues on the rise. The 1999 Monitoring the Future Study reported that daily cigarette use among U.S. eighth grade girls jumped from 6 percent in 1991 to 16 percent in 1996.

Smoking levels are also high among college students at 29 percent, compared with 25 percent of adults.

Smoking has its own powerful industry promoting nicotine as a method of weight control. In magazines targeted to girls and women, cigarette ads nearly always use a thin model and the word *slim* in a subliminal way, such as *Capri Superslims,* or *slim price.*

The jump in girls' smoking began during the late 1970s, "to the point where for almost two decades teenage girls have been puffing away at rates exceeding or equal to those of teenage boys," mourns Joseph Califano, Jr., former secretary of Health, Education and Welfare. He says he regrets not dealing with the fear of weight gain early in the fight against smoking.[31]

The irony is that 30 years later, smoking programs still fail to address the issue, because the health community refuses to acknowledge that people smoke to control weight. This irony exposes the hypocrisy of the current U.S. health policy, which supports the thinness obsession and the diet industry, seemingly at any cost to health. The only way to deal with this problem is to admit that the drive for thinness is a major reason girls smoke. In my opinion, anti-smoking efforts that ignore this are insincere and will be ineffective.

Targeting women in cigarette advertising began in the late 1960s, and in the next 20 years, death rates from lung cancer increased 500 percent for female smokers. And girls and women are not as likely to quit as males.

With teenage girls leading the way, 3,000 American adolescents become regular smokers every day. "Virtually all will be sicker than the rest of the population, most will never quit, and more than a third face early death as a consequence of their addiction," says Califano. (Eventually, they will also find that smoking ages the face, causing deep vertical wrinkles and a muddied or purplish complexion.)

Califano says the nation's obsession with thinness is a great boon for tobacco companies who play shrewdly on the fear of weight gain. "That's what makes Virginia Slims and Capri Superslims — with their names, slim cigarette outlines, and extremely thin models — so attractive to teenage girls."

Young people are smoking earlier. Of high school students who have ever smoked, about one-quarter first smoked by sixth grade. It's harder to quit when kids start early, and they are more likely to become heavy smokers and develop a smoking-related disease.[32] Tobacco companies deny targeting children, yet advertise heavily in magazines they read, sponsor sporting and concert events that attract young people, and get wide exposure as accepted background for televised sports events.

Tobacco is responsible for more than one of every six deaths in the U.S., and smoking during pregnancy accounts for up to 30 percent of low birth weight babies and 10 percent of infant deaths, according to the Healthy People report.

And it's true: research confirms the popular belief that smoking helps keep weight down, and upon quitting smoking, most people gain some weight.[33] This effect is well-known to teenage girls. In national studies, smokers who quit gain an average of about six to 10 pounds, but their weight does not differ much from that of persons who never smoked. This is consistent with studies that show people who quit smoking catch up with their peers who never smoked.

Thus, nicotine acts much like prescription diet drugs. People keep off six to 10 pounds and regain them when they stop smoking. The weight control effect is not much compared with the economic and health costs. However, instead of pretending there is no effect, we need to help kids realize how foolish it is to smoke for weight control.

Healthy People 2010 goals are to decrease smoking from 36 percent of high school youth to 16 percent, and to increase the average age of first use to 16 from 14 years in the next decade. But if Healthy People and other federal policies continue their pressures for thinness, meeting these goals will probably be impossible.

Miracle diets and quick fixes

Other weight loss methods include an array of fad diets and gimmicky ways of restricting food. There are liquid diets in a can, fruit diets, rice and grapefruit diets, the cabbage diet, low carbohydrate diets, and other faddish food combinations. Most are severely unbalanced and lack variety, but luckily, are so boring kids don't stick with them long. There are also ways to "detoxify" the body, a quack notion that usually involves a fast of several days.

The simple answer to why restricting food doesn't work is that our bodies don't want it to. The human body wants to restore its normal weight, and does this through a highly regulated internal system. Most nutritionists no longer believe in a simple numbers game, in which calories are counted in and out to figure pounds lost. It doesn't work that way long term — and if not long term, then why bother?

Other quack weight loss methods are herbal teas and mushroom tea, which have been linked to deaths. The FDA warns of at least four deaths and adverse effects ranging from diarrhea, cramps and fainting to permanent loss of bowel function related to herbal weight loss teas. Many contain large doses of stimulant laxatives, but since they are sold as food supplements, they're not regulated and contain unknown amounts. Potency varies widely with growing season, amount used, and steeping time.[34]

Also in the quack arena are numerous gadgets such as slimming insoles, vacuum pants, appetite-suppressing earrings, appetite patches, passive exercise tables, electrical stimulators, acupressure devices, battery-driven spot-reducing belts, body wraps, hypnotism, meditation, mystical panaceas, aroma therapy, seaweed soap, spot reducing creams and lotions. Most of the gadgets are probably harmless, yet they involve scams or deception. The voice of the quack is seductive in enticing youngsters to waste money on worthless schemes.[35]

Medically monitored programs

While kids often choose self-directed methods to lose weight, many are treated within the health care system. Thus, they are medically monitored, but this does not mean they are without risk.

Most physicians care about their patients, and understand that weight loss programs seldom give lasting and safe results. Many others, however, favor quick fixes or get-rich-quick plans. Still others are well-intentioned, but misinformed. They seem convinced a pill or diet will do the trick; if not, the patient is at fault.

The medical community has become tainted during the last decade by its misplaced enthusiasm for two lucrative weight loss treatments that turned out to be failures and even harmful: very low calorie liquid diets and fen-phen/Redux pills. Twice burned, will physicians and their patients think more carefully before launching the next round? We can hope so — but don't count on it.

Prescribed widely in the early 1990s, the very low calorie diet of under 800 calories, has the highest risk for sudden death syndrome, warn researchers at the National Institutes of Health Obesity Research Center in New York. Sudden death can come without warning or follow cardiac arrhythmias when the heart muscle itself loses size during large, rapid weight loss. Gallbladder disease is another risk. Children rarely develop gallstones, but one 13-year-old girl had to have her gallbladder removed after losing weight through a weight loss center diet. Her mother, Loretta Pameijer, told a congressional subcommittee at the 1990 weight loss industry hearings, "We're angry because it never occurred to us to be suspicious of a doctors' clinic."

A New York City investigation also turned up numerous health problems from dieting, including the case of a 15-year-old Long Island girl who had to have her gallbladder removed after losing 72 pounds in six months.[36]

The federally funded 1995 book, *Weighing the Options*, recommends very low calorie diets for large children, suggesting liquid diets of 600 to 800 calories, with part of the calories made up by two to four cups of low-starch vegetables. This is called a "protein-sparing modified fast," meaning fat will be lost but not muscle, a theory long ago proven false. *Options* recommends this diet be reserved for high-risk kids, the "more serious cases of childhood and adolescent obesity, for which rapid weight reduction is essential." It fails to explain why a diet that does not work and is unsafe for healthy kids should be used on those who are at high risk.[37]

Yet, it seems no child is too young: "In children, the protein-sparing modified fast has been used on children as young as six and by children whose weight ranges from 120 percent to greater than 200 percent of ideal . . . (However) in England, (it) is not recommended for children under 13."

Not until 1998, after years of endorsing VLCDs, did policy makers at the National Institutes of Health tell the truth. The NIH Guidelines now admit that diets of 800 calories cannot be recommended because they are unsuccessful, usually more weight is regained than lost, and they increase risk of gallstones and nutrient inadequacies.[38]

Drugs for weight loss

About six million adults and children in the United States took the weight loss drugs fenfluramine in combination with phentermine, and dexfenfluramine or Redux when it was made available in 1996. Then abruptly the drugs were pulled from the market in September 1997.

At the time the pills were banned, the FDA had reports of more than 100 patients with heart valve disease, and three had died. There were also 55 confirmed reports and nine deaths of primary pulmonary hypertension related to these drugs. The FDA says up to one-third of people who took them may have developed leaky heart valves, a finding later confirmed by investigators at five medical centers.[39] Primary pulmonary hypertension, long linked to the fenfuramine drugs, is considered fatal within four years for nearly half its victims. Most who died from the two conditions were young healthy women. Some had used the pills less than a month. Brain damage was also documented in more than 80 animal studies, and evidence of brain effects showed up in some patients as sleep disturbances, depression and psychotic reactions.[40]

Ironically, the popular fen-phen pills kept off less than 10 pounds.

But, prescribed with a diet that brought on temporary weight loss, they seemed effective.

Today's approved prescription diet pills don't work very well either. Average weight loss over placebo is only seven to 11 pounds for sibutramine, sold under the brand name Meridia, by Knoll, and 8 pounds for orlistat, sold as Xenical, by Hoffman-LaRoche.[41] Patients demand better results than this — thus a weight loss diet is prescribed to go along with the pills. The patient loses weight for a few weeks or months from the diet, then gains it back.

Meridia works on brain chemicals to suppress appetite. But it tends to raise blood pressure, speed the heart rate, and is advised only for severely obese patients — but not if they suffer from poorly controlled hypertension, heart disease, or irregular heartbeat, or if they have survived a stroke, according to the FDA.

Only one-year studies of safety and effectiveness are available, which means it is foolish to take Meridia for more than one year. Yet, in Catch 22 fashion, weight is regained when the pills are discontinued. On the other hand, weight loss is not assured even if pills are taken continuously; in the past, one-year data has usually meant that longer term results were not good.[42]

Orlistat, sold as Xenical, acts on the intestine, blocking up to 30 percent of the fat absorbed into the intestines. Orlistat has been criticized for having unpleasant side effects of soft stools and oily leakages as it sends undigested fat out of the body, but marketers say this purging effect teaches the patient to eat less fat.[43]

It's hard to believe people will spend money indefinitely on such pills, just to keep off eight or 10 pounds. Will it really benefit the person who weighs 250 pounds? We don't know of any health benefits to this treatment. Nor do we know the long-term risks.

Amphetamines are no longer recommended because of potential addiction risk, but are still available and being prescribed by some doctors. In their youth, many of today's large people were prescribed amphetamines and struggled with addictions.

In the book *Real Women Don't Diet,* a woman named Gloria says she was prescribed her first diet pills at age 12. "They weren't called 'yellow jackets' or 'uppers' back then. They were just some little yellow pills given to a physically healthy 12-year-old to lose weight . . . Withdrawing from years of diet pills, which meant having vivid hallucinations and periods of extreme paranoia and finally becoming bulimic, were the most dangerous, physically damaging aspects of my war with my body, but the psychological damage and pain have been far more lasting."[44]

Marcia G. Hutchinson, a psychologist and author of *Transforming Body Image*, recalls, "From a very early age, I was subjected to state-of-the-art diet methods — amphetamines at age six, a 10-day hospitalized water fast at 15, and a dizzying array of restrictive regimes in between."[45]

Yes, sometime in the perhaps-distant future we may have weight loss drugs that are safe and effective for most people. But not yet. Our vulnerable children have time to wait. They need not be victims of these experiments.

Stomach stapling

Weight loss surgery such as stapling of the stomach carries real risks and is not recommended for children under age 17, according to the 1991 Gastrointestinal Surgery Consensus Development Conference. Yet children are having the surgery, and do die from it. A review of gastric weight reduction surgeries at the University of Florida Department of Surgery, Gainesville, showed three deaths within the first year among 11 children who had jejunoileal bypasses. Three others had severe complications requiring reanastomosis or a reopening. Thirty-nine surgeries for weight loss were performed on adolescents from age 11 to 19 at that institution during the previous 11 years.[46] Nationwide, an estimated 15,000 people have weight-reduction surgeries each year. Of these, about 180, or 1.2 percent, are listed as being age 18 to 19.[47]

Death rate for this elective surgery is up to 2.5 percent in published studies, or as many as five patients for every 200 who undergo the surgery.[48]

Even liposuction can cause death and lasting injury, particularly when the provider has little specialized training. A study released by the American Society of Plastic Surgeons reveals 95 deaths between

1994 and 1998 in liposuction procedures performed by board-certified plastic surgeons, a rate of one death for every 5,000 surgeries. "Choose your surgeon carefully," warns Rod Rohrich, MD, plastic surgeon and co-editor of Plastic and Reconstructive Surgery, the journal that published the study.[49]

Summer camp

In the hope they will lose weight, many parents send their children to summer weight loss camps. But how good are these camps — and what are their long-term results?

"Most camps are costly, stress excessive weight loss and fail to include an intensive family component," warns Laurel Mellin, RD, Director of the Center for Adolescent Obesity, San Francisco.[50] Mellin says that the typically severe dietary restrictions actually stimulate binge eating after camp is over. And since the family has not made changes to support a new lifestyle, the youngster's weight loss does not last long. Such camps, Mellin points out, "are most likely to attract families that are desperate about their adolescent's weight and want to have their child "fixed." The overweight adolescent becomes the victim as parents first delight in initial weight loss, then despair and blame him or her as weight regain predictably occurs."

Kids at summer camps may be especially vulnerable to unfortunate weight loss experiences. While some camping programs recognize the vulnerability of young people and hire qualified health professionals, many others do not. They may focus on restrictive diets and strenuous exercise which cannot be maintained.

A doctor in China seems to have taken the weight loss camp idea to the extreme. An Associated Press story tells of a 10-day weight loss camp for 60 children, ages eight to 14, directed by Dr. Yan Chun, chief endocrinologist at Beijing Children's Hospital. Yan restricted his young campers to an 800 to 1,000 calorie, high protein, low starch, no-sweets diet. He exercised them four to five hours per day, and medicated them with a "new appetite suppressant." Appallingly, the visiting reporter wrote that the program "seems to be working," because "the children's main topic of conversation was how much fat they'd shed."[51]

Making weight in sports

Athletes in appearance sports and those in which performance is related to weight often bring together several dangerous techniques for quick weight loss. Wrestling is at the top of this list. "If there's a way to lose weight, a wrestler will find it," warns Don Herrmann, associate director of the Wisconsin Interscholastic Athletic Association. "I've seen vomiting, laxative abuse . . . even a self-induced bloody nose."[52]

A Pennsylvania study found 42 percent of high school wrestlers had lost 11 to 20 pounds at least once in their lives. One-fourth were losing six to 10 pounds every week. They used a variety of aggressive methods including dehydration, food restriction, fasting, vomiting, spitting, laxatives and diuretics. Seven percent were using vomiting on a monthly basis, 1 to 3 percent had used diuretics or laxatives.

A study of college wrestlers found food intake was extremely chaotic. One 118-pound wrestler ate 334 calories the day before the match, 4,214 calories in the evening after his match, and 5,235 the next day. His weekly loss was 12 pounds, followed by rebound after each match. Many were deficient in needed nutrients, which was more severe because of their strenuous training.[53]

The wrestlers had five hours between weigh-in and match to consume food and fluid, but this was judged too short a time to restore electrolyte balance or replenish muscle glycogen concentration. Many competed with greatly reduced carbohydrate stores, leading to premature fatigue and poor performance.

Dehydration used by wrestlers in this college study included saunas (51 percent), wrestling in a heated room (74 percent), wearing rubber or plastic suits while exercising (42 percent), and restricting drinking (58 percent). Parents often feel helpless in the face of such determination to "make weight."

Competing or training while dehydrated is an extremely hazardous practice. It inhibits sweating and increases risk of body temperature problems and heat stroke. Dehydrated wrestlers also lose stamina. Muscle endurance in these studies dropped 31 percent after a 4 percent loss of body weight from dehydration. Even four hours after rehydration, endurance was depressed as much as 21 percent.

The deaths of three college wrestlers within six weeks in 1997 shook the sport of wrestling. All three were restricting food and fluid and were trying to dehydrate in supervised training sessions when they died. They included a University of Michigan student who was wearing a rubber suit and riding a stationary bike while trying to lose six pounds in three hours to reach 153 pounds; a University of Wisconsin La Crosse student who also was riding an exercise bike in a rubber suit, aiming at 153 pounds and trying to shed the last four pounds; and a wrestler from Campbell University in North Carolina who died while trying to lose 15 pounds over a 12-hour period to compete at 195 pounds. In the wake of these tragedies, the National Collegiate Athletic Association revised the guidelines to prohibit hot boxes, hot rooms over 79 degrees, saunas, steam rooms, vapor-impermeable suits, use of laxatives, emetics, diuretics, excessive food and fluid restriction, and self-induced vomiting.[54]

The rapid weight loss wrestlers undergo can cause kidney and heart strain, low blood volume, electrolyte imbalances, increased irritability, depression, inability to concentrate, and increased vulnerability to eating disorders. Severely restricting food and fluid can also affect metabolism, body composition, performance, body temperature and overall health. Fluid losses and resulting electrolyte disturbances can increase risk of cardiac arrhythmias, renal damage, impaired performance and injury. For young wrestlers, concerns are also raised about stunting of growth at a time in their lives when growth should be active and natural.

The loss of three or four pounds is a big loss for the smaller 103-pound wrestler, compared with the same amount for a 189-pounder, but it is often treated as the same by the coach. The average young man, with normally 14 to 16 percent body fat, will often strive for 5 to 7 percent fat if he is serious about sports in which leanness can be a factor, says the U.S. Olympic Committee's Division of Sport Medicine and Science. A study of elite high school wrestlers at the Iowa State Wrestling Championships found 30 percent had only 5 percent fat or less. Girls, too, may try for extremely low body fat, even though they might normally have body fat of 20 to 22 percent. Body fat measurements are notoriously inaccurate, with a 5 to 7 percent error factor by even recommended methods, so there's added risk when body fat readings are this low.

Severe dieting affects both the mind and body, but young athletes may not realize this, experts say. Athletes may fear that the symptoms they experience — poor concentration, moodiness, irritability, anger, depression, feelings of inadequacy, anxiety, obsessional thinking, poor decision making and social withdrawal — are signs of deeper emotional disturbances.[55] Instead, these are the natural effects of severe food restriction, and can be expected.

Making weight was associated with fatigue, anger and anxiety in the Pennsylvania study. After a match, 30 to 40 percent of wrestlers reported being preoccupied with food and eating out of control. One specialist in wrestling research warns that a sign of losing too much weight is loss of concentration and "a skinny kid walking around in a daze."

Working with a sports nutritionist throughout the season is strongly recommended for athletes in sports in which weight is a concern, especially wrestling and gymnastics.

Higher mortality with weight loss

Even when successful, most large, long-term studies show that losing weight is a risk factor for death at an earlier age. The NIH Conference on Methods for Voluntary Weight Loss and Control first compiled this evidence in 1992. It showed that weight loss is associated with increased risk of death, rather than the other way around, as was expected.[56]

During 18 years of follow-up in the large Framingham Heart Study, both men and women who lost weight through 10 years had the highest death rates. Similar findings were reported from other long-term comprehensive studies including the Harvard Alumni Study, MRFIT, CARDIA, a follow-up to the NHANES I study, and a 10-study review by Reubin Andres, MD, clinical director of the National Institute on Aging. All exhibited higher mortality with weight loss, even though they controlled for early deaths that could have resulted from existing illness.

The question is *why?* Why, when short-term studies show benefits from weight loss, do long-term studies show the opposite? The answer may involve muscle loss. A recent study that separately analyzed two large studies — the Framingham Heart Study and the Tecumseh Community Health Study — found that loss of lean body mass increased death rates, even though fat loss seemed a benefit. The majority of people may have lost an unfavorable ratio of fat to lean, losing too much muscle, bone and organ tissue. On average, the harmful effects of losing weight outweighed the benefits.[57]

David Allison, of the Obesity Research Center in New York, concluded, "Past research has shown people who lose weight don't live as long, on the average. This suggests they may be losing an undesirable ratio of fat to lean."

Perhaps it is time to up the ante. Not only should we demand that weight loss be safe and effective, but also that people will be healthier afterward. Or certainly not *less* healthy, or with lives cut short.

Wait two years

For those eager to try each new weight loss miracle, "just in case it works," my basic advice holds: wait two years after the media and doctors and your friends are enthusiastically promoting this great new miracle. In two years you'll know the truth, and will have saved yourself a lot of grief. So far it has proven good advice. Certainly, for children and adolescents, it seems wise to delay those two years. These kids have time to wait, and many years to regret a harmful decision.

The real successes I'm seeing for both children and adults aim at improving lifestyle habits in lasting ways, making gradual changes toward active living, moderate eating, relieving stress, and letting weight come off as it may, naturally, the result of changed habits. Weight lost this way stays off because both habit and one's metabolism support the change.

But, unfortunately, consumers are continually lured into weight loss treatments by the promise of a quick fix. Our children need help to avoid being victimized by all this.

CHAPTER 6

Eating disorders
shatter young lives

■

An eating disorder is an unpleasant full-time occupation, terrifying in the way it takes over a child's life and that of her or his family's. Yet we have reached a point in modern society where young women eye the skeletal forms of anorexic students hovering at the edges of their classes and murmur in envy, "Wish I could control my eating like she does. Wish I could be that thin!"

While eating disorders may carry a certain aura of glamour for some, highlighted by the veil of "heroin chic," in truth they offer not sophistication, but the deadening opposite. They expose the raw state of advanced starvation, a human being at her lowest survival level, losing even her sense of humanity, compassion and love. How can this be called attractive or desirable?

As American adults continue to obsess about weight and diet, it is hardly surprising that eating disorders among their children have risen to crisis levels.

"I have many regrets. I lost a number of friends, hurt a lot of people I care about," laments one young woman, recovered from anorexia nervosa and bulimia nervosa. "My memories of the last 16 years are spotty and dim. In fact, there have been many major events, such as my sister's wedding, that I have no recollection of. Eighty to 90 percent of my time was spent in [disordered] behaviors. My behaviors overtook my life and I essentially lost 16 years of living — years that I can't have back."[1]

While overweight may carry health risks over a lifetime, eating disorders can be deadly and take but a few years to kill. Sometimes less. It took only 13 months for Andrea Smeltzer, a college sophomore from Napa, Calif., who struggled with bulimia, then died suddenly when an electrolyte imbalance led to heart failure.

In a poem, Andrea wrote, "I have an eating disorder. It is not *had* or *did* or *used to*. It is present tense. I am accepting . . . food as a necessity not an enemy. I am alive . . . fighting to remain that way. . . . I am on a journey . . . laughing, crying, cartwheeling, eating. It is ok. I am ok." But she was not okay, and her mother and father are responding to their loss with a personal crusade to bring Andrea's story to college campuses, and to promote changes in a culture that fosters such tragedies as this.[2]

Eating disorders steal time and energy from fun, relationships and growing-up activities. They can be associated with alcohol or drug abuse, increasing medical and mental complications. Sufferers lose energy, irritate easily, are lonely and driven to keep their disorder a secret. The father of one girl said, "She has withdrawn into her own world. She's lonely and is missing out on all the fun and exciting things during her teenage years . . . I have cried many times over this."[3]

Families of eating disordered youth are in a difficult situation. They see their child behaving in destructive ways and feel helpless and frustrated. They may try to gain control over what she eats. Some police washrooms and search through drawers for diet pills or laxatives. Moms and dads struggle not only with the child's immediate problem eating and concerns over lasting injury, but also with guilt that they must somehow be to blame. The eating disorder tends to take over and dominate family life.

Sufferers of this illness can be extremely rigid, determined to keep their own small rituals and rules. They become manipulative, often exasperatingly stubborn. In many ways, those who are caught up in eating disorders are not sympathetic figures. They have a desperate need for love, yet are not always easy to love.

The sister of a girl who died from anorexia confesses her feelings of anger. "At times I felt overcome with anger at my sister and blamed her for the painful discord my family was experiencing. Stronger though was the sadness I felt for my parents as I watched them be blamed, suffer, and hope, only to be repeatedly disappointed.[4]

Eating disorders have gone global. For the first time they are known in third world countries that are more used to battling natural starvation. They've spread to girls and women of all socioeconomic and ethnic backgrounds in Seoul, Hong Kong and Singapore. Many cases are reported in Taipei, Beijing and Shanghai, and even in countries such as the Philippines, India and Pakistan. First documented in Japan in the 1960s, anorexia now afflicts an estimated 1 percent of young Japanese women, about the same as in the United States.

"Appearance and figure have become very important in the minds of young people," says Dr. Ken Ung of the National University Hospital in Singapore. "Asians are usually thinner and smaller-framed than Caucasians, but their aim now is to become even thinner."[5]

Widely regarded as only a modern problem, eating disorders have been known for centuries, often as fasting in a religious context. Earlier it was believed that eating disorders struck only upper and mid socioeconomic levels. But it is now clear they know no barriers, affecting both females and males, all ages, races, religions and economic backgrounds.[6]

Prevalence

An estimated eight million people in the United States have eating disorders, including 10 percent of high school and college-age youth, 90 to 95 percent of them female, according to eating disorder sources.

Anorexia nervosa affects about one to four of every 400 girls, according to figures recently compiled by Michael Levine,[7] while the Canadian Eating Disorder Information Centre gives a higher figure of up to 3 percent for North American women. Bulimia nervosa affects 1 to 3 percent of high school girls, and 1 to 2 percent of community samples in Levine's figures. In the third category called *other eating disorders*, he finds prevalence rates of 2 to 13 percent of middle school and high school girls, and 3 to 6 percent of post puberty women in the community.

In Norway, where statistics appear to be based on stronger data, eating disorder prevalence was recently estimated at 15.5 percent of high school girls. Highest rates were among girls who were physically active and members of fitness clubs, but not athletes.[8]

A Canadian review finds that anorexia more than tripled among women in their 20s and 30s between 1950 and 1992, and increased 10 percent for teenagers.[10]

Among college-age youth, anorexia affects close to 5 percent, bulimia affects 20 percent of women, and 12 to 33 percent of women use vomiting, diuretics and laxatives on a regular basis, reports Russell Marx, Princeton Eating Disorders Program in New Jersey.[9]

Eating disorders appear to have increased over the last few decades, although this statistic is somewhat controversial. Statistics are sketchy, and there is resistance from the diet industry and supporters to obtaining clearer national data.

Harold Goldstein of the U.S. National Institute of Mental Health suggests that both anorexia and bulimia have doubled in the past decade. And a study in Scotland found the incidence of anorexia increased over six times between 1965 and 1991 in that country.

Most convincing are the Rochester, Minn., studies which looked at all community cases of a first diagnosis of anorexia over 55 years. In the most vulnerable group of women, age 15 to 24, there was a steady increase throughout all the years, and the trend has been an increase for all groups. Overall, the incidence was 8.3 per 100,000 person-years, with a yearly increase over this time of 1.03 per 100,000 person-years. Since Rochester is a major medical center, most diagnoses are made locally.[11]

Many experts believe the figures are actually much higher, that eating disorders are striking at ever younger ages, and affecting many more boys and men. Unfortunately, eating disorder statistics are based on small, incomplete and non-representative studies. The Canadian review reported in 1998 that the largest published study included only 166 cases, and not a single large population-based study had been reported in scientific literature.[12]

Death rates

Eating disorders have relatively high death rates, suggesting the severity of these disorders. The Canadian National Eating Disorder Information Centre in Toronto warns that 10 to 20 percent of anorexia and bulimia cases can be fatal.[13] Michael Levine puts the mortality rate at between 15 and 20 percent.[14]

In his 2000 book, *Eating Disorders,* Richard Gordon reports that at least half the deaths result from complications associated with extreme starvation — while a significant percent are from suicide.[15]

Eating disorder survivors find the road to recovery long and difficult. There are severe physical and mental effects, sometimes irreversible damage. There are the losses: while in the grip of the disorder, health, jobs, school and relationships all suffer — and rebuilding can seem a nearly insurmountable challenge. Less than half of patients with severe disorders, about 44 percent, recover well, according to these sources. About 31 percent are intermediate, and 25 percent have poor outcome.

With a disorder this severe, why are there no adequate statistics? Why are eating disorders not at the forefront of national health priorities? I have often asked these questions, and found the answers unsatisfactory.

Granted, compiling eating disorders statistics may be difficult because of sufferers' denial and the extreme measures they take to hide their disorder. Yet screening on campuses and in malls during Eating Disorder Awareness Week is very successful in measuring eating behavior and in bringing many new cases to treatment. Deaths from eating disorders could also be compiled if states would keep track.

The reason it isn't happening seems to be due to resistance from the powerful diet industry, as well as apathy on the part of health officials and the public. Neither health agencies nor the public has come to grips with the severity and extent of eating disorders.

This may be in part because the victims are nearly all women. Therapist Susan Wooley, PhD, has charged that the field of eating disorders would be very different if it were young men instead of young women who were being hospitalized and dying at the height of their educational and career aspirations.

Eating disorder diagnosis

■ Anorexia nervosa

Patients with anorexia nervosa refuse to maintain weight at what is minimally normal for age and height (they weigh less than 85 percent of expected weight), and have an intense fear of weight gain or becoming fat. They have disturbance in body image, causing undue influence on self-esteem, and amenorrhea if female, defined as the absence of at least three consecutive menstrual cycles.

Two types are:

- **Restricting type:** severely restricts food without regularly binge eating or purging.

- **Binge eating/purging type:** severely restricts food and binges or purges (vomiting, laxatives, diuretics, enemas).

■ Bulimia nervosa

In bulimia nervosa, the individual has recurrent episodes of binge eating. An episode includes eating, in a discrete period of time, an amount of food larger than most people would eat, and a sense of lack of control over what or how much one is eating during the episode. It includes recurrent inappropriate compensatory behavior to prevent weight gain, such as induced vomiting, misuse of laxatives, diuretics, enemas or other medications, fasting or excessive exercise. Both binge eating and the compensatory behavior occur on average at least twice a week for three months. Self-evaluation is unduly influenced by body shape and weight.

Two types are:

- **Purging type:** uses regular purging behavior (induced vomiting, misuse of laxatives, diuretics, enemas).

- **Nonpurging type:** uses other inappropriate compensatory behaviors, such as fasting or excessive exercise, but does not regularly engage in purging.

Source: Diagnostic criteria for eating disorders. Diagnostic and Statistical Manual, Fourth Edition, 1994. American Psychiatric Association, Washington, DC.

■ Eating disorder not otherwise specified

The largest category is *Eating disorder not otherwise specified.* Individuals in this category do not meet the definitions for either anorexia nervosa or bulimia nervosa.

Examples are:

- All criteria met for anorexia nervosa except amenorrhea.
- All criteria met for anorexia nervosa except, despite weight loss, current weight is in normal range.
- All criteria met for bulimia nervosa except frequency of binges is less than twice a week or for a duration of less than three months.
- An individual of normal body weight who regularly engages in inappropriate compensatory behavior (such as induced vomiting) after eating small amounts of food.
- Repeatedly chewing and spitting out large amounts of food without swallowing.

■ Binge eating disorder

A subtype under the category *Eating disorder not otherwise specified,* binge eating disorder is defined as recurrent episodes of binge eating, which includes eating in a discrete period of time an amount of food larger than most people would eat, and a sense of lack of control over eating it. The individual has marked distress regarding binge eating, and engages in binge eating at least two days a week, on average for six months. (The binge eating is not associated with regular use of inappropriate compensatory behaviors and does not occur exclusively during the course of anorexia nervosa or bulimia nervosa.)

At least three of the following must be part of the binge episode:

- Eating much more rapidly than normal.
- Eating until uncomfortably full.
- Eating large amounts of food when not hungry.
- Eating alone because of embarrassment about how much is eaten.
- Feeling disgusted with oneself, depressed, or very guilty about eating.[1]

Certainly we would have better statistics by now if eating disorders had not been kept off the nation's Healthy People 2000 agenda in 1990. Now Healthy People 2010, a huge two-volume report, sets forth 467 objectives in 28 major focus areas in this nation's most serious health areas, and again, eating disorders are mysteriously absent. No hint of any need for prevention. Nothing on the urgent problem of undernutrition and malnutrition of teenage girls. Nothing on the hazardous ways kids are using to lose weight.[16]

Unbelievably, the *only* mention of eating disorders — which severely affect the health of 10 to 15 percent of girls and young women, or more, and cause many deaths — is a brief two-paragraph mention that hospital treatment of eating disorders should not relapse. And this is buried in the mental health section, not upfront in nutrition where problem eating and malnutrition issues belong.

Bizarre behaviors

One of the most important advancements in the understanding of eating disorders is the recognition that severe and prolonged dietary restriction can lead to serious physical and psychological complications, says eating disorder specialist David Garner.[17]

The bizarre behaviors common to anorexia nervosa, once thought to be caused by pre-existing psychopathy, are typical of those described under other starvation conditions, such as the Minnesota Starvation study. Chronic dieters and people who severely restrict their food intake are familiar with such behavior.

Some people develop odd eating rituals, cutting up food into small pieces, chewing a certain number of times. One of the most striking features of eating disorders is how intently the person is preoccupied with food, often to the exclusion of other interests or time spent with friends.

Eating disorder pioneer Hilde Bruch observed, "Food thoughts crowd out their ability to think about anything else."[18]

Feelings related to this kind of behavior are explained by a woman who had recovered from anorexia nervosa and bulimia nervosa, in *Eating Disorders*. "While anorexic, my body not only anticipated eating, it reveled in it. Being starved and hungry makes the experience of eating more intense — almost sensual. The feeling is analogous to what is experienced when drinking water when extremely thirsty, sleeping after being totally exhausted, or urinating after one's bladder has become overly full. What is usually somewhat ordinary becomes exciting — something to look forward to in an otherwise painful and lonely world. This made changing behaviors so that I no longer experienced intense hunger extremely difficult."[19]

Common symptoms of eating disorders include fatigue, lethargy, weakness, impaired concentration, nonfocal abdominal pain, dizziness, faintness, sore muscles, chills, cold sweats, frequent sore throats, diarrhea and constipation, according to Allan Kaplan and Paul Garfinkel in *Medical Issues and the Eating Disorders.*[20]

Warning signs that a person may have an eating disorder include highly-controlled behavior, eating little while denying hunger, hyperactive exercising, mood swings, hiding feelings, and sudden weight loss or weight changes.

While some patients drink copiously to feel full, others restrict fluids, although this is less often documented. In a study of seven fluid-restricting patients in Australia, researchers said once this behavior began it progressed rapidly, with patients refusing to drink anything within a few days. In all patients, food restriction was severe prior to fluid restriction, and all denied the symptoms of dehydration. Two common reasons given was that restricting fluids made them feel bloated, and that they believe even water contains calories, through its impurities. They said it gave them a strong sense of control.[21]

Eating disorders are disproportionately common among vegetarians. Perhaps some of the same traits that put one at risk for an eating disorder may be involved in the vegetarian choice, such as perfectionism, guilt, and the need to do penance or be perceived as "good." Some specialists are seeing so many vegetarian girls in their practices today that they consider it a marker for an eating disorder. They suggest that being vegetarian seems to be an acceptable way to have an eating disorder, or perhaps a step along the way.

Because food choices are so restrictive and limiting, the girl who is both eating disordered and vegetarian is most likely to be malnourished, and to have the most severe effects. The more rigid the vegetarian behavior, the more severe the individual's psychopathology often turns out to be, says Monika Woolsey, a dietitian who specializes in eating disorders in Glendale, Arizona.

Restoring full nutrition to release the body from its closed-down, protective state brings dramatic improvement to sufferers of anorexia nervosa, as it does in starvation.

Roots of eating disorders

Eating disorders are complex. They arise out of both emotional problems and eating disturbances related to food, body image and relationships, within a culture that puts great emphasis on thinness and appearance, and complicated by the effects of starvation and purging.

Factors that increase a dieter's vulnerability to eating disorders are believed to be genetic, biological, psychological, sociocultural and familial, as well as have a history of sexual or physical abuse.

Often sexual abuse or trauma will be a triggering event to an eating disorder. Puberty is a critical time. Some specialists see eating disorders as survival strategies developed in response to harassment, racism, homophobia, abuse of power, poverty, or emotional, physical or sexual abuse.

Some problems may be rooted in families that are overly controlling or disengaged, or who have problems they are unable to acknowledge or deal with openly. Parents can thus be a strong influence. Pressure from parents on daughters to lose weight links to eating problems during late childhood. In some studies, mothers of eating-disordered teenagers show greater eating disturbances and dieting than other mothers.

Even during early childhood, dieting parents affect their sons and daughters. Mothers who diet, restrict food, are dissatisfied with their bodies, and have bulimic symptoms are more likely to have children who exhibit eating disturbances during their first five years of life. These very young children are at risk for inhibited eating, secretive eating, overeating and vomiting, a San Francisco Bay area study found.[22]

Yet experts say that eating disorders may not be so very different from the dysfunctional eating of so many other girls. It may be only a matter of degree. It is no longer possible to dismiss patients with severe eating disorders as having pathological roots, as was often done in the past. Girls who suffer from eating disorders may be simply expressing what many other girls and women are feeling.[23]

In less than two decades, the "ideal" female body has been cut by one-third, not just by the media but also by what I consider ill-advised health policy. Most women no longer fit that size, and trying to do so takes up more and more of their lives. Some are pushed to an apparent point of no return by "our era's culminating demand that women give up nourishment and a large share of their bodies," write Patricia Fallon, Melanie Katzman and Susan Wooley, editors of *Feminist Perspectives on Eating Disorders.*[24]

For some girls, entering adolescence and accepting their rapidly-changing bodies becomes nearly impossible when placed against this cultural backdrop. Not only are their female role models extremely thin and usually dieting, but males they know openly denigrate large women and praise thin women for their bodies alone.

Strong evidence of the media's powerful influence comes from the island of Fiji. Within 38 months of the time that satellite television came to the island in 1995 and began beaming in images of thin female celebrities, the number of teens at risk for eating disorders more than doubled to 29 percent. Five times as many girls were vomiting to control their weight.[25]

Society and the health community have to take responsibility for the tremendous impact of idealizing an increasingly thin female body.

Does dieting cause eating disorders?

There is debate over whether dieting may lead to eating disorders. Specialists who support the weight loss industry or promote dieting, argue that it does not.

Yet, dieting is increasingly being regarded as an important risk factor. Many experts in the field are convinced that the current high rates of eating disorders in the U.S. are the inevitable result of 60 to 80 million adults dieting, losing weight, rebounding, and learning to be chronic dieters. The majority of chronic dieters are women, as are most who suffer from eating disorders.[26]

A study of 15-year-old girls in London linked dieting to the development of eating disorders. Those initially dieting were significantly more likely than nondieters to develop an eating disorder within one year.[27]

"The onset of an eating disorder typically follows a period of restrictive dieting; however, only a minority of people who diet develop eating disorders," says the American Dietetic Association in its position paper on eating disorders.[28]

ADA warns against promoting weight loss to persons with binge eating disorder or other eating disorders. When youngsters request help with weight loss, the ADA paper recommends counseling on body image issues and how to stop the pursuit of thinness, rather than helping them try to lose weight. It may be healthier, ADA says, to help young people accept themselves at or near their present weight, stop binge eating and learn how to prevent future weight gain.

Anorexia nervosa

"When I first started to eat strangely, all I would eat were sweets, and that wasn't any good. Then I got into just eating salads, just lettuce and diet pop, and that wasn't any good. Then I got into pretty much not eating at all, and that wasn't any good," said a former anorexic patient.[29]

Anorexia has had some high-profile victims. Singer Karen Carpenter. Actress Ally McBeal. Gymnast Christy Heinrich.

Actress Tracey Gold, of the ABC sitcom "Growing Pains," was only 12 when her pediatrician first diagnosed her anorexia. Four months of psychotherapy seemed to get the problem under control and she gained weight, up to 133 pounds by the time she turned 19 in 1988. It was too much, she thought. To lose weight her endocrinologist put her on a 500-calorie-a-day diet and in two months she had dropped to her goal of 113. But during the next three years her weight kept dropping, until in January 1992 at 80 pounds, she was hospitalized and fought for her life. Two years later, claiming to feel "healthy enough to know I don't want to lose any more," she was still keeping her weight at 92 pounds and panicking at the thought of going up to 100 pounds.[30]

In explaining what it is like to be a male with an eating disorder, Michael Krasnow writes that he began to feel fat as early as age 11, but it was as a high school freshman that "fat feelings" began to take over his life. He dropped swiftly from his normal weight of about 135 pounds. Now 27, he maintains 75 pounds on his 5-foot-9 frame.

"When I first got this anorexia, I tried to get better, but now I just don't care," says Krasnow. He does not get together with friends, "I haven't had a friend in 10, 15 years."

He refuses to drink water and says he fears if he let go of any of the rules he makes for himself, he would lose control. "It would all fall apart. If I took one cup of water a day, I'd be drinking two gallons a day. Pretty soon I'd be a compulsive eater — that's what goes through my mind — I won't be able to stop."[31]

Female athletes and dancers are at high risk for anorexia nervosa also. As many as 13 to 22 percent of young women in selected groups of elite runners and dancers have the disorder. Two studies of female dancers cited by Jacqueline Berning and Suzanne Steen, authors of *Sports Nutrition for the 90's,* found between 5 and 22 percent had anorexia nervosa, with a higher incidence among young women competing in national versus regional performances.[32]

In anorexia nervosa, by definition, the individual is more than 15 percent under expected weight; she fears gaining weight, is preoccupied with food, has abnormal eating habits, and has amenorrhea. If male, sexual drive or interest decreases. There are two types of anorexia: one restricts food; the other restricts food and either purges regularly, or binges and purges both.[33]

As the malnourished body shuts down, changes occur in behavior, perception, thinking, mood and social interaction. A sense of heightened control and control over food seems important to the person with anorexia. Pleasure and enjoyment during eating are replaced by guilt, anxiety and ambivalence. They grow depressed, irritable, anxious and unstable, often leading to increased social isolation. Compulsive exercise may be part of the disorder.

Symptoms are usually evident: emaciated appearance, dry skin, sometimes yellowish, fine body hair, brittle hair and nails, body temperature below a normal 96.6 degrees, pulse rate usually below 60 beats per minute, subnormal blood pressure, and sometimes edema, say Kaplan and Garfinkel.

Initially, these are similar to symptoms associated with a restrictive diet: light-headedness, apathy, irritability, and decrease in energy. Then the consequences of prolonged semi-starvation begin to set in and effects worsen. Duration of the disorder may range from a single episode to a lifelong illness.

Hospitalization may be required, depending on body weight, the amount and rapidity of weight lost, severe metabolic disturbances, certain cardiac dysfunctions, syncope, psychomotor retardation, severe depression or suicide risk, severe bingeing and purging (with risk of aspiration), psychosis, family crisis, inability to perform activities of daily living, or lack of response to outpatient treatment programs. Most severely underweight patients, under 20 percent below average weight for height, and those who are psychologically unstable require a residential health care setting.[34]

Families as well as patients usually need therapy for this debilitating illness.

Bulimia nervosa

"I can't stop throwing up. I try, I really do. Yesterday, I promised myself I wouldn't do it anymore. I tried to keep myself busy. I cleaned house, played with the cat, prayed . . . But I don't want to gain weight. I can't do that! I never want to be fat again. I'll never go back there. Nothing is worse than that pain . . . My joints even hurt. I feel so old. My hair looks horrible; and it keeps falling out. I find it all over the place. My mouth is so full of sores, it's gross! I can't even walk around the house standing straight any more. I'm in a daze. I can't focus. But I can't stop. I feel so trapped. Please help me . . ." said a patient from Lemon Grove, Calif.[35]

By definition, the person with bulimia nervosa goes on an eating binge at least twice a week, eating a large amount of food within a discrete period, and then tries to compensate by purging (vomiting, using laxatives or diuretics) or other means. As the disorder progresses, it develops into a complex lifestyle that is increasingly isolating, with depressive mood swings and low self-esteem. Up to one-third of anorexic individuals develop bulimia nervosa, also.

Vomiting is the most common form of purging. Some bulimics binge and purge many times a day. They may be of normal weight and seem physically healthy — except for the tell-tale signs of vomiting behavior: finger calluses or lesions on the dominant hand from stimulating the gag reflex (especially in early stages when stimulation is needed to induce vomiting), "chipmunk" cheeks from stimulation of the salivary glands, erosion of enamel especially on the surface of the upper teeth next to the tongue.[36]

The consequences of this self-abusive behavior become increasingly obvious as the frequency and duration increase; they include hair loss, fatigue, insomnia, muscle weakness, edema, dizziness, sore throat, stomach pain or cramping, bloating, bad breath and bloodshot eyes. Cardiac arrhythmias affect 20 percent and require emergency treatment. Ipecac syrup abuse may lead to death through cardiomyopathy, myocarditis.

Bulimia was only recognized in 1980, and in 1987 was given the term bulimia nervosa. It is unclear whether the disorder has long been a hidden syndrome.

Other eating disorders

Some eating disorders don't fit neatly into the diagnostic criteria of anorexia or bulimia. They may have many of the same features or involve other behaviors, such as repeatedly chewing and spitting out, but not swallowing, large amounts of food.

Binge eating disorder, first described in 1959, is included in this group. It meets the criteria for bulimia nervosa except that those with binge eating disorder do not regularly purge and are not unduly concerned with weight and shape. They eat large amounts of food at least twice a week, in a relatively short time, with a sense of loss of control. They may be of average weight, but most often are overweight.

Excessive exercise

One of the fastest growing eating disorder behaviors in the past few years is excessive exercise — known as activity disorder or exercise dependance — aimed at losing weight or sculpting the body.

Eating disorder warning signs

Anorexia nervosa

- Significant or extreme weight loss (at least 15 percent with no known medical illness)
- Reduction of food intake
- Ritualistic eating habits such as:
  a. Cutting meat into extremely small bites
  b. Chewing each bite a great number of times
- Denial of hunger
- Critical and less tolerant of others
- Excessively exercising (hyperactive)
- Chooses low-to-no-fat and low-calorie foods
- Says he/she is too fat, even when this is not true
- Exhibits highly self-controlled behavior
- Does not reveal feelings

Bulimia nervosa

- Makes excuses to go to the restroom after meals
- Exhibits mood swings
- May purchase large quantities of food, which suddenly disappears.
- Unusual swelling around the jaw
- Weight may be within normal range
- Frequently eats large amounts of food (a binge), often high in calories, and does not seem to gain weight
- Laxative or diuretic wrappers found frequently in the trash
- Unexplained disappearance of food in the home or residence hall setting

Binge eating disorder

- Frequently eats a large amount of food, larger than most people would eat during a similar amount of time
- Eats rapidly
- Eats to a point that is uncomfortably full
- Often eats alone
- Shows irritation and disgust with self after overeating

Additional signs of related eating disorders

- Makes excuses to skip meals and does not eat with others
- Develops a tendency to be perfect in almost everything
- Focuses conversation on foods or around body shape
- Often listens to others problems but does not share own
- Is highly self-critical
- Worries about what others think
- Thinks about weight and body shape most of the day
- Begins to isolate more from friends and family
- The odor of vomit is in the bathroom regularly
- Repeatedly chews and spits out food — does not swallow large amounts of food
- May purge and yet not binge[2]

NOTE: The more warning signs a person has, the higher the probability that the person has or is developing an eating disorder.

National Eating Disorders Organization 1994
Children and Teens Afraid to Eat 2001, 1997

The girl with an activity disorder follows rigid patterns, insists on continuing exercise even when it aggravates a serious injury, and may suffer withdrawal symptoms if unable to exercise. It is especially harmful when severe calorie restriction is combined with excessive exercise.

Activity disorder can be defined as excessive, purposeless, physical activity which goes beyond any usual training regimen and ends up being a detriment rather than an asset to health and well-being.[37]

Karin Kratina, MA, RD, an exercise physiologist and dietitian at the Renfrew Center in Florida, says at least half the anorexic and bulimic patients she sees probably deal with some form of exercise dependency.[38] "Stress injuries are common, and frequently the person exercises right through an injury so it can't heal properly." Kratina describes the typical scenario of a young woman with exercise dependence. "She rises each morning at 5:30, hits the pavement for a brisk three miles, rain or shine, works out 45 minutes at the fitness center on lunch break, and goes to another health club after work for an hour of aerobics, half an hour on the Stairmaster and a half hour on the Lifecycle. She appears to be a motivated, fit and happy person but her legs ache constantly as she continues to work out, despite shin splints. When she stops for a time her depression and anxiety become so overwhelming, she can't wait to get back to her workouts."

Anorexia and bodybuilding have many similarities, points out David Schlundt, PhD, an eating disorder specialist at Vanderbilt University in Nashville. "There are special diets, use of diuretics, steroid use, obsessive exercise, very low fat diets, and so on. An obsession with changing size and shape of the body leads to extreme and sometimes dangerous changes in diet, exercise and substance abuse."[39]

Boys are responding to a new emphasis on body sculpting and muscle building. Many express an intense desire to alter their appearance, conforming to advertising that is now teaching body dissatisfaction to males. Experts say this is one of the reasons eating disorders are increasing among boys and men.

Links to sexual abuse, violence

Childhood abuse violates the boundaries of the self, and increases the risk for eating disorders. Violence, physical or psychological abuse, trauma and sexual abuse are invasions of self that can have extremely harmful effects, one of which may be eating disorders.

Sexual abuse is a common experience of many eating disorder patients, says Susan Wooley, PhD, professor of psychology and co-director of the Eating Disorders Clinic at the University of Cincinnati Medical College.[40] Until very recently, the importance of a history of sexual or physical abuse was ignored or minimized by the mostly male therapists who dominated the field, and who reported the research in journals and at conferences. Wooley calls sexual abuse the "concealed debate" which women therapists long held in conference hallways, and is now finally recognized.

The National Women's Study, a national random sample of 4,008 adult women in the U.S. who were interviewed at least three times over the course of one year, found that women with bulimia nervosa were twice as likely to have been raped (27 percent vs 13 percent) or sexually molested (22 vs 12 percent), and four times as likely to have experienced aggravated assault (27 vs 8 percent) as women without an eating disorder.[41]

Over half the women with bulimia reported a lifetime history of some type of criminal victimization event compared to less than one-third of women who did not have an eating disorder (54 vs 31 percent). Twelve percent of women with bulimia nervosa had been raped as children, at age 11 or younger, compared with 5 percent of women without an eating disorder. The age at the time of rape pre-dated the age of the first binge episode in all cases, suggesting child-hood sexual abuse as a causal factor.

Even so, the true extent of sexual abuse is unknown due to the silencing of victims and their reluctance to disclose abuse even to therapists trained to help them in this area. Wooley cites one report that 33 percent of patients who later disclosed their abuse had denied it during five weeks of hospitalization at a center highly experienced in abuse treatment and sensitized to its importance. Another of the few clear findings of the past decade is the extremely long delay that may precede disclosure even among patients in extensive therapy, reports Wooley.

She says underestimation is virtually unavoidable; yet critics express most concern with overestimation and false reports, despite lack of evidence for the latter and much evidence that estimates are low. The accusation that the patient or therapist made it up holds sexual abuse to a test not customarily applied to clinical data, she charges.

Wooley reports that the predominantly female patients more often disclose histories of sexual abuse to women therapists. Male therapists as a whole have not recognized the extent and consequences of sexual abuse until recently. Now that it is realized, she says there is a polarization over how to deal with it in the eating disorder field. The controversy involves medical versus sociocultural models, technical versus humanistic approaches, and apolitical versus feminist analyses.

Wooley notes that the unmasking of sexual abuse at long last was largely due to the persistence of feminist writers and clinicians, in the face of patriarchial resistance.

In a similar way, Freud's suppression of his discovery of sexual abuse among his women patients was not revealed until the early 1980s. And it is only in the past 20 to 25 years that the social institutions that now help female victims of sexual abuse and domestic violence have developed.

Until quite recently, childhood sexual abuse was believed to be rare and likely harmless. In their book *Sexual Abuse and Eating Disorders,* Mark Schwartz and Leigh Cohn point out that the rate of sexual abuse was estimated at only one in 1,000 in a major psychiatric textbook of the 1960s. Yet by the 1980s, publications were reporting sexual abuse as high as one in three females and one in seven males.

They suggest that, like Freud, male clinicians have sometimes needed not to know and not to see, in order to maintain their own illusions. "The fundamental question is: Why has it taken so long to recognize the association if, as has been reported by one major center, 80 percent of their sample of eating-disordered patients have a history of sexual abuse? Why then has there been such resistance to knowing and believing?"[42]

Steven Levenkron, MS, author of *The Best Little Girl in the World,* suggests male therapists can be more effective if they are "parental" rather than "paternalistic" in their feelings toward patients.

"I don't think there is anything problematic about men treating women with eating disorders if they understand the dilemma many women face in today's culture. This dilemma concerns how much to value their femininity while maintaining a level of assertiveness in order to compete with men."[43]

Much progress has been made in the last decade in male therapists recognizing the conflicting messages adolescent girls are given in modern culture. Male therapists say they have learned how important it is to be silent and listen to girls and women, without taking the role of "male expert."

"Many if not most of the patients we treat have been traumatized either physically, sexually or simply in relationships where they've experienced some disappointment in others," says Craig L. Johnson, a clinical psychologist and co-director of the eating disorders program at the Laureate Psychiatric Clinic in Tulsa.

At the same time it needs to be made clear that many eating-disordered clients were *not* sexually or physically abused, and many abused youngsters do not develop disorders.

This abuse information is all so new that there is wide variation in reports. Further investigation is needed to clarify the issues. What should be considered sexual abuse? How can it be assessed in a reliable way? How can experts cope with the difficulty of disclosure?

Complications of eating disorders

Following are mental and physical complications or traits commonly associated with anorexia nervosa and bulimia nervosa, adapted here from Kaplan and Garfinkel.[44]

Mental complications

Anorexia nervosa

Many of the mental and emotional symptoms common to anorexia nervosa are directly related to the physical effects of starvation. Other traits have to do with attitudes and behavior toward eating and weight.

- **Energy level.** Fatigue, weakness, lassitude, lethargy, apathy, decreasing energy, persistent tiredness, dizziness, faintness, light-headedness; yet compulsively exercises (hyperactive).

- **Mood, attitude and behavior.** Moodiness, often depressed, mood swings (tyrannical); anxiety and ambivalence; irritability; critical and intolerant of others; depression; low self-esteem, self-esteem controlled through weight loss; invulnerability and success dependent on weight loss; feelings of lack of control in life; hopelessness; rigidity, highly controlled behavior; does not reveal feelings; perfectionist behavior; fantasy that weight loss can cause or prevent some life event (prevent parental divorce, attract romance); denies hunger; denies problem of weight loss (sees self as fat); denies eating disorder; body image distortion, overestimates body size and shape, "feels fat" despite emaciated appearance; ritualistic habits.

- **Mental ability.** Inability to concentrate, decreased alertness; difficulty with reading comprehension, diminished capacity to think; loss of memory; extreme narrowing of interests; decline in ambition.

- **Social.** Social withdrawal, isolates self from family and friends, becomes increasingly aloof and withdrawn; lonely; feelings easily hurt; avoidance by peers; worsening family relations, fights with family, cost of treatment may be a family financial drain.

- **Weight.** Increasing preoccupation with body; frequently monitors body changes (may check with scale and/or mirror many times per day); compares size and shape to others, envious of thinner persons; heightened control, feelings of having control over body.

- **Food, eating and hunger.** Misperception of hunger, satiety and other bodily sensations; hunger and increasing hunger; fears food and gaining weight; eats alone; guilt when eating; may secretly binge; dieting and weight increasingly important focus; unusual food-related behaviors (makes rules for specific foods, placement on plate, time of eating, size of bites, number of chews per bite); progressive preoccupation with food and eating (may begin to cook and control family eating); need to vicariously enjoy food (may collect recipes, dream of food, hoard food, enjoy watching others eat, pursue food-related careers — as dietitians, chefs, caterers).

■ **Other.** Hypersensitive to cold and heat, hypersensitive to noise and light; sleep disturbance.

Bulimia nervosa

The person with bulimia nervosa is often normal weight and may not experience the effects of starvation. However, if she has nutrition deficiencies due to purging, she may have starvation symptoms. When a patient with anorexia becomes bulimic, she or he experiences symptoms characteristic of both eating disorders.

Typically, these mental and emotional symptoms may be associated with bulimia nervosa.

■ **Mood/attitude/behavior.** Anxiety, depression; mood swings; low self-esteem, self-deprecating thoughts; embarrassment, shame related to behavior; persistent remorse; paranoid feelings; unreasonable resentments; makes excuses to go to bathroom after meals; may buy large amounts of food, which suddenly disappears; impulsive as compared to anorexics who are overcontrolled.

■ **Mental ability.** Loss of ordinary willpower, poor impulse control, self-indulgent behavior; recognizes abnormal eating behavior.

■ **Social.** Depends on others for approval; feelings of isolation; unable to discuss problem, others are unhappy about food obsession; social isolation; distances self from friends and family; fear of going out in public; family, work and money problems.

■ **Weight.** Feels that self worth is dependent on low weight; constant concern with weight and body image.

■ **Food, eating and hunger.** Eats alone; eats when not hungry; preoccupation with eating and food; fears binges and eating out of control; increased dependency on bingeing; binge eating of large amount of food in a short time, feeling out of control, cannot stop eating.

■ **Purging.** Feels need to rid body of calories consumed during binge (through vomiting, laxatives, diuretics, enemas, fasting or excessive exercise); experimentation with vomiting, laxatives and diuretics often leads to regular abuse.

■ **Binge/purge cycle.** Spends much time planning, carrying out, cleaning up after bulimic episode; eliminates normal activities; complex lifestyle may develop with episodes occurring several times a day; worsening of symptoms during times of emotional stress; feels soothed and comforted by binge/purge cycle — it may serve to relieve frustration, anxiety, anger, fear, remorse, boredom, loneliness.

■ **Other.** Dishonesty, lying; stealing food or money; drug and alcohol abuse; suicidal tendencies or attempts.

Physical complications

Anorexia nervosa

■ **Electrolytes.** May be low in potassium, sodium, chloride, calcium, magnesium, and high or low bicarbonate. Electrolyte imbalance more likely when there is dehydration and/or purging.

■ **Gastrointestinal.** Constipation is likely, may promote laxative use. Commonly there is vomiting, feelings of fullness and bloating, and abdominal discomfort. There may be ulcers, and pancreatic dysfunction. Excessive laxatives over time may result in gastrointestinal bleeding and impairment of colon functioning.

■ **Cardiovascular.** Commonly present are chest pain, arrhythmias, hypotension, edema and mitral valve prolapse. Electrocardiogram (EKG) changes. Heart rates lower than 40 beats per minute are common and as low as 25 reported in severe starvation. Prolonged QT intervals can lead to sudden death syndrome.

■ **Metabolic.** Abnormal temperature regulation and cold intolerance are common. Abnormal glucose tolerance, fasting hypoglycemia, high B-hydroxybutyric acid, high free fatty acids, hypercholesterolemia, hypercarotenemia are common. Diabetic patients with an eating disorder may have fluctuating blood glucose levels leading to serious long-term consequences.

■ **Bones.** Decreased bone mineral density may lead to fractures, growth retardation, short stature and osteoporosis.

■ **Renal.** Elevated blood urea nitrogen, changes in urinary concentration capacity, and decreased glomerular filtration rate are common.

■ **Endocrine.** Amenorrhea is 100 percent for females, by definition, although many anorexia nervosa patients menstruate over time. Amenorrhea related to weight loss but may precede weight loss (in one-third); may cause delayed puberty, contributes to osteoporosis, breast atrophy, infertility. Hypometabolic state resulting in cold intolerance, dry skin and hair, bradycardia, constipation, fatigue, slowed reflexes. High plasma cortisol, decreased cortixol response to insulin.

■ **Hematologic.** Anemia, leukopenia, bone marrow hypocellularity, common; these effects are usually mild, but can include bleeding tendency.

■ **Neurological.** EEG and sleep changes are common; epileptic seizures affect up to 10 percent.

■ **Musculocutaneous.** Muscle weakening, muscle cramps. Hair loss, brittle hair and nails, lanugo hair, dry skin and cold extremities are common.

Bulimia nervosa

■ **Electrolytes.** Low potassium, low chloride, dehydration and metabolic alkalosis are common. May lead to cardiac arrest, renal failure. Dehydration is common along with hypotension, dizziness, weakness, muscle cramps. Cardiac arrhythmias affect 20 percent; unpredictable, may require emergency treatment. Hypochloremia is common; limits kidney's ability to excrete bicarbonate.

■ **Gastrointestinal.** Constipation and increased amylase common. Rarely gastric and duodenal ulcer, acute gastric dilation and rupture. Frequent abdominal pain. Severe abdominal pain may lead to rigid abdomen and shock which may result in death. Abuses of laxatives may lead to iron deficiency anemia, rectal bleeding and cathartic colon.

■ **Pulmonary.** Aspiration pneumonia possible from aspiration of vomitus.

■ **Cardiovascular.** Peripheral edema is common along with EKG changes and QT changes, which can lead to serious arrhythmias and congestive heart failure. Uncommon is sudden cardiac death. Ipecac syrup abuse may lead to death through cardiomyopathy, myocarditis.

■ **Metabolic.** High B-hydroxybutyric acid, free fatty acids. Less common edema, abnormal temperature regulation and cold intolerance.

■ **Renal.** Possible changes.

■ **Endocrine.** Menstrual irregularities with low body weight, dexamethasone nonsuppression common.

■ **Hematologic.** May be anemic with nutrition deficiency.

■ **Neurological.** EEG changes common. May have epileptic seizures with malnutrition and electrolyte imbalance.

■ **Musculocutaneous.** Calluses on dorsum of dominant hand are common from inducing gag reflex. Muscle weakening with ipecac abuse.

■ **Dental.** Enamel erosions with vomiting.

CHAPTER 7

Size prejudice
punishes large children

■

Large children and teens often live with vicious prejudice from classmates, parents and teachers, which can interfere with their ability to grow into self-assured, successful adults. Disrespect for their size can be painful for youth who are taller, shorter, or thinner than most, but it is especially cruel and abusive to larger kids.

Echoes from his youth, writes Dan Davis of Salinas, Calif., in *Radiance*, are the shouts: "I don't want you on my team. You're too fat to run." "Look at the fat tub." "Your belly looks like a watermelon." Today he says, "My stomach still knots when I remember . . . I'll carry the scars to my grave — (but) today's kids have it worse."[1]

Her first experience in public humiliation came when she was a 185-pound high school sophomore, recalls Terry Nicholetti Garrison, author of *Fed Up!*, when she heard one of a group of school jocks call out, "Hey, fat ass!" as she walked down the hall. Hoots of laughter followed.

"I turned, my face flaming . . . I shrunk with shame and slinked to the cafeteria, where I nursed my pain with a lonely lunch. I was sure that Billy was right. I should feel ashamed of my body. I was fat and bottom-heavy."

Research confirms what we all know, that there is strong prejudice, harassment, and even oppression against obese youngsters regardless of age, sex, race and socioeconomic status. Many struggle with discrimination in education, employment, health care and social relationships.

Even young children feel the stigma of obesity and fear being a target. In one study children as young as six described silhouettes of an overweight child as "lazy, dirty, stupid, ugly, cheats and lies." When shown drawings of a normal weight child, an overweight child, and children with various handicaps, including missing hands and facial disfigurement, children rated the overweight child as the least likable. Sadly, this bias even afflicted the larger children who felt the same prejudices.[2]

Large children and teens can be healthy, eat normally and live active lives, but the stigma may be overwhelming. It may be difficult for them to develop confident, healthy attitudes about themselves because of the devastating prejudice practiced by their peers, their parents and their teachers.

"Clearly obese children are blamed for their condition. It is an unusual person who does not fashion this into serious self-doubt and a persistent concern with dieting," says Kelly D. Brownell, an obesity researcher and professor of psychology at Yale University.[3]

Oppression against large children can be a form of persecution. They are teased on the playground, called names and chosen last to play on teams. But it is during puberty when the problems of obesity become most painful. Despite the discrimination against them, studies show that large children's sense of self-worth is similar to that of average-weight children. But in adolescence, the powerful social messages become internalized and a lifelong negative self-image can develop.[4]

Harassment is illegal, no longer allowed in many schools, but is often ignored by the staff.

"For me, living is literally hell," said one teenage girl. "The insults I must endure, the pity, the loneliness, the self-hatred and the loathing are all punishments I would not wish on anybody. I didn't do anything wrong. I am fat. . . . My life is a Catch-22. I'm lonely and don't have friends because I'm fat, and I eat because I'm lonely. Nobody wants to be seen with me — including some of my family. . . . Whenever there are people walking behind me, I am afraid they are making fun of me. Sometimes they are. . . . I have dreams about what it would be like to be thin. There is nothing I would not give to be thin."[5]

Gaining a strong sense of self-worth is especially difficult for large teenagers in modern countries, where both feminine and masculine ideals have become very thin. Male stars of movies, television, sports and pop music are not only lean, but usually appear muscular and fit.

"All this results in a distressing position for an obese adolescent who has to face up to negative attitudes at school . . . or even in the family. Clumsiness, unattractiveness to the opposite sex, are serious problems at this age," notes William Dietz, an obesity specialist.

One study shows that large adults who were obese as teens are more likely to develop negative body image and low self-worth than those who gained their excess weight later.

Obesity is the last socially acceptable form of prejudice, charge Albert Stunkard and Jeffery Sobal, in *Eating Disorders and Obesity:* "Obese persons remain perhaps the only group toward whom social derogation can be directed with impunity."[6]

Teachers reinforce prejudice

Discrimination has been shown in the way teachers interact with large students and the grades they give for comparable work. Acceptance into prestigious colleges is lower in one study for large females, even when they do not differ in academic qualifications, school performance or application rates to colleges.[7]

In 1993, the National Education Association launched an investigation into size discrimination against students and teachers in the schools as a human rights and civil rights issue. This is the nation's largest teacher organization — the professionals who see the worst examples of size prejudice daily and potentially have the power to bring about change.

The next year, NEA published its 27-page "Report on Size Discrimination," which describes size discrimination in schools at every level.[8] The report says the school experience is one of "ongoing prejudice, unnoticed discrimination and almost constant harassment" for large students, and "socially acceptable yet outrageous insensitivity and rudeness" for large teachers.

"At the elementary level, children learn that it is acceptable to dislike and deride fatness. From nursery school through college, fat students experience ostracism, discouragement, and sometimes violence. Often ridiculed by their peers and discouraged by even well-meaning education employees, fat students develop low self-esteem and have limited horizons. They are deprived of places on honor rolls, sports teams, and cheerleading squads and are denied letters of recommendation."

A member of the investigating team sympathized with large teens who are uncomfortable in showers and don't want other students to stare at or ridicule them. Another told of a high school drill team that for 10 years excluded overweight girls from the team. Those who were progressing toward their goal weight were allowed to practice at school, but not perform in public.

My friend Carol Johnson, a Wisconsin therapist who founded Largely Positive support groups for large women, writes in her book, *Self-Esteem Comes in All Sizes,* how her cheerleading ambitions came to an abrupt end.[9] "One of my dreams was to be a cheerleader. When tryouts were announced in the seventh grade, I signed up immediately and practiced night and day. After tryouts, I knew I had given a flawless performance. However, the physical education teacher who was judging the competition took me aside and gently told me that although I was one of the best candidates, she simply could not choose me. The reason? I was too chubby. My body was unacceptable for public display.

"Shortly thereafter, I became intrigued by the baton and decided to take twirling lessons. You would have thought the cheerleader episode would have deterred me forever, but somehow it didn't. I dreamed of leading the marching band down the football field, and adept as I was, I thought there was good chance this dream would become reality. Reality did set in, but not the one I had dreamed about. Once again I was trying to do something chubby girls weren't supposed to do — put themselves on display. This time I was told not to bother because the uniforms wouldn't fit me. I didn't even try out. And the message pierced deeper: You're not acceptable.

"The truth is that my weight in high school exceeded the weight charts by no more than 30 pounds. Now, when I look at my high school pictures, I don't think I look at all heavy. Yet at the time those extra 30 pounds felt like the weight of the world on my shoulders. Losing weight had become the most important thing in my life."

Johnson says her parents were always loving, supportive and proud of her, but they couldn't protect her from the outside world. "I truly believed, deep in my heart that I was not as good as the thinner girls. Only by losing weight could I become their equal."

The NEA report quotes a *New York Times* article about a girl named Aleta Walker as an example of the "outrageous behavior" to which large children are subjected in schools. Aleta never had any friends during her childhood and adolescence in Hannibal, Mo. She was ridiculed and bullied every day. When she walked down the halls at school, boys flattened themselves against the lockers and cried, "Wide load!"

But the worst was lunchtime. "Every day there was this production of watching me eat lunch." She tried to avoid going to the school cafeteria. "I would hide out in the bathroom. I would hide out behind the gym by the baseball diamond. I would hide in the library."

One day, schoolmates started throwing food at her as she sat at lunch. Plates of spaghetti splashed onto her face, and the long greasy strands dripped onto her clothes. "Everyone was laughing and pointing. They were making pig noises. I just sat there," she said.

Another friend of mine through the size acceptance movement is Cheri Erdman, now a 42-year-old therapist and college teacher. She was actually sent away from home at age five, on the advice of a kindergarten teacher, to live for more than a year in a residential weight treatment facility for children with "special nutritional needs." In her book, *Nothing to Lose: A Guide to Sane Living in a Larger Body*, Erdman, describes the sadness of being separated from her family for so long.[10]

Prejudice in health care

Unfortunately, humiliation often has been the chief outcome of encounters with health providers for large children.

Sally Smith, editor of *BBW (Big Beautiful Woman)*, recalls, "When I was seven, I was sent to a dietitian for my first diet. There were weekly weigh-ins. . . rare praise and more often, scoldings. When I was nine and alone with my pediatrician in the examining room, he told me to take off my gown, get off the table, stand up and bend down and touch my toes, 'so I can see how fat you are.' There I was, a naked nine-year-old, being degraded and humiliated by my doctor."

Invariably, Smith's weight was always a doctor's focus, even though she was generally healthy. "I remember public weighings where the nurse would make derogatory comments about my weight, and the doctor scolding me. When I was 16, my doctor told me that I was so fat I'd never live to see my 18th birthday. When I was 20, another doctor told me I'd never live to see 21."

No safe haven at home

For some children, fat oppression, teasing and ridicule comes from inside the family circle, so there is no escape from tormentors.

Pat, 34, describes her father's disdain of her size in *Real Women Don't Diet*. "My experience of prejudice for being fat started at a very young age. The sadness and teasing I went through then was not from individuals outside my family; it was from within my family, by the people who are supposed to most love you. At the age of nine, I did not consider myself overweight, but in my father's opinion I was not only overweight but also a 'fat cow' and a 'fat pig.' His ridicule and teasing continued as I grew older and larger. High school was the worst. I not only had to tolerate the hatefulness of my classmates calling me 'fat Pat,' but then I would go home and hear my father threaten to send me to Missouri. He wanted to have his mom lock me up and feed me bread and water so that I could lose weight.

"My father's threats were always at the tip of his tongue. One time he had a new idea: 'If I tie you to the back of my truck and make you run around the block a few times, you'll really lose weight.' Although he never did, just the horror of knowing it might happen was never far away. During all the years of growing up, I never was able to defend myself. I felt like I was a leper or something very bad, just for being overweight. I spent years taking drugs. I overdosed many times. Why should I care? My life wasn't worth that much. After all, I was different. I was fat."[11]

Effects of this stigma carry over into adulthood, especially for women. Women who are overweight as adolescents or young adults earn less, are less likely to marry, complete fewer years of school, and have higher rates of poverty than their normal weight peers. Fewer of these effects occur for overweight males.[12]

One study shows adults who were overweight as children, but of normal weight as adolescents, had a body image comparable to that of individuals who had never been overweight. But adults who had been obese as adolescents had an extremely negative body image and feelings of low self-worth.

Some of them experience a great deal of unresolved anger and rage. Jean Rubel, 36, describes turning this anger against herself.

"Under my loneliness simmered a lake of molten rage. Sometimes I turned it loose when I felt ignored, criticized, misunderstood, or unloved. Most of the time, though, I held it in the pit of my stomach, where it became the only defense I could find against my belief that I was flawed in some critical way that kept me from joining the human race. Unfortunately, I too often turned this hateful energy against myself in storms of self-criticism and loathing. I began to blame my body for all my problems. If I weren't so ugly, so big, so soft and flabby, I would be happy and popular. I was six feet tall and 145 pounds. According to yearbook pictures I was slender and reasonably attractive, but I couldn't see it. I wanted to be thin, admired, and loved. Instead I felt awkward, shy, fat, defective and extremely lonely."[13]

Too much pain

Large kids often experience the pain and humiliation of size prejudice from an early age. At times it may seem unbearable, such as in the following example.

The Fort Lauderdale Sun-Sentinel in Florida reported a tragedy on August 27, 1996, that took place the day before school opened in the fall.[14] To 12-year-old Samuel John Graham, starting at the new middle school meant being called fat and getting teased by kids again. Broward County Sheriff's detectives said Samuel so dreaded the idea of walking into the first day of classes on Monday that he got up in the middle of the night and hanged himself from a tree in the back of his Fort Lauderdale-area home.

As they got ready for the first day of school, his younger brothers, 8 and 10, looked outside and saw Samuel hanging by a rope from a tree. They called their father, who cut his son down, called paramedics, and tried to resuscitate him, but it was no use. He was pronounced dead at the scene, and his father went out and chopped down the tree his eldest son had used to take his life.

The last time the family saw Samuel was about 10:30 Sunday evening, when they had prayed together. Then Samuel went to bed. At 2:30 a.m. his grandmother heard Samuel stirring and thought he had gotten up for a snack. They found a flashlight and step-stool beside his body the next morning.

Samuel, 5-feet-4, 174 pounds, had talked of suicide before and his humiliation at the teasing from kids at school. He was sensitive, and when they chased him down the street or smacked the back of his head, he sometimes cried. A reporter observed that photos in the family living room showed him as the fat kid, who didn't have any friends. "The easy target. The mark. It's all there in his eyes: The sweetness. The shyness. The hurt."

His parents had tried. They had met with his teachers, showered him with affection and love, took him to physicians and counsellors, sent him to Jamaica that summer to spend time with an uncle, a fitness buff, hoping he would build muscle and self-esteem. Now they are setting up a center where shy, overweight children can swim without shame. Sammy loved to swim, they said, but only after dark. He was too ashamed to let anyone see him in his bathing suit.

Invisible behind a stony mask

Charisse Goodman recounts the unfairness of her childhood experiences in *The Invisible Woman*.[15] "I was always 'the fat kid.' I wasn't me. I wasn't a name or a person, just an object described by an adjective. If I was naturally shy, I became doubly so.

"To make things worse, my family moved several times during my childhood. I found out early that I'd be lucky to have one or two friends who didn't care what I looked like. I learned that no matter what anyone says, it really doesn't count if you're smart, kind, funny, sweet, generous, or caring because if you also happen to be heavy, you may find yourself on the receiving end of more cruelty than you even knew existed.

"I learned that keeping to myself and minding my own business didn't help because people would seek me out to ridicule and humiliate me. I learned that 'ignoring it,' as I was nonchalantly advised to do by my emotionally disengaged parents, usually just made me a greater challenge to bullies, so that I inevitably became 'the one to get.' I learned that adults are often indifferent to the suffering of a fat child, perhaps because on some level they agree with her tormentors, or maybe it's just convenient for them to believe that an abused child will somehow emerge unscathed into adulthood, magically free of emotional scars.

"I discovered that anytime I moved my body, people would laugh at me, and that even if I sat still and quietly read a book they would point and laugh. I learned that if they saw me cry or show any weakness, they would laugh at me even more. And so I learned to cry alone, and laugh alone, and live alone inside my head. I learned that the word 'pretty' never included me.

"Even those times when I lost weight to try and fit in, it was never enough, and I grew to realize that when it was time to choose teammates for a game, or dates for a dance, I was invisible; but when someone needed a cheap laugh or a quick ego boost at my expense, people saw me, all right. I learned my place. I tried to learn not to care.

"As I grew up, I assumed a stone-faced mask in order to deprive people of their sickening delight in hurting me, a mask which in later years I would find extremely difficult to remove. I became a tense child with a perpetual air of bewilderment. But I was not angry. Any anger on my part was met by adults with the huffy insistence that I had a hostility problem. What other people did to me was natural and normal, while I was neither.

"Now I am a grown woman. I know without a doubt that in every town and every city, in every state in America, countless other fat children are learning the same heartbreaking, soul-destroying lessons that I was forced to learn. My pain and the pain of others like me has been conveniently invisible to thin people for far too long. They have been too comfortable with the price that we have paid for their imaginary superiority.

"At long last, I am angry."

Venting feelings

Nancy Summer, another leader in the size acceptance movement, presents workshops in anti-violence and anti-prejudice programs to sixth-grade girls in schools.[16]

She encourages the girls to vent their worst prejudices against large people and get all the negative things out in the open right away. "I invite them to insult me. 'What do you think when you see a person as fat as me? What words come to mind? You can be honest.' (I weigh more than 400 pounds.)

"After the initial giggling and squirming in chairs, the responses are never the same. In one class, a rambunctious thin girl looks me dead in the eye and calls me a horse! 'Good!' I say. I smile and write horse on the flip chart and then ask if they can think of other animals that are associated with fat people. Soon horse is joined by suggestions from other girls: cow, elephant, pig, hippo, buffalo and whale. Then we discuss how beautiful these animals are in their own right. My calm response to the challenge sets the tone for that workshop.

"Whether the girls are polite or candid, aware of the issues or not, we always manage to bring out many of the stereotypes and negative language that they've heard (and use) about fat people. They especially enjoy talking about their larger teachers in a setting where they can 'get away with it.' One girl actually admits that she teased a teacher until she made her cry. She is proud of this revelation until she hears her classmates define this as being mean.

"When a group is too polite, I ask what the boys say to or about fat girls, and that often brings lots of responses: 'Shamu,' 'bubble butt,' and 'lard ass' are favorites. We also discuss the many stereotypes people believe about fat kids and adults. 'Fat and lazy,' 'Fat people eat all the time,' and 'Boys don't think fat girls are pretty,' are just some of the responses I get.

"I always counter the negative stereotypes with facts and personal stories. For example, when one girl says that fat people are stupid, I counter with the fact that when I was in sixth grade, I was invited into a program where I could skip eighth grade.

"But always I stress my basic message: bias against fat hurts people of all sizes. 'Imagine that you are sitting in the lunchroom and a bully starts making fun of a fat kid a few tables away. How does that make you feel?' I ask them. 'We can imagine that the fat kid feels bad about being picked on, but what about all the other kids who hear it?'

"'I'd be afraid he'd pick on me next,' one girl responds. Another says, 'I'd be afraid that if I got fat, people would pick on me, too.' 'I wouldn't eat my dessert.' 'I'd probably laugh, too,' one candid soul admits, but goes on to tell us about a fat boy in her school who always laughs when people pick on him. One brave girl says, 'I'd tell him to shut up.'

"I explain that it isn't just large kids and adults who are hurt by size discrimination. Everyone else is hurt, too, because as long as fat is hated, everyone will be afraid of becoming fat. Fear of fat makes everyone unhappy and dissatisfied with their bodies. And that makes us have lower self-esteem and less self-confidence. And sometimes it can lead to dangerous diets and eating disorders."

Clearly size prejudice is a potent force for these youngsters and sixth grade girls understand it well.

CHAPTER 8

Weights continue to rise

■

When is a child overweight? What causes it? And what can we do about it?

These are old questions and yet ones so new that before 1980, many believed obesity to be simply a problem of too many calories. As a result, the solutions offered by experts have often been simplistic and ineffective.

Faced with the failure of the old approaches, researchers are asking new questions? What are the hallmarks of obesity? Does it start in childhood through excess fat cell development, or even in the womb? Is it most likely to be triggered at high-risk points during a child's development? How powerful are genetic factors? And if heredity is the important determining factor, why are we seeing such steep increases in childhood obesity in just the past decade?

While there have been advances, intense debate continues and much remains unknown. The bottom line is that researchers and many health professionals now recognize obesity as a complex condition that resists intervention. The fact is, there is much we don't know about childhood obesity — or what to do about it.

"Obesity continues to humble the scientific community by eluding effective understanding and intervention in many important respects," says Shiriki Kumanyika, associate professor of nutrition epidemiology at Pennsylvania State University.[1]

Prevalence of overweight

While researchers and health professionals ponder childhood obesity, its causes and outcomes, one thing is clear: The prevalence of overweight has increased sharply in the last two decades for both children and adolescents. Not only are more American youngsters overweight, but they are more severely overweight than ever before.

The striking evidence for this comes from the Third National Health and Nutrition Examination Study (NHANES III) which gathered data from 1988 to 1994, measuring a large national sampling of youth, and comparing it to data from 1963.[2]

To define the cutoff point of overweight and obesity, researchers now use the sex- and age-specific 95th percentile of body mass index from the year 2000 U.S. Growth Charts.[3]

Using this definition, at the 95th percentile, 11 percent of children age six to 19 are overweight or obese. This is more than double the five percent baseline set in the 1960s. At the 85th percentile and above, 22 percent are considered at risk. It's a big increase in a public health sense, yet at the same time, we need to keep these figures in perspective. Most kids — nearly 90 percent — are not overweight or obese, and well over three-fourths are not at risk of it.

What alarms public health officials is that rates of overweight and obesity were fairly stable during the 1960s and 1970s, but since the early 1980s, both children and adults have gained weight, particularly at the upper end (*figure 1*). The heaviest children are now heavier than children in earlier studies — and more of them have moved above the cutoff point. But at the other levels, percentages have remained fairly constant for the past three decades.[4] The Healthy People target for the year 2010 is to reduce these percentages to 5 percent.[5]

Another study that documents increases in overweight for children is the long-term Bogalusa Heart Study. During 14 years, this survey of 2,500 to 3,500 youth measured dramatic increases in overweight for ages 5 to 14. At each age level, children were five and a half pounds heavier in 1984 than 1973. Again percentages at the lean and average weights tended to remain constant, with most increases in the heavier categories. It did not appear that heavier children were eating any more calories than leaner children, the researchers said.[6]

Higher rates for minorities

African American children tend to be taller, heavier, and mature earlier. Even by age 10, African American girls were 11 pounds heavier, 1.6 inches taller, had more body fat, and reached puberty earlier than white girls, in a study of black Harlem youth.[7]

The NHANES III study found more minority children than white children overweight at all ages, except for younger toddlers *(figure 2)*. About 8 percent of all kids are overweight at age four and five, compared with 3.5 percent at age two and three. Of African Americans, 8 percent of boys and 11 percent of girls in that preschool group (age 4-5) are overweight. Of Mexican-Americans, this figure is 12 percent of boys and 13 percent of girls.[8]

Overweight prevalence is also high for American Indian children.[9]

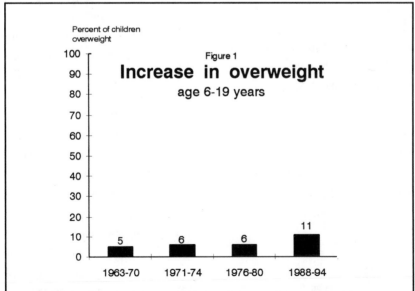

Percent of children overweight

Figure 1
Increase in overweight
age 6-19 years

The prevalence of overweight has increased from 5 to 11 percent since 1963 for boys and girls age 6-19, at the 95th percentile. NHANES III (1988-1994).[1]

HEALTHY PEOPLE 2010/ CHILDREN AND TEENS AFRAID TO EAT 2001

A look at Zuni children found that more than half of girls and one third of boys ages 11 to 20 were overweight. A study of Cherokee teens found that gender trend reversed — half of boys and one-fourth of girls were overweight.[10] Among the Pima, who suffer extremely high rates of type 2 diabetes associated with obesity, about half of youth exceed the 95th percentile.[11]

Figure 2 **Prevalence of overweight** by sex, age and race/ethnicity	
Boys	95th percentile
6-11	
Total	14.7
White, non-Hispanic	13.2
Black, non-Hispanic	14.7
Mexican American	18.8
12-17	
Total	12.3
White, non-Hispanic	11.6
Black, non-Hispanic	12.5
Mexican American	15.0
Girls	
6-11	
Total	12.5
White, non-Hispanic	11.9
Black, non-Hispanic	17.9
Mexican American	15.8
12-17	
Total	10.7
White, non-Hispanic	9.6
Black, non-Hispanic	16.3
Mexican American	14.0
NHANES III, PHASE I/ AFRAID TO EAT 1997	

Fat patterning

The location of fat on the body can indicate if children and adults may be at higher risk for health problems. Excess fat concentrated on the upper body or abdomen, in a centralized pattern (apple shape) rather than in the lower body (pear shape), increases a person's risk factors for chronic disease.[12]

Genetic factors are important in determining this. African American and Mexican American children tend to have more upper body fat (apple shape) than white children, which increases with age, particularly for boys (figure 2).[13]

Defining obesity

Some experts say

obesity should be defined as the level at which health risks begin, and that it differs for individuals, depending on fat distribution, genetics, family and culture, dieting history, lifestyle and physical activity. Family history needs to be considered to determine what may be normal for a particular child.[14]

Currently overweight and obesity are defined for youth at the 95th percentile of body mass index (BMI). This is a more conservative definition than the 85th percentile, often used in the past, and is less likely to mislabel children who are muscular, or in the midst of puberty fat changes and growth spurts. At the 85th percentile, youth are being called at risk for overweight, although often they are not. (Phase 1 of the NHANES III study placed 22 percent of youth age 12 to 17 in these two higher categories.)

Children grow and develop at every age in widely differing ways. The problem with using BMI, a measure of weight and height, to identify health risk is that it doesn't work for individuals, although it is often used and abused in this way. It works for population groups, because *on average* people with higher BMIs have the higher body fat that translates to risk.

Swedish research shows clearly that risk is related to body fat, not weight. In a study that followed 735 men over a lifetime, Swedish researchers found that weight was not very important in longevity; instead, body fat was the determining factor. In every weight category the men who had the lowest body fat and highest percent of lean mass lived longer. They warn that BMI does not give an accurate indication of body fat, and therefore does not accurately predict risk. While higher mortality was linked to higher body fat in a linear direction, BMI showed a "U" relationship (higher mortality with both low and high BMI).[15]

Body fat varies widely in each weight category — from 13 to 42 percent at a BMI of 30 in one community study, and some professional basketball players carry only 5 percent body fat at that weight.[16]

For both children and adults, using BMI often mislabels risk. For example, one-fourth of children labeled as "at risk" (BMI at or over the 85th percentile) turned out to have normal body fat, in a USDA study of 979 children age 3 to 18. There were also errors in under-identifying kids with high body fat: one in six with a normal range BMI had high body fat, and the range was 10 to 40 percent. Mislabeling of this many children is a major concern when using BMI, the authors say.[17] (High body fat has sometimes been defined as 25 percent body fat for boys and 30 percent for girls.)[18]

To compare a child's weight with national norms, health providers use the 2000 growth charts from the Centers for Disease Control and Prevention. These charts define weight levels for ages 2 to 20 at the various percentiles with a series of curved lines. Using these charts, children with a BMI at the 5th percentile are considered underweight and at the 95th percentile, overweight. (When used to track an individual's growth, the charts are best used by professionals, taking into consideration the child's history and other factors. A problem in relying too heavily on weight alone is that early maturing children weigh more at earlier ages, so will usually top the charts.) The growth charts reveal the ways body fatness changes over the years as children grow, with a decrease between age 2 and 5, followed by a normal adiposity rebound about age 5 to 7. They show how girls and boys differ as they mature, and how a child's growth can be plotted.[19]

Standards for children are in general agreement with those of adults, for which the official definitions are: overweight, BMI of 25 to 29.9; obesity, BMI of 30 or more. This puts 55 percent of American adults in these two categories (32 percent overweight, and 23 percent obese).[20] Setting the overweight category this low has been criticized because it suggests that health risks begin at levels much lower than is supported by research. It ignores the body fat issue altogether.

What happened?

Although we knew it was coming from many smaller studies all pointing to obesity rate increases, the nationwide statistics that came out in the mid-1990s sent a shock wave reverberating through the health community. What happened? Why did obesity rates jump across the board for young and old, for boys and girls, for every ethnic and racial group?

Perhaps the simplest explanation is that children today are less active, even sedentary. Other answers are more complex: genetic vulnerability; kinds and amounts of food eaten; disruption of normal eating and disregard of satiety signals; more weight gain in pregnancy; larger babies; higher population increases in groups with "thrifty genes," the genes that help bodies conserve fat.

The interplay of genetics, food supply, physical activity, culture, socioeconomic and psychological factors all have an effect on the regulation of appetite and satiety, and how calories are used and stored as fat.

The tendency to gain excessive fat varies from one person to another, even in the same family, and even when food intake, physical activity and lifestyle appear to be the same. It is likely that genetic tendencies route more fat into storage for some individuals, and that they have extraordinary ability to protect that stored fat and restore supplies quickly when depleted.

Genetic factors

Weight is highly influenced by genetic factors. Studies of identical and fraternal twins indicate that the genetic contribution of obesity in children may be as much as 80 percent. In recent research that looked at 66 pairs of twins, age 3 to 17, genes accounted for about 75 to 80 percent of differences in body fat between twins, and 70 percent of differences in BMI, with an overlap of 30 percent. The environmental has far less effect. Shared environment had no significant effect on differences between twins, and only 20 to 25 percent was attributed to nonshared environmental influences.[21]

A child with two overweight parents has an 80 percent chance of becoming overweight, compared with 14 percent for the child of two average weight parents.[22]

The "thrifty gene" theory helps explain why obesity rates are so high for children of African, American Indian, Mexican or Pacific Island descent. This theory holds that certain genetic traits helped ancient people survive under harsh conditions. It was survival of the fittest: people with thrifty genes were most likely to live and pass them on to their children. The closer modern people are to their subsistence roots, the more likely they retain thrifty genes, while those of us whose ancestors came from agricultural areas where food was more plentiful,

Ethnic differences in fat patterning

Ethnic differences in body build and fat patterning were analyzed by William Mueller of the School of Public Health, University of Texas Health Science Center, using data on national and other studies of children and adolescents. His studies show ethnicity accounts for about one-third to one-half of the variance of sex and maturation. His findings are independent of average fatness levels. However, Mueller cautions some of the variance may still result from the differing obesity levels.

Comparing statistics on black, Mexican American and white children, he reports the following:

1. **Children, ages 1 to 5**
   - Preschool children are much more peripheral in fat distribution (less centralized/ abdominal) than older children.
   - Black preschool children have more centralized or upper body fat patterning than white preschoolers.

2. **Adolescents**
   - Mexican American children have higher skinfold measures at triceps, subscapular and suprailiac, but lower at medial calf site, compared with white children (more centralized fat).
   - Black children have lower skinfolds at both arm and leg sites than white children; their fat is more centrally distributed.

3. **Girls, ages 12 to 17**
   - Black and Mexican American girls have a more central distribution of fat than white girls.

   - Fatness increases with age for all three groups.

4. **Boys, ages 12 to 17**
   - Centrality of fat increases with age in all three groups.
   - Black and Mexican American boys have more centralized fat than white boys.

5. **Other differences, ages 6 to 17**
   - Black children tend to have more centralized fat patterning at all ages, with less arm and leg fat, compared with white children.
   - Black children have the broadest shoulders and narrowest hips, compared with Mexican and white children.
   - Mexican American children have more upper body fatness with less leg fat, compared with white children.
   - Mexican Americans tend to have the narrowest shoulders of the three groups.
   - Sex differences emerge at puberty, but ethnic differences remain.
   - Youth with type 2 diabetes (age 14 to 17) tend to have broader shoulders and narrower hips than nondiabetic youth of same sex and age.
   - Circumference ratios of waist-to-hip show less ethnic difference than skinfolds, yet consistent sex difference. Thus circumferences may be measuring muscle and bone development, not fatness levels.[3]

Bouchard, Johnston
Healthy Weight Journal
AFRAID TO EAT 2001, 1997

such as northern Europe, may have lost them.

Thus, having thrifty genes is like driving a highly efficient sports car with good gas mileage, compared to an old "gas guzzler." Those with thrifty genes conserve fuel in fat cells for later use; others who stay thin "waste" a lot of fuel by burning it off. In primitive times having the thrifty genotype was beneficial, but in our modern world of sedentary living and abundant rich food, it promotes obesity.[23]

Genetic factors can affect metabolic rate, thermogenesis, endocrine function, fat storage, appetite and satiety.

Still, Claude Bouchard, Laval University, Quebec, who has done extensive research comparing twins, adoptees and nine types of relatives, cautions against putting too much blame on genetics. Many factors are involved, and there's "A lot of chaos in the body system we're working with. . . . We are seeing big increases in obesity worldwide. This has to be the result of environmental factors."[24]

Inactivity prevails

It's hard to measure activity, but most experts agree there has been a continuous decline in general physical activity.

Our streets are perceived as unsafe, and fewer kids walk or ride bikes to school. More stay indoors watching television, playing video games or surfing the Net. In a climate of decreasing budgets, schools have cut physical education programs. In 1995, only 25 percent of U.S. school children attended daily physical education class.

American teens are sadly inactive, and African Americans, Hispanics, and Asians are at greatest risk. Girls, especially older ones, tend to be the least active of all.

The more time spent watching television, the higher children's risk for becoming overweight, no matter what their race, according to some studies. Spending so much time in front of the TV can mean they are less active or snack more in front of the small screen, or both, or that television itself may have a lulling effect by lowering metabolism, as some evidence suggests.

African American girls watched an average of 36 hours a week compared with 24 for white girls, in one study. And almost twice as many reported that they usually ate while watching television. The

African American girls were also more overweight, as were girls of both races who watched more television. Girls who said they usually ate while watching television consumed more calories than others.[25]

A University of North Carolina study of more than 13,000 seventh to twelfth graders across the nation found among boys, time spent watching TV was 14.4 hours a week for whites, 15 for Asians, 17 for Hispanics and 21 for blacks. Among girls, average weekly TV viewing was 12 hours for whites, 13 for Asians, 15 for Hispanics and 20 for blacks. For both sexes total inactivity hours ranged from 19 for whites to 30 for African Americans, with Asians and Hispanics in between. Only one third said they were moderately to vigorously active five or more times a week, and one third failed to meet minimum public health recommendations for physical activity. Overweight was highest among African American girls at 39 percent and lowest among Asian girls at 11 percent.[26]

In Japan — where obesity for children increased from 5 percent in 1974 to 11 percent in 1995 at the level of 120 percent or more of standard body weight — researchers blame a shift from outdoor to indoor games, more private schools allowing less playing time after school, and more cheap, high-calorie snack foods.[27]

Food intake and fat content

The kinds of food children are eating may also make a difference in weight increases. Today kids eat more snack foods (crackers, chips, dessert foods and candy) and less of the foods that seem to provide more satiety (meat, eggs and milk).

Eating patterns have changed, too. Children are eating fewer meals at home, and more often eating at fast-food restaurants where increasingly larger quantities are being served, often of high-fat, high calorie foods. Some specialists believe the disruption of normal eating brought by these and other changes may be part of the problem.

It has been thought that the increase in obesity reflects consumption of foods too high in fat and calories. Certainly this seems a likely factor for many youth today. Yet, on average, children as well as adults are eating less fat today than a decade ago and calorie increases, if any, appear to be small. Fat consumption has dropped from 36 to 33 percent of total calories in the last decade, according to USDA nutrient intake surveys.

In one large study, African American and white girls ages 9 and 10 kept food diaries for three days. The African American girls ate more calories and fat and tended to be heavier. They ate less meat, milk and cheese and snacked more on high-fat foods. For the white girls, eating more high-fat foods was associated with overweight.[28]

Eating a high-fat diet has been blamed as a major culprit in obesity and its rising rates. But it's not this simple. Many experts are rethinking low-fat advice.

At first it seemed to make sense, back in the 1980s when those first studies came in showing fast weight and fat gain for lab rats fed Crisco-laden diets. It became clear that dietary fat is easily stored in the body. And it is not regulated, with more being burned when more is available, as happens with protein and carbohydrate. (However, even with lab animals there are wide individual and strain differences in how much they gain from high-fat diets.) Fat has more calories per gram (nine calories per gram compared with four for protein and carbohydrate), and makes food taste good, so people often overeat.

Americans responded to this news by dropping their fat intake from a high of about 42 to 44 percent of total calories in 1965, to 33 percent in 1996. Health gurus urged a still lower drop to 30 or even 20 percent of total calories. But while this was happening, obesity rates skyrocketed. The same thing happened in other countries, where obesity rates went up as fat intake went down.

Was it because of the advice to eat less fat? Or in spite of it? Either way, there is growing realization that decreasing the amount of fat one eats is not the answer that had been hoped for.

"Diets high in fat are not the primary cause of the high prevalence of excess body fat in our society, nor are reductions in dietary fat a solution," concludes Walter Willett, of the Harvard School of Public Health.

Fat intake studies for humans are less convincing than for lab animals. People seldom eat pure sources of fat. In mixed meals it doesn't seem to make much difference whether people eat much or little fat as long as they do not overeat, according to research by

Andrew Prentice, of the MRC Dunn Clinical Nutrition Centre, Cambridge, England. Unless calorie intake is high, he reports, there's little difference in fat storage — even when diets range from 10 percent to 80 percent fat. Only when people eat more than their bodies can use, are more of the excess calories from high fat diets than low fat diets stored as fat.[29]

Lowering fat intake by itself has not been a successful weight loss method. For instance, women lost weight the first year when reducing their fat intake from 38 percent to an extremely low 20 percent in the Women's Health Trial, a treatment study of women with breast cancer. However, by the end of the second year, they had regained it all and weighed about the same as the control group, even though they had carefully followed the low-fat diet.[30]

Another problem with low-fat diets is that they are not necessarily low in calories. Many low-fat processed foods are very high in sugar and calories, including many of the fat-free cookies, cakes, chips and candies that now crowd supermarket shelves. As an example, adding chocolate powder to a glass of milk can double the calories but reduce the *percent* of fat so that it counts as a low-fat food.

Alcohol is often forgotten when we talk about calorie intake, yet it accounts for about 6 percent of calories in the average American

Figure 3

Parental food prompts
Average number per meal[4]

	Normal weight child	Overweight child
Encouragements to eat	4	16
Food presentations	11	20
Offers of food	3	7
Total food prompts	18	43

Klesges/Healthy Weight Journal/ Afraid to Eat 1997

diet and can be as much as 10 percent for regular drinkers.

Alcohol may promote fat storage in a special way, by allowing more of the energy from fat to be stored as fat. Therefore, it has additive effects in a higher-fat diet.[31] Drinking is also associated with increased risk of abdominal fat — the proverbial "beer belly."[32]

Family control and disruptive eating

What you do, what you say and how you eat in a family counts. Simple things, like urging a child to clean her plate can have a direct effect on overweight.

Fourteen families with young children ages one to three were observed several times at meals in a psychology study at North Dakota State University in Fargo. The researchers found that the overweight toddlers were urged both verbally and nonverbally to eat twice as often as normal weight children. They received an average of 43 prompts per meal compared with 18 for the normal weight children *(figure 3)*. All children usually ate more when urged to do so. When they refused, parents almost always encouraged them to eat more, and 70 percent of the time they did. The researchers concluded that many parents encourage overeating in their very young children in ways that override satiety signals and may lead to excess weight gain.[33]

On the other hand, being underfed and encouraged to eat less than satisfies a child's needs can also promote overeating, binge eating, secret eating and excessive weight gain.[34]

Ellyn Satter says young children can regulate their own food intake, but a controlling, authoritarian parenting style impedes their ability to do this. Moms and dads often believe it's their job as parents to get their children to eat the "right" amount. Their strategies can be coercive and controlling. When parents focus too much on what to eat, when to eat, or how much food is left on the plate, their children don't learn to respond to natural hunger and satiety signals. A parent who is dieting may be overconcerned about a child's weight and eating, and kids feel this anxiety.

Diets are not helpful, especially for kids. Several studies suggest that their dieting can lead to excess weight gain. In a northern California study, 692 ninth-grade girls from three high schools were studied over a period of three years, using actual measurements and behavioral questionnaires. At every weight, girls who tried to lose were at greater risk for obesity.

Their initial weight made no difference — thin girls were just as susceptible to weight gain as girls who were overweight or average at baseline. Restricting food made the difference. The risk for obesity was over three times as great for dieters as for those who lived diet-free. Girls who reported the more strenuous dieting, exercise for weight control, and radical weight loss efforts such as use of laxatives, diet pills, vomiting and fasting gained even more weight over time, and they also binged more. The researchers concluded that weight loss efforts can lead to "dysregulation of the normal appetite system," resulting in excess weight gain.[35]

Poor family communication can also contribute to overweight. If children are isolated in a disinterested or disengaged family, they may be at a higher risk of overweight, reports Laurel Mellin, MA, RD, San Francisco. Her study of 254 obese adolescents found that four factors accounted for most of the weight differences: family cohesion, adolescent communication, age of obesity onset and the mother's weight.

Surprisingly, the major environmental factors were not diet or exercise, but instead were related to relationships, family cohesion and communication. As families were less engaged and the child less involved with family, childrens' overweight increased. Mellin suggests that targeting family communication and teaching family interactional skills may be more effective in preventing obesity than targeting diet and physical activity.[36]

Quitting smoking

Smoking a cigarette induces an acute rise and perhaps longer-term rise in metabolic rate, and tends to reduce food intake, so there is some weight loss when kids take up smoking.[37] Then, if they quit, as nearly all say they intend to, they usually "catch up" with others who did not smoke.

Recently, Williamson studied a national sample of smokers and non-smokers and found that on average men gained six pounds and women eight pounds on quitting smoking (about the same amount that smoking keeps off). Younger people and heavier smokers, however, tend to have higher weight gain when they quit, up to 28 pounds.[38]

When a significant portion of the population quits smoking, this can cause a small rise in overall obesity rates. However, it is important for youth to understand that the benefits of quitting smoking far out-weigh any risks of overweight.

Vulnerabilities throughout the lifespan

Six periods in life are identified by the World Health Organization as vulnerable times for the development of obesity:

1. **Prenatal.** Nutrition during fetal life may affect development of size, shape, body composition and the way the body handles nutrients.
2. **Adiposity rebound.** (Age 5 to 7.) Early pre-school years are a time of lower body fat, followed by a rapid rebound in fat.
3. **Adolescence.** Body changes at puberty promote increased fat deposition, especially for girls. This may also be a time of irregular eating and inactivity.
4. **Early adulthood.** (Age 15 to 19 for women; several years later for men.) There may be marked reduction in physical activity and often weight gain.
5. **Pregnancy.** Net weight gain for mothers averages about one pound with each child. But the range is wide, and with more pregnancies, higher gains are more likely.
6. **Menopause.** The reason for weight gain at mid-life is likely hormonal, a metabolic slowdown, and possibly reduced activity.[39]

Bigger babies

Since 1989, U.S. Public Health directives have called on women to produce larger babies by gaining more weight in pregnancy. The goal of this policy is to increase average birthweight to 8 to 8.5 pounds in a perhaps-misguided effort to reduce the numbers of small, premature babies. But there is evidence that larger babies are more likely overweight later in life, especially for minority children. And gaining more weight in pregnancy clearly increases obesity risk for mothers.

Ray Yip, MD, MPH, Centers for Disease Control, reports that CDC surveillance programs show birth weight influences later growth: heavy babies are four times as likely to become heavy 5-year-olds.[40]

Another federal analysis of height and weight at age 6 to 11 showed similar results: children with higher birth weights were heavier and taller. However not all fat babies are at risk.[42]

Being taller early is also related to earlier maturity, which in turn is related to obesity.[41] Some researchers have observed that infants who are quiet, inactive and placid tend to become overweight even with moderate intakes of food.

From birth, babies born to overweight mothers seem at higher risk of obesity. Studies of British and Canadian children show that even if the babies of larger women are normal weight at birth, by 6 months they are heavier and growing faster than other infants.

Infant feeding

Breastfeeding seems a healthy course for both mother and baby, but its link to weight is unclear. Some studies in the 1970s suggested that bottle-feeding and the early introduction of solid foods contribute to childhood overweight, but more recent studies refute that claim.

A 16-year longitudinal study followed 180 children from age 6 months to age 16, in Berkeley, Calif. The type of infant feeding or when solid food was introduced made no difference in weight. Neither did the kinds of food eaten for meals or snacks, or whether the child had a "sweet tooth."[43]

Another four-year study in Maine found no relationship between formula feeding or the early introduction of solid foods and preschool overweight. Solid foods were given earlier to babies who were bottle-fed, while babies who were breast-fed usually started solid foods later. After four years, 12 percent of the children were overweight, with no relationship to their feeding practices.[44]

Pregnancy weight gains

Women have long recognized that gaining too much weight during pregnancy can trigger obesity, but this is largely ignored by the medical and health communities. Many doctors shrug off any concerns, saying any excess weight can be taken off later. Unfortunately, this is not true.

Early teen and preteen mothers-to-be are urged to gain more weight during pregnancy, and to have heavier babies than a couple of decades ago, in an effort to reduce the number of low-birth-weight babies. However, it's clear this bodes higher risk for obesity, especially for low-income and ethnic minority girls who are already at risk.

There is evidence that it is normal for African-American women to gain less in pregnancy than white women and have smaller babies, who then grow faster in their early years than white babies. By age 1 to 4, growth is accelerated for black children over that of white children, according to Kumanyika. Small babies are common in Africa, she says.[45]

American Indian babies, too, were known to be smaller in earlier times and childbirth was easier, in what may be genetic survival traits. The recent insistence by health officials that minority babies be large may not be as beneficial as hoped. This advice is paralleled by a steep rise in obesity for both minority women and their children.

At the same time, many young pregnant girls are so poorly nourished that they don't gain enough weight to support both their own healthy growth and that of the infant. They often give birth to tiny, high-risk or premature babies. Thus, it is urgent that pregnant teens and preteens get early nutrition counseling and regular prenatal care.

Having more pregnancies is also linked to obesity.

Early puberty

The age of puberty for American and European boys and girls has dropped steadily during the last 100 years. Instead of reaching menarche at age 15 or 16 and their adult height at 20 to 21 years as they did 100 years ago, American girls now reach menarche at an average of 12.8 years and complete growth by age 16 to 18, according to Rose Frisch, PhD, Harvard Center for Population Studies.[46]

Their first menstrual period comes even earlier for African American girls, age 12.2 on average, and half are beginning to develop sexually by age 8. For white girls, only 15 percent develop sexually this early.[47]

Why is this happening?

Frisch suggests this trend is related to higher body fat and inactivity. Girls need about 22 percent body fat to reach menarche, she says, and mean weight at puberty is 105 pounds. Average body fat for young women is 25 to 30 percent, according to the American Alliance for Health, Physical Education, Recreation and Dance, 1984. "Children now are bigger sooner. And girls on average reach the mean weight at menarche . . . more quickly," says Frisch.

Early puberty is a largely-unrecognized risk of overweight. Being sexually mature at these very young ages is a factor in the high rates of preteen pregnancy in the U.S. And it increases the risk of reproductive cancers later in life, according to Frisch's research. At the same time there are also risks, particularly to bone health, in delaying menarche too long.

Female athletes average 15.5 years at menarche, about the same as all girls a century ago. Girls who train or exercise heavily often delay this much longer. In one study, female college athletes who began training before menarche started their periods about three years later on average than those who began after menarche, Frisch says.

Is obesity contagious?

Can obesity, or some part of it, be caused by a virus? Don't rule it out. University of Wisconsin scientists have found an intriguing virus — called *avian adenovirus* — that fattens chickens, and a related virus that causes them to develop an unusual amount of visceral fat.

In screening human adenoviruses that cause respiratory infections, they found one type that can cause obesity when injected into chickens and mice. When they tested 154 obese and 45 average-weight men and women, they found that 15 percent of the obese adults carried antibodies for this virus, while none of the average-weight controls did.

They advise skeptics to keep in mind the analogy with stomach ulcers, whose infectious cause was only discovered in 1983, drastically altering treatment.[48]

Tracking overweight

In the controversy about action to take concerning childhood overweight, one factor is its impact on later life. Does overweight track into adulthood? Is an overweight child charting a course that will lead to lifelong obesity and perhaps related health risks, which could be altered by making early changes? Or will young children outgrow their fatness? If they do, being wrongly labelled as obese may contribute to psychosocial difficulties. Growth may also be affected by weight loss attempts.

Two important factors are age and severity of condition. Severe overweight at any age is more likely to continue. Yet it is important to recognize that most large infants and preschoolers will outgrow their fatness. Interfering may distort their natural growth and development.

In a University of Iowa study, over half of children and teens in the highest of five weight categories remained in the highest category as adults. However, nearly one-third dropped down into the lowest three quintiles.[49]

Data compiled from four studies suggests the likelihood of overweight tracking into adulthood increases with age, as seen below. Risk is low at age 5 1/2, is somewhat higher by age 7 when 41 percent are likely to become obese adults, and becomes much higher by age 10 or 12, when 70 percent of overweight children are likely to become obese adults.[50]

Age of overweight child	Percent who become obese adults	Relative risk
0-6 months	14	2.3
6 months - 5.5 years	20	3.4
7 years	41	3.7
10-12 years	70	6.0

However, it's important not to overreact. In these figures, about 60 percent of obese 7-year-olds will *not* be obese as adults. And a 22-year follow-up of 151 obese youngsters in Japan, ages 6 to 14, found two-thirds were no longer obese by the age of 20.[51]

Overweight that starts in adolescence tends to be more severe than adult-onset, and most severely obese people were overweight as teens, one review says. It suggests this is especially true for women: about one-third of all adult obesity in women began in adolescence, and obesity is more likely to continue for women than men.[52]

Risks of overweight

Overweight children may be at increased risk for future diabetes and cardiovascular problems. And since the social stigma of being large is so strong, they're also at increased risk of using dangerous weight loss methods and developing eating disorders. Increasingly, health problems from hazardous weight loss attempts and ill-advised treatment are being recognized as risks of overweight for children and adults.

Health risks related specifically to adolescent overweight, as given by Pauline Powers, MD, at the NIH Strategy Development Workshop for Public Education on Weight and Obesity, include:

• Increased blood pressure
• Increased total cholesterol and abnormal lipoprotein rations
• Hyperinsulineamia[53]

It should be noted that physical fitness is related to blood pressure in 5- and 6-year-old children, independent of weight, in both cross-sectional and longitudinal studies, says Steven Shea, MD, Columbia Presbyterian Medical Center. Activity may be the key, but because of mobility or social reasons, some large children tend to be sedentary, which can increase risk factors and even be their root cause.

Being overweight as a child may influence adult health. Tufts University researchers found that men who were 20 pounds or more overweight as teenagers were twice as likely to have died or developed heart disease by age 70. They were also more likely to suffer colon and rectal cancer and gout. Men who had been overweight as teens but not as adults had lower risk.

However, they found no added risk at age 70 for women who had been overweight teens. They did have double the risk of arthritis and eight times as much difficulty in walking a quarter of a mile, climbing stairs and lifting heavy objects. The study looked at health records of students and tracked their weights and health for 55 years.[54]

In the Bogalusa Heart Study, a clustering of three risk factors correlates highly with overweight, and especially with centralized overweight, in children. These are: systolic blood pressure; fasting insulin; and ratio of low density lipoprotein cholesterol to high density lipoprotein cholesterol (the "bad" LDL vs "good" HDL cholesterol). Children in the upper third weight category showed increased clustering of these factors, compared with lean children. The Bogalusa team suggests preventing overweight early in life may be important in reducing later heart disease.[55]

Obstructive sleep apnoea is another complication, which can cause hypoventilation and even sudden death in severe cases.[56]

Powers also suggests these psychological risks:

- Poor body image, "imprinted" in adolescence
- Low self-esteem, including fear of overweight and increasing preoccupation with size and shape
- Cultural stigma, since both children and adults devalue overweight children

Some child specialists suggest the greatest problems of childhood overweight may be emotional and psychological, such that when children are labelled and stigmatized as obese they may have long-term damage to self-esteem and body concept.[57] Thus, they view overweight as a severe social handicap.

Yet others point out that while this is true, cultural stigma is not a reason to change the child, but rather to change the culture.

CHAPTER 9

Lifestyle choices increase problems

■

A yellow school bus pulls up to the convenience store and out pours a hungry load of junior high students traveling directly from their last class to a sporting event. What foods do these youngsters bring up to the counter? One after the other, they lay out: candy, chips, large bottles of soda pop. More of these foods will be eaten during the game, and the bus will probably stop again on the way home.

What are kids eating today — the other aspect of how and what? How active are they? How are they dealing with the stress in their lives? Some of their lifestyle choices may mean they're not as healthy as they could be.

It's not that there is anything wrong with eating candy, chips, or soft drinks. They're not bad foods. But they are tip-of-the-pyramid foods — low in nutrients and high in sugar and fat — snack foods, not meant to sustain anyone for long.

Kids are making these kinds of choices at earlier ages, in a world that has changed dramatically in recent years. They are more likely now to be children of divorce, live with one parent, or have parents unavailable. Children thus spend more time away from home, eat more meals out and on their own, and spend money as they choose.[1]

The problem of their food choices goes far beyond the dinner table, though. So do the problems of sedentary living. How children eat and the activity habits they develop now will affect them the rest of their lives.

What are teens eating?

Many children start out eating healthy diets. But as they reach their teens, diets change. In the government's Healthy Eating Index, teens do not score well. Their scores are only in the low 60s out of 100 points.[2]

The Bogalusa Heart Study of children in the American South documents this trend. The percent who get less than two-thirds of recommended nutrients increases for teens. Food choices shift more toward higher-calorie, lower-nutrient food, toward more dessert and snack foods, and more soft drinks.

Compared with 20 years ago, young people are eating twice as much food like crackers, popcorn, pretzels and chips, and more pasta, rice dishes, tacos, burritos and pizza, the all time favorite — more grain-based foods from the bread and cereals group. They are drinking three times as much soda pop and consuming more desserts and candy.[3]

What's missing? All of the other four food groups — fruits, vegetables, milk and meat. Teens are coming up short in four out of five.

Boys are more likely fully nourished than girls, mostly because they eat more, not better. Teenage girls have the poorest diets in the nation, and are most at risk from nutrient deficiencies. Younger teen girls from age 12 to 15 are even worse off than older teens, due to their tremendous growth needs.

Missing foods

Few American kids eat the recommended five-a-day servings of fruits and vegetables, except for younger children. Only about one in four high school students gets five — boys more than girls, white kids more than black or Hispanic, 9th graders more than 12th graders.[4] Their favorite veggie is potatoes — a good starchy food, but only one of several important categories, and too often eaten as high-fat chips or french fries. Low on the list are green beans, corn, green peas, lima beans, the nutrient-packed dark greens and deep-yellows, and the cancer-fighting vegetables from the cabbage family. Variety is important in both vegetables and fruits because they provide so many different nutrients in varying quantity. Also, they are important sources of fiber, notably low in teen diets. But many kids avoid all but two or three kinds of veggies, and eat no fresh fruits at all.

Many teens do not eat meat, mistakenly believing this is a healthy choice. Only one-fourth of girls eat recommended amounts from the meat group, including alternates. Their painfully low levels of iron and zinc reflect this. Overall, kids eat less meat, fish, poultry and eggs, and not much of the bean and nut alternates. Often what they do eat comes in combination dishes with only small amounts of meat, such as those thin slices of pepperoni on pizza.

As milk drops, soda jumps

Milk consumption, too, has dropped off drastically in the last 20 years. Only half of teenagers drink milk, compared with three-fourths in the 1970s. Those who do, drink only about one and a half to two cups a day on average, not the three glasses recommended.[5] Thus calcium intake is declining rapidly at a time when there is growing concern that it needs to increase.

Why this devastating drop in milk? Experts say teens have a new perception that milk is "just for little kids." They are responding to aggressive mass marketing of soft drinks as "fun" foods, and switching over from milk. More sobering are school policies that promote higher-profit beverages rather than milk.[6]

Soft drink consumption has nearly tripled since 1967, and now adds more than one-third of all refined sugars in the diet. One out of four teen boys who drink soda has five or more cans a day; one of ten has seven or more. Teen girls are not far behind. By contrast, 20 years ago the typical soft drink consumer had only two-thirds of a can per day. Now teenage boys drink twice as much as milk (averaging two and two-thirds cups a day compared with one and one-fourth cup milk).[7]

Heavy soft drink intake is associated with low intake of calcium and other nutrients, and with a diet high in calories and fat. A national study shows children and teens who drink milk at their noon meal are more likely to have high quality diets.[8]

Unlike cave man diet

An odd thing about the way kids eat today is that it's almost directly opposite what our early ancestors ate — diets high in meat, fruits and vegetables (after weaning from mother's milk at age 4 or 5). They ate almost no grain, say anthropologists.

In Europe, big-game hunters of 30,000 years ago were tall and strong with massive bones. They grew six inches taller than their descendants who settled down to farming, raised grains, and seldom had animal products to eat. And it took their descendants until the Industrial Revolution, when they again ate more meat, eggs and milk, to gain back that height.[9]

Today our children are shifting away from the five food groups, and even farther from that ancient diet, to relying mostly on grains — bread, pasta, cereals, baked goods, crackers. Plus, they are pulling down those niche foods from the tip of the pyramid — desserts, candy, high-fat snacks, soft drinks — and expanding them into a major part of their diet. Teen boys consume especially high levels of fat, saturated fat, cholesterol and sodium. More than 90 percent of teenage boys exceed Dietary Guidelines levels of these.[10]

This is a significant departure from five groups eaten in moderation, balance and variety *(see Food Guide Pyramid in Chapter 13).* It's extremely limited. How can it be healthy? Why are parents allowing it? Can it be because many parents are also eating this way? And what of the next generation who will be taught by these kids?

Teenagers also eat more food outside the home, and this contributes to their often unbalanced food choices. Foods eaten at home or school tend to be higher in nutrition and lower in fat and sugar. One-third of students get nearly half their calories away from home, way up from the 1970s. Teen boys report eating more often at fast food restaurants than at the school cafeteria.[11]

Even at home, more food comes from take out vendors, and less is "made from scratch." Thus, improvement in children's diets will need to focus on restaurants, as well as home and school, experts say.

Supplementing

People are taking a lot of supplements today and giving them to their children, hoping to fill gaps in their nutrition with pills. But they may be fooling themselves. It's real food that counts in a healthy diet.

For example, take phytochemicals, one of the hottest new areas in cancer research. It's estimated there may be over 100 different phytochemicals in just one serving of vegetables. We haven't identified them all, much less which ones are most effective against cancer. This is why a balanced diet with variety is so important in food choices, to ensure getting the needed nutrients. If you take a pill instead of real food, you lose out.

Even with regulated fortification and supplements there are questions over how well they are absorbed and used by the body. *Tufts University Diet and Nutrition Letter* reports that the type of iron sprayed on breakfast cereals is "additive iron" which "passes through the digestive tract largely unabsorbed."

The natural fiber and phytates in the cereal also inhibit the absorption of zinc, as does the calcium in milk. Richard Wood, head of Tufts mineral laboratory, says, "If you supplement a breakfast cereal with 100 percent of the daily value of zinc and then add milk, not a bit of the zinc will be absorbed by your body." Further, since nutrients are sprayed on cereals, many end up in the milk; when kids throw out the milk, as often happens, there go the nutrients.[12]

Worse, herbal supplement companies have begun aggressively targeting children and their parents with untested, unregulated products of unknown potency, some of them powerful drugs alleged to treat illnesses, improve mood, or help kids gain strength and energy. One survey found almost 20 percent of parents were giving their children supplements.

The surge in herbal supplement use by children is causing rising alarm among pediatricians, children's health advocates and medical officials. In 1998, the American Association of Poison Control Centers reported 704 adverse experiences involving kids age 6 to 18.[13]

Supplements may help to meet special nutritional needs but are usually not needed by people who eat well. Large amounts can be harmful.

Calorie intake stable

While children have been getting heavier, they seem not to have increased their calorie intake. Several studies suggest they may eat less. In 20 years of NHANES studies, 1971 through 1991, children's average calorie intake has declined slightly for most age groups.[14]

It's puzzling that even though the children in the Bogalusa study are heavier than those studied 14 years ago, they eat fewer calories and less fat and cholesterol.[15] This trend is seen in other countries, too. A French study found that in 1995 10-year-olds ate fewer calories, less total fat, and lower percent of fat than in 1978. Yet they had more than double the rates of obesity, at 14 percent, and a more dangerous abdominal fat distribution. What's going on here? Researchers say this puts the origins of obesity into question: overeating and fat intake may not be the culprits in weight gain, after all.[16]

Recommended intake is about 2,000 calories for younger children, increasing by age 15 to 2,200 calories for girls and 3,000 for boys.[17] Most eat considerably less than this, especially girls. Therefore, many experts are saying that to reduce obesity, children probably should not cut calories, but instead, increase activity.

Missing out on meat

That children and adolescents are missing out on meat is a serious matter that needs to be addressed by pediatricians, nutritionists and health policy makers.

Somehow it has become common in the media and certain health circles to denigrate the contribution of meat to the American diet, to regard it as unhealthy, and to call for low-meat diets. But it's an "urban rumor," an idea that gets passed around, seems logical and could be true, but is not, says eating expert Ellyn Satter.

It's not supported by mainstream nutrition; there is no credible evidence that eating lean red meat is unhealthy in any way, and volumes of scientific evidence that meat is health-promoting, especially for children and women. But this trendy notion has been around long enough to have a profound impact on the health of children and women in America today.

Many youth, especially girls, are turning to vegetarianism, rejecting most or all animal products. Vegetarianism can be healthy, but when diets are planned by children, especially those on restrictive weight loss diets, often it is not. We need to respect children's decisions on food choices, yet this can be a serious health issue. When they choose to give up meat, there is concern about how they are doing it and to what extremes they might go.

From coast to coast, eating disorder specialists tell me they are seeing many new young vegetarians — small children with eating problems, stunted growth, fragile bones, and stress fractures, who are responding to a frightening message brought by animal rights activists into their schools. Other new vegetarians they see are eating disordered girls who fear meat is fattening.

"This is very dangerous for kids," says William Jarvis, PhD, Loma Linda University, president of the National Council Against Health Fraud. Jarvis says ideologic vegetarian extremism has caused mental and growth retardation in children, is linked to nutritional rickets and scurvy, and in some cases, death. They often suffer the stomach distress common in vegetarians.

After many years of living and teaching in a Seventh-Day Adventist academic community and having been a practicing vegetarian himself, Jarvis questions the motivation of the new young vegetarians. "As a religion, vegetarianism attracts the guilt-ridden. It attracts masochists because it gives guilt a boost. And it seduces the unskeptical by causing guilt and/or by instilling false guilt. Guilt leads to self-denial, even asceticism . . . Vegetarianism is riddled with delusional thinking from which even scientists and medical professionals are not immune."[18]

Today, many impressionable children and teens are being influenced by this kind of delusional thinking. They come under the spell of fringe groups of two types that come into the schools and exert tremendous pressure on youth of all ages, including college students. They are overzealous environmentalists who falsely teach that grazing livestock wastes land, and radical animal rights groups who seek to persuade kids to stop eating animal foods, as well as to abolish pets, zoos, research and farm animals, and silk and leather clothing.

They have been surprisingly successful in manipulating the media in this effort. "The AMA continues to marvel at how effectively a fringe organization of questionable repute continues to hoodwink the media," says the American Medical Association. The AMA denounces the misinformation campaigns, laboratory bombings, maiming of scientists, and threat to the future of biomedical research associated with these groups.[19]

Theirs is a dangerous agenda that calls for investigation by the media, rather than promotion. Patricia Hunt, a registered nurse in Mukilteo, Wash., whose daughter Jennifer became a vegan after an animal rights group came into her school, recently told the *Wall Street Journal* she was "angry with the schools and the propaganda." Hunt says her daughter even refuses to take vitamins prescribed by her doctor because they are made from animal products. "She has a hotline number that she calls before she'll take anything."

Parents from Maine to California complain about animal rights activists and the teachers who invite them into the classroom to push the vegan lifestyle. No longer able to influence their children's healthy eating, these parents are further frustrated by being harangued about family foods, compelled to fix two sets of meals, and lectured about their own eating.

"There is a sense that these kids have been traumatized . . . influenced by the message that the animal rights people are taking into the schools. When children see these gory pictures about mistreated animals, they really don't have the ability to stop and say, 'Wait a minute, is there another side to this story?'" explains Monika Woolsey, MS, RD, a nutrition consultant and eating disorder specialist in Arizona.

Woolsey has noticed a trend in her practice in which youth often give up meat soon after having watched a graphic animal rights movie in school. "These films may be inappropriate for children who are not equipped to handle the trauma they may inflict." She says vegetarianism seems to be a politically correct way to have an eating disorder. "Many of these children have suffered from emotional, physical or sexual abuse or trauma, and it's almost as if they've made a vow not to hurt animals as they have been hurt."[20]

They struggle with self worth, says Woolsey. "They believe their self-esteem comes from what they do, not who they are, and part of what they do is eat. So they are trying to eat perfectly, and they get this black and white sense of what is perfect: 'If I'm a nice person I'll be a vegetarian, and if I'm not a nice person I'll eat meat.' That's how black and white their thinking gets when you talk to them." Woolsey has developed a self-test to help vegetarians understand whether their choice is reasonably considered or eating disordered *(see appendix)*.

In Kentucky, where schools have been targeted by animal rights activists, dietitians launched an educational campaign to inform educators and parents about the threat of misinformation and deception in programs brought into the classroom. Nancy Tullis, RD, chair of the Reliable Nutrition Information section of the Louisville Dietetic Association, says, "Self appointed 'nutritionists' should not be allowed to go into the schools to present an emotional diatribe about society's shortcomings in the areas of nutrition, air, soil, water and animal cruelty, place blame on certain groups, and then irresponsibly teach the new vegan diet pattern, leaving some inadequate brochures behind. The children will go home short on facts and long on anger. We do not believe in setting children up for this emotional confrontation with their families."

Cutting fat

High fat intake combined with overeating contributes to obesity, and is a risk factor for chronic disease; yet, low-fat eating has its own risks.

All things being equal, fat is stored as body fat much more easily than other nutrients. One-fourth is wasted in converting excess carbohydrate to fat and, even in excess, protein is seldom stored as fat. Before discovering this, Americans were eating about 42 percent of total calories in fat — plus 25 percent in sugars. This left only about one-third of calories for more nutritious foods.

Teenage boys still eat particularly high levels of fat, saturated fat, cholesterol and sodium. More than 90 percent of teen boys exceed the Dietary Guidelines in these.[21]

However, much progress has been made in reducing fat intake. During the past decade, Americans reduced fat intake to an average of 34 percent of total calories, bringing them closer to the goal of 30 percent fat and 10 percent saturated fat.

But unfortunately the new awareness has led to a deep fear of fat. At one extreme, fearful kids with "fat phobia" are deficient in needed fat and at the other, kids eat still eat high-fat diets. What happened to moderation?

Some experts believe dropping fat to 30 percent is too low for children. Diets this low in fat are not appropriate for either children or the elderly, argues Alfred Harper, PhD, professor emeritus of biochemistry at the University of Wisconsin. Harper faults the Dietary Guidelines for use in children. "These guidelines represent a sharp change in direction in health policy and dietary guidance, away from dietary advice to ensure that growth and development of children will not be impaired — and toward a program of dietetic medicine to prevent chronic and degenerative diseases," he told attendees at the Southern California Food Industry Conference in Costa Mesa, Calif. Harper said research does not show that limiting fat intake in children will mean they have healthier lives as adults.

Why has the current drop in fat not been accompanied by a decrease in overweight, as expected, but rather by a sharp increase? Harper argues that low-fat foods may make people fatter because they lose their satiety cues. They may not feel as satisfied with today's highly processed, prepackaged foods, as when they ate mostly home-cooked foods in family meals at home.

Harper also argues that blaming fat for the increase in chronic disease is a myth. The increase in chronic disease is the natural consequence of a healthier aging population that has overcome acute infectious diseases with improved medicine. He's probably right. Most Americans no longer die young. They die in old age of heart failure or other diseases they live long enough to get.

Confusing the public

Today there's great confusion over what to eat. People are intensely caught up in an obsession with bad foods versus good foods. They ignore *how* to eat, but seem convinced that *what* they eat can kill or save them.

Key factors in healthy food choices are still moderation, balance and variety. We need to affirm these principles. In Canada, kids and adults are encouraged to enjoy eating well, be active and feel good about themselves, clearly the best way to prevent weight and eating problems. But we in the United States don't always get that message. Often family choices make the difference. But parents, too, often swing from one extreme to another, rejecting the sane moderate course. It's all or nothing.

Can we forgo the drama of this mentality? Can we find peace with food and let this misplaced excitement flow into other interests?

The media urges us on. It adds confusion and barriers to reasonable food choices. Parents are fearful over the many supposed risks they read about daily in newspaper headlines. Children reflect this confusion and fear.

The problem is, in this time of instant communication, we get an overload of insignificant information. Newspapers can't resist bringing us the *health terrorist message of the day*. Scare headlines warn of the risks of white bread, or movie popcorn, or peanuts, Mexican or Chinese food, mad cow disease or alar treated apples. People take in this startling news and, while it is actually insignificant, here today and gone tomorrow, they are left more shaken and fearful.

On a recent flight from Chicago, where I was a guest on the Oprah show, I sat next to a Kentucky businessman who told me he travels often. "I was on a plane when the morning headlines in *USA Today* read, 'Coffee raises cholesterol,'" he said. "No one drank coffee. On another flight the headlines said coffee might prevent suicide, and everyone was calling for coffee. Another time it was orange juice, and everyone drank orange juice. We're crazy, aren't we?"

Right. And headlines sell papers. Yet the media needs to be more responsible in keeping the story in perspective. Also, some sources quoted are barely credible. Others seem to be irresponsible, headline-grabbing scientists, shoring up grant funds. Professionals today are often chagrined by "health terrorist" messages beamed out by scientists who should know better.

Headline seekers and groups with a political agenda have learned to manipulate the media to their own ends. Much of the fear they engender deals with non-risks. If these risks make any difference at all, they might affect a person's life span by days at the most. Studies may be preliminary, or represent one unorthodox view of an obscure controversy. They'd be better left to scientists talking to scientists, rather than headlined on the front page.

The paradox is that our national panic over food and health comes at a time when Americans are healthier and living longer than ever before, and when the U.S. food supply is the best it's ever been, and without doubt, one of the safest and healthiest in the world.

Some of this fearmongering about food may be a deliberate smoke screen laid over other issues, such as smoking, charges Elizabeth Whelan, president of the American Council on Science and Health. She claims the nearly $6 billion spent yearly by the tobacco industry on advertising and promotion, plus the deep roots the tobacco industry has forged throughout corporate America, and the financial support it gives members of Congress "clearly buys silence and diversion" to hide the fact that half of all premature deaths before age 80, a half million each year, are directly and causally related to tobacco. She says nothing could make "this killer advertiser more content than having the word 'carcinogen' used so often it loses all its meaning. Remember: when everything is dangerous, then nothing is. These purveyors of one of the nation's leading causes of death — lung cancer — have enough clout to keep the legislative and publicity spotlights off the cigarette — and on the multitude of nonrisks around us."[22]

So, instead of clear health messages, what we get is scare-mongering, an endless parade of good foods/bad foods, food as medicine that heals or toxic hazard that shortens our lives. It's not true. Instead it's important to restore confidence in the basic principle that health depends on the total diet, not on single foods.

Stress — measures of despair

Healthy living helps kids feel good about themselves. But if suicidal thoughts are an indication of how our youngsters are faring, they're not doing well. Girls especially are in trouble. Every year, one in 13 high-school students attempts suicide. Girls make the attempt more often than boys, but boys succeed more often, perhaps because they are more likely to use firearms.

In the U.S., youngsters are twice as likely to commit suicide as in other developed countries. The rate is 55 in 10 million children, compared with 27 for the rest of the industrialized world. Suicide rates quadrupled among U.S. children under age 15 between 1950 and 1993.[23] Teen suicides have declined somewhat in recent years, but are still staggering — boys have triple the rate of 30 years ago. It is the third leading killer of young persons between the ages of 15 and 24.[24]

Nearly one-fourth of high school students nationwide report they seriously considered suicide during the past year in the 1995 Youth Risk Behavior survey, a slight increase over 1993 *(figure 1)*. The rates are twice as high for girls, and are especially high for Hispanic girls. Of Mexican American girls, 34 percent reported seriously considering suicide, 26 percent had made a suicide plan, 21 percent attempted suicide, and 7 percent made an attempt that required medical attention, all in the past year. For white girls these figures are 32, 22, 10 and 3 percent, and for African American girls, 22, 16, 11 and 4 percent, respectively.

Figure 1

Suicide thoughts and behavior
percent of high school students[1]

	Thought seriously about attempting suicide	Made a suicide plan	Attempted suicide one or more times
Female	30%	21%	12%
Male	18	14	6

Suicide-related thoughts and behavior of U.S. high school students during 12 months preceding the survey, as self-reported.

1995 YOUTH RISK BEHAVIOR SURVEY/ CHILDREN AND TEENS AFRAID TO EAT 2001, 1997

For white high school boys, the suicide behavior rates are: 19 percent seriously considered suicide, 15 percent made a plan, 5 percent attempted suicide, and 2 percent made an attempt that required medical attention. For African American boys, the figures are 17, 13, 7 and 3, and for Mexican American boys, 16, 13, 6 and 3 percent.

Younger girls were more likely to have considered, planned or attempted suicide; freshmen more than seniors. This trend was somewhat reversed for boys.

What's going on with girls that these rates are so high? What part does malnutrition-induced low moods and depression play? What about their struggle with body image and low self-esteem? Does sexual abuse play a role? What's happening to Mexican American girls to cause such despair? We need answers to these questions.

Activity levels need to increase

Young children are the most active and physically fit of all Americans, averaging one to two hours of moderate or vigorous physical activity each day. But they're less active than their parents were as children — and are developing habits that could turn them into inactive, unhealthy, overweight adults. And the less active they are, even at age 3 or 4, the less active they will be later on. Most kids become less active each year.

There's a strong link between the drop in physical activity and the increase in obesity. It's difficult to measure physical activity, or its relationship to obesity, but many experts believe this is the crux of the problem. What is clear, is that both children and adults live less active lives than even two or three decades ago.

Many families have changed their lifestyles in response to violence or fears that they're unsafe in their communities. More parents work longer hours. More conveniences and remote controls save us the effort of getting up to switch channels or open the garage door. There are more TV channels, more computer games, video games, movies, and hours of Internet to surf.

And as the 21st century unfolds, it only promises more, not less, of these kinds of sedentary recreation.

Sedentary living

Watching television, playing video games, listening to music, and surfing the Net have become full time occupations for the typical American child, according to a new study by the Kaiser Family Foundation.

The study shows an average kid age 2 to 18 spends nearly six hours, seven days a week, this way. Most is in isolation — in bedrooms fully media-equipped, with no parental supervision. The study found most kids age 8 and older (65 percent) have television in their rooms, and that most parents (61 percent) have no rules about TV watching. Most of these kids (70 percent) had computers, but spent less time using them (21 minutes compared with 2 hours, 46 minutes watching TV). Thankfully, kids are still reading — 82 percent read for fun each day and spend about 45 minutes on non-homework material.[25]

Another national study of 13,000 seventh through 12th graders found boys watch more television than girls, and African Americans more than whites, with Asians and Hispanics in between. Among boys, weekly time spent watching TV is 14.4 hours for whites, 15 for Asians, 16.6 for Hispanics and 20.8 for blacks. Among girls, average weekly TV time is 11.9 hours for whites, 12.8 for Asians, 14.6 for Hispanics and 20 for blacks. Total inactivity hours for both sexes ranges from 19.3 hours for whites to 29.7 for blacks.[26]

Healthy People 2010 has set the goal of reducing time spent watching TV to only two hours or less per day for 75 percent of children and adolescents (baseline 60 percent).

Goal of 30 minutes activity

Only one-fifth of high school students are *moderately active* for at least 30 minutes on five or more days a week. This drops from 28 percent at grade 9 to 15 percent at grade 12. Two-thirds are *vigorously active* for 20 minutes, three or more days a week. For boys, this figure is 73 percent of whites, 69 percent of Hispanic or Latinos, and 67 percent of African Americans. For girls, the figures are 58 percent of whites, 50 percent of Hispanic or Latinos, and 41 percent of African Americans.[27] Lower income students tend to be less active.

Thus, one-third are not vigorously active at recommended levels. Only a few combine that with moderate activity for a longer period of 30 minutes at least five days a week. Goals are to increase both kinds of activity in the next decade.

Boys are more active than girls, and the gap widens through high school and college, says researcher James Sallis, PhD, of San Diego State University. He found that both boys and girls think they are more active than they really are (so do adults). Girls may be at higher risk of inactivity-related health problems because of their sedentary lifestyles, warns Sallis.

Activity drops with age

Physical activity of all types declines strikingly with age, especially for girls. Many girls already lead very sedentary lives by age 15. Girls experience a steep drop in activity from their freshman to senior year

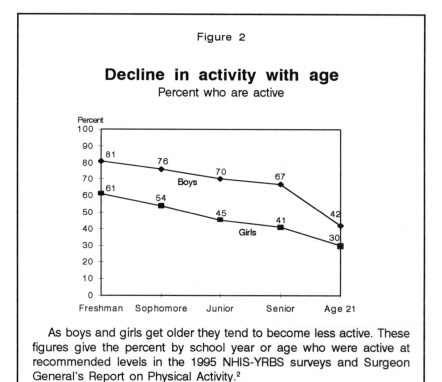

Figure 2

Decline in activity with age
Percent who are active

As boys and girls get older they tend to become less active. These figures give the percent by school year or age who were active at recommended levels in the 1995 NHIS-YRBS surveys and Surgeon General's Report on Physical Activity.[2]

NHIS-YRBS, 1991-1995/CHILDREN AND TEENS AFRAID TO EAT 2001, 1997

— from 61 percent who are active as freshmen to 41 percent as seniors *(figure 2)*. However, this drop was even more severe in 1990, when fewer girls were active; decline then was from 31 percent to 17.[28] Others stay active, but focus only on weight loss, as if burning calories is their sole reason to move.

Boys mark a similar decline from 81 percent active as freshmen to 67 percent as seniors. By age 21, activity drops further; only 42 percent of boys and 30 percent of girls are active.

Lifetime skills in PE class

The reputation of physical education class was never stellar. Despite many recent improvements, research shows that in many classes, students still spend more time standing in line or watching others than being active themselves. One study found that a 40-minute physical education class provided youngsters with an average of less than three minutes of vigorous activity.[29]

"It appears that a major opportunity to influence favorable physical activity is being missed in schools," says one Public Health report. It points out that PE classes seem to have little effect on the students' fitness levels or in increasing their lifelong physical activity.[30] The goal to have kids be active for at least half of PE class time is met by fewer than one-third of students nationwide (defined as more than 20 minutes of actual activity in class three to five days a week).[31]

PE classes are further criticized for what they teach. Games and competitive team sports are the major focus of most programs. The Children and Youth Fitness Study found less than half the PE curriculum is based on *lifetime activities*, which are those that require only one or two people and are readily carried into adulthood, such as biking, swimming, jogging, dancing and racquet sports. Competitive sports and children's group games don't count.[32]

Nonathletic and less fit youngsters are the ones who need PE the most. Yet they are most neglected, especially in classes that feature competition. One in six U.S. children is so weak or uncoordinated as to be considered physically underdeveloped by the President's Council on Physical Fitness and Sports. "That cold statistic barely hints at the personal trauma and social problems behind it. Such a child is likely to become a sedentary, overweight adult with all of the added health risks those conditions entail," says the Council.

Kinds of activity

Half of all students play on at least one school sports team, with girls almost as likely as boys (42 vs 58 percent). But boys are more likely to play on sports teams outside of school — 46 percent compared with 27 percent of girls. About half of high school students work on weights and toning activities at least three days a week. Boys are more likely than girls, white students than African American, and freshman girls more than older girls.

Walking or biking 30 minutes at least five days a week is used as a measure of light to moderate physical activity. This declined from 26 percent of high school kids to 21 percent between 1992 and 1995. African American and Mexican American students, both boys and girls, are more likely than white students to have walked or biked.

Seven additional types of activity were surveyed in the Fitness study: aerobics or dancing; baseball, softball or frisbee; basketball, football or soccer; housecleaning or yard work; running, jogging or swimming; skating, skiing or skateboarding; tennis, racquetball or squash. Boys are more likely to engage in these activities, except that girls are more likely to dance, do aerobics, house cleaning and yard work. All decline as kids get older, except for cleaning and yard work.

Nearly two-thirds of girls said the reason they exercised in the month before the survey was to lose or maintain weight. So did one-third of the boys.

Girls discouraged from sports

Girls are involved in sports more than ever before, yet they have a long way to go. Sallis says we need to reevaluate why girls are less fit than boys. Girls have lower muscle mass as they mature; maybe this is not natural, but occurs because they are so inactive. Sallis urges research of this, and warns that girls need effective programs to prevent this drop.

Girls are still neglected in physical education activities. Often their enthusiasm is dampened by family, friends, the institutions in charge of sports and health, and media neglect. They get far less encouragement to stay involved than boys.

Historically, women's sports were thriving during the 1920s and 1930s, and most high schools fielded girls' basketball teams. But incredibly, these were dropped in the late 1940s, as men returned from war and a changing national mood sent "Rosie the Riveter" back to the kitchen. In the ensuing "feminine mystique" era, sports were said to be too strenuous for girls, potentially harmful. Most states did not reinstate girls' basketball until Title IX required it, in the 1970s.

Yet most girls still drop out of sports in their teens, and studies show their self-esteem drops at the same time. Melpomene, a Minneapolis-based women's sports research group asks why this happens, and how girls can be helped to continue their interest in sports. A recent Melpomene study finds younger girls, age 9 to 12, enjoy sports and describe them as a way they feel good about themselves.

But older girls, age 12 to 17, while agreeing that they enjoy sports, cite major obstacles. Among these are the behavior of boys and systems that favor male athletes.[33] These girls said boys on mixed teems control the games. Typical comments: "Boys like to hog the basketball." "Even if you're right there, they won't pass the ball." "In soccer we have half the girls standing out most of the time because all the boys are playing."

Some said they hesitate to play on mixed teams for fear of male criticism or of making a mistake. This male control is evident in picking teams. The girls said boys are chosen first, and girls last. The girls also describe a system in which boys have more team choices, better equipment, and are taken more seriously by the school and fans.

An illustration that girls are not being taken seriously is the flippant attitude toward stress fractures. It is known that female athletes are at greater risk of stress fractures than males, for three reasons: women athletes are often undernourished, getting inadequate calcium, protein and total calories; they have smaller bones; and they may have weak bones if they diet or exercise excessively, dropping estrogen levels.

The solution? Instead of insisting that women athletes stop dieting and fully nourish themselves, it seems that coaches and trainers are recommending they learn an odd little three-step hop to help protect fragile bones in jumping![34]

Sports coverage

Despite shining examples in the Olympics every two to four years, girls have relatively few athletic role models. Media coverage tends to ignore women's teams and women athletes.

When the media does focus on women in sports, it is often in a confusing way that sends mixed messages to girls. Female athletes may be portrayed in ways that emphasize their femininity, rather than their athletic skill and excellence in their sport. This can cause much ambivalence for girls, uncertain whether their role is primarily athletic or looking attractive on the field.

Amy Terhaar Woodcock, a graduate student in sports management at the University of Minnesota, says reporters watch for female weaknesses and often exploit that in photos and stories. She explains that the media tries to find a way for female athletes to fit into feminine ideals by pointing out that women are too frail for contact sports, citing references which document how the media focuses on "sex specific rather than sport specific conditions or injuries" for women but not men. When a male athlete is injured, the injury is attributed to the sport, but for female athletes, the injuries are blamed on female weakness.

Sports magazines, such as *Sports Illustrated,* avidly read each week by sports-minded girls and women as well as men, typically devote far more space to swimsuit editions, pinup calendars, and cheerleaders and the clothes they wear than to women athletes. One study of *Sports Illustrated* covers from 1957 to 1989 found a decline in the number of times women were featured in active poses over these 22 years. Men graced the cover 782 times and women 55 times, but only two of the women were pictured in active poses.

Another study found photos of female Olympic athletes were often suggestive, emotional, or in poses where the women were away from their sport. Many focused on the female athlete's body in sexually suggestive ways. Emotional shots showed the athlete crying and being comforted by male coaches and family. Most of the photo captions mentioned feminine characteristics, rather than pointing out athletic skill and achievements.

When a female hockey player was chosen athlete of the week, she was pictured sitting on a bench holding her stick and gloves. An article headlined, "Small Stature, Big Talent," ran a photo emphasizing the girl's small size by cutting off her teammates' heads, and referred to her as the "tournament darling." In a more positive portrayal, a rival newspaper focused on her athletic talent, mentioned her size once, and ran a photo of her shooting a puck.

Women's sports are vastly under-represented in television, newspaper and sports magazines. A look at four daily newspapers found that women were the subjects of only 3.5 percent of all sports articles, and men, 81 percent. Men were pictured in 92 percent of all sports.

This unequal coverage is reflected in sports books — even picture books for very young children. A 1993 Melpomene study found girls portrayed only half as often as boys in picture books on sports. Often the girls were shown watching boys play. They are major improvements, however. During the 1950s and 1960s, no girls at all were shown in the same series of books.[35]

When exercise takes over

At the other extreme from sedentary living are young people who exercise obsessively, and develop an activity disorder that takes over their lives.[36] Many girls try to "fix what's wrong" with their bodies through exercise. Boys join them, driven by today's emphasis on muscles and body sculpting.

Activity disorder is closely linked to eating disorders. Eating disorder patients need to be closely monitored for signs of overtraining

A warning sign that exercise is becoming a problem is when goals shift from enjoyment and becoming fit, to body shaping. It is critical that coaches emphasize health-promoting goals, and question weight loss and excessive muscle building.

Female athlete triad

Everywhere girls are taking part in athletics as never before. But there's a dark thread running through women's sports. It's the vulnerability for the female athlete triad and its separate components: eating disorders, amenorrhea and osteoporosis. Any of these can impair health and performance; together they compound the risk.

Amenorrhea is associated with scoliosis and stress fractures in young ballet dancers. Delayed menarche, as late as age 19 or 20 for very thin female athletes and ballet dancers, usually with a restrictive diet, is linked to osteoporosis and bone fractures. (At the same time, a somewhat later puberty, well over today's young average of 12.8 years, appears beneficial in reducing reproductive cancer risk.)[37]

Avoidance of meat, which is common among female athletes, is highly linked to menstrual abnormalities, warns a recent article in *The Physician and Sportsmedicine*.[38] One study cited finds less than 5 percent of nonvegetarian women had menstrual irregularities, compared with over 26 percent of vegetarian women. Another found among women runners that nearly half of menstruating runners ate red meat, but none of the amenorrheic runners did. Another showed that even though their iron and calorie intake were the same, female runners who ate less meat had lower iron levels compared with those who ate more meat. Protein levels were also compromised.

Struggling to be best at a sport while coping with adolescent changes is difficult for young people, and is compounded by social pressures promoting thinness. Trying to control weight while focusing on training and performance can lead to a sense of frustration, guilt, despair and failure, and to undernourishment and eating disorders.

Bodysculpting

Weight training increases strength, endurance and bone density and is a valuable part of high school athletic programs.

Yet working on the weights can become detrimental when boys or girls focus on reshaping their bodies for the sake of appearance. Coaches may also get caught up in muscle building, to the extent their influence can be harmful to youth. Athletic directors, coaches and parents need to be aware that the new emphasis on muscle building and body sculpting is strongly influencing teenage boys and adults through advertising, television shows and muscle magazines.

Joe McVoy, PhD, a Virginia eating disorders specialist, says he is seeing more eating disordered boys caught up in bodybuilding. "This has become more epidemic . . . in our society. There's a great increase in fitness and muscle magazines, fitness spas, and home exercise equipment all with a focus on shape and muscle building."

Bodybuilding contests as featured in muscle magazines are not really about skill or strength. Rather, they are a form of modeling for both men and women, of reshaping the body so it is "right." The emphasis is all on appearance. Often they involve profound alterations to the natural body, extremely restrictive ways to eat so as to deplete fat under the skin, and dehydration so severe that skin is thin as paper. This defines rope-like muscles and makes blood vessels stand out like veined leaves just under the surface. Bodybuilders call this being "ripped" or "sliced."

Some teenagers, along with hours of high-intensity training, turn to illegal steroids and other drugs as a shortcut to building muscles. Anabolic steroid effects may be permanent. For boys, steroids can reduce sperm, shrink testicles, and cause impotence and irreversible breast enlargement. Girls can develop irreversible masculine traits. Dangers include stunted bone growth and potentially permanent damage to heart, liver and kidneys. There are reports that steroids may increase aggressive behavior and violence. Dependency is another risk, according to Jim Wright, PhD, an editor of *Muscle & Fitness*.[39] He cites a study indicating that at least one-fourth of high school users of steroids are dependent on the drugs.

Red flags for athletes

Obsession with a sport may be a "red flag" that an athlete is overtraining in unhealthy ways. Athletes at risk tend to talk and think constantly about their sport, often spending hours upon hours in the gym perfecting their workout at the expense of school activities, friendships and hobbies.

Experts call for mandatory training for coaches to help them become more aware of obsessive exercise and its connection to eating disorders, and learn to watch for warning signs.

Nancy Thies Marshall, chair of the USA Gymnastics's task force on eating disorders, who has herself struggled with disordered eating, offers these "red flags" to watch for:

- **Obsession with the sport.** Devotes self to sport at the expense of family, friends, hobbies and school activities.
- **Preoccupation with food and weight.** Thinking or talking often about food, fat and calories, frequent weighing, skipping meals and binge eating. Motivation for exercise may be a belief that losing weight will improve performance or appeal to a judge's eye.
- **Drinking an overabundance of fluids,** in the effort to feel full.
- **Laxative or diet pill use.**
- **Bathroom visits after meals.** Such visits may suggest a potentially fatal binge-purge cycle of vomiting food after eating.
- **Menstrual dysfunction.** Missing periods or delayed menarche raises concerns of premature osteoporosis and bone fractures.
- **Wearing baggy clothing.** Clothing may be used to hide weight loss.
- **Dramatic weight loss.**
- **Physical deterioration.** Malnutrition may cause chills, apathy, irritability, dry and pale skin, hair loss. Vomiting may cause callused finger, and sores on lips and tongue.
- **Withdrawal from relationships.** Feeling depressed, moody and lonely.
- **Overexercising.** Compulsive exercise beyond regular workouts may be a sign the athlete is trying to compensate for eating.[40]

PART II

HELPING

YOUTH

IN A

WEIGHT-

OBSESSED

WORLD

Health at Any Size
for kids

Guidelines for parents:
- *Be active together with your children. Have fun in a variety of activities.*
- *Promote communication and sharing of feelings.*
- *Teach positive self-talk. Praise and support each other.*
- *Promote self-acceptance, self-respect, respect for others, and appreciation of diversity.*
- *Promote normal eating. Avoid dieting.*
- *Eat family meals together at least once each day, if possible, and with the television off.*
- *Be a role model of normal, healthy eating and lifestyle.*
- *Avoid focusing on weight or shape, or talking about it in a negative way — every body is a good body.*
- *Help children develop interests and skills that lead to success, pleasure and fulfillment, apart from appearance.*
- *Encourage friendships with caring neighbors and other adults.*

CHAPTER 10

Health at Any Size

■

As these problems claim more and more children, it's time for a new approach. It's time to move ahead with vision and direction, to focus on more positive ways of living. The traditional ways of dealing with weight and eating must be replaced by a new paradigm, a new philosophy that helps children and does not harm them. This is an urgent challenge for America and countries around the world today.

Health at Any Size is an approach that deals with the weight and eating crisis in a better way. It frees adults and children from diets by helping them to be healthy at the size they are now. It's a movement that meets people where they are in their health journey.

Today's policies are not working. Our children are afraid to eat. More are eating abnormally. More live with eating disorders. More struggle with overweight. More contemplate suicide. They live in a culture that tells them their bodies are wrong, and promotes destructive values through media, advertising and entertainment. In the obsession with thinness that grips our culture, many young people are making their bodies their life's work.

We can do better than this. We can help them live up to their rich potential as strong, capable, loving, generous individuals.

Health at Any Size affirms that beauty, health and strength come in all sizes, that good health is not defined by body weight, but by a state of physical, mental, and social well-being, by wellness and wholeness. It recognizes that people are healthiest at the weight that results from a healthy lifestyle.

Ellyn Satter, registered dietitian, family therapist, and well-known authority on feeding infants and children, explains that the difference is trusting our bodies. This new way of living accepts that fatness may be normal for some people, unlike what she calls "the current control paradigm" that assumes all obesity is harmful and must be fixed.

"The task for the growing child is not to remain slim, but to maintain energy balance in response to variations in caloric density of the diet, activity level and growth," says Satter.

This new philosophy leaves restrictive thinking behind, and frees us from size constraints. It furthers the idea that large people and thin people are a normal part of the human spectrum, and all deserve respect and consideration. It celebrates diversity as a positive characteristic of the human race. And it declares that everyone can be healthy, regardless of size.

"It means listening to your body," writes dietitian Linda Omichinski, author of *You Count, Calories Don't* and *Teens and Diets: No Weigh.*[1] "It means discovering individual patterns for food and activity levels that keep you energized. It means finding the strength to accept yourself just as you are and get on with life."

What we need to do is consider all the eating and weight problems together as interrelated issues. We need to understand how they affect each other, and we need to be wary of the harm so easily done to vulnerable children and teens. The six problems — dysfunctional eating, undernutrition of teenage girls, hazardous weight loss, eating disorders, size prejudice and overweight — are not separate issues; they're all part of the same problem and they're all influenced by our unnatural drive for thinness. Simplistic solutions won't work.

Understanding this helps us realize we can't rush in to "fix" one problem without affecting others. We can't diet without disturbing normal eating patterns — and once disturbed, eating habits are not easily restored, even after dieting ends.

This new approach asks: How can we gradually shift to healthier habits that will last a lifetime? How can we prevent the onset of eating and weight problems?

Following these three principles will help us make this shift:

1. **Eat well.** Think of food as a friend — celebrate, enjoy, taste, savor. Eating well has two aspects: *what* and *how* we eat. For healthy nourishment choose foods from all five groups — fruits and vegetables, whole grains, meats and meat alternates, and milk, which give a good balance of the many nutrients we need for health, energy, and empowerment of our immune system. Take pleasure in eating a variety of fruits, vegetables, and other foods. Eating moderately, an amount that feels "just right," reminds us to avoid extremes, neither undereating or overeating. It helps us understand that all foods can fit in a healthy diet, so we neither overeat high-fat, high-sugar foods nor fear to eat these foods.

   Normal eating means eating at regular times, usually three meals and one or two snacks to satisfy hunger. It means listening to our bodies, so we eat when hungry and stop when full and satisfied. If we encourage children to do this, trusting their natural tendencies, we can prevent many eating and weight problems. Normal eating enhances our feelings of well-being, promotes clear thinking and mood stability; it furthers normal growth in children and stable weights for adults.

2. **Live actively.** Help children celebrate activity as a natural and joyful part of their lives. This comes naturally to all children. Encourage them with plenty of time for active play, especially outside. Some kids will normally be more active and others less. Parents can help by limiting television to less than two hours a day and breaking up long periods of inactivity. Fitness feels good. Share the benefits by having active fun together as a family — it's the natural way for kids to grow. Be a good role model by keeping active your own way, every day, and reject the goal of weight control as a major reason to be active. Live actively for better health and because it's a great and wonderful way to live.

3. **Feel good about yourself and others.** Celebrate and enjoy every child's special traits and talents. Accept and trust the child, supporting each as a unique individual. Children who

are raised in homes that are accepting, emotionally safe, and filled with unconditional love, will feel good about themselves. Good communication means they will be encouraged to talk about their feelings. Parents set a good example, too, by being accepting and respectful of diversity in others. They can insist on zero tolerance for size bias in school and the workplace, and make it clear that every person of every size deserves acceptance, respect, and a sense of well-being, peace and tranquility.

With this approach, we can shift from thin-at-any-cost to a positive focus on health and well-being. Helping youth to eat well, live actively, and feel good about themselves and others allows them to get on with their lives.

Instead of struggling against a child's natural weight, parents and health professionals need to recognize and work with it. A change in attitude toward acceptance can be liberating. It frees a child (and parents) from "waiting to be thin," and helps that child move on with health-centered changes that make his or her life infinitely better. Children grow at different rates and through numerous growth spurts, so it's important that adults not overreact, but reassure them that their growth is normal, and expect them to "grow into" their natural size.

Goal: healthy children of all sizes

The goal of Health at Any Size is the well-being of children and adults of all sizes, furthering their physical, mental, emotional, social and spiritual health.

The Health at Any Size diagram in the first chapter of this book illustrates this model (*page 25*). For us to raise healthy children of all sizes (in the center), children and teens need to receive consistent messages that encourage them to eat well, live actively, feel good about themselves and others. When these positive messages come from health providers, teachers, family, peers and the media (around the outside of the circle), then weight and eating problems can be diminished or prevented. Negative aspects of the culture are dealt with more easily.

This is an approach that does no harm. It maintains a healthy perspective, while challenging the harmful effects of policies aimed at size alone.

Defining healthy weight

Healthy weight may be defined as the natural weight the body adopts, given a healthy diet and meaningful levels of physical activity.[2] Each of us has a natural weight at this time in our lives that our bodies want to weigh. For some this will be higher, and for others, lower.

Health policy makers have defined healthy weight narrowly in terms of body mass index (weight related to height). But this reliance on the scale can be limiting and deceptive.

Many health experts are calling for a new, broader definition that takes other factors into consideration. Some even question whether health has a weight component. If fitness, not weight, is the key to health and longevity as current research suggests, perhaps setting weight targets has little relevance for most people. After all, the critical risk factors seem to be healthy lipids, glucose levels, blood pressure, and even healthy nutrition and physical activity. Why not measure these instead?

Metabolic fitness does this. Defined as a measure of metabolic or biochemical risk factors for chronic disease, its goals of reducing risk factors are reachable for large people, independent of weight loss.[3] It also recognizes the good health of many very large persons.

Satter also proposes a new definition of obesity as fatness that is abnormal or unnecessary for the individual. Fatness may be just as normal for children at the highest 5 percent as thinness is for the lowest 5 percent, provided they grow in a consistent and predictable way, and any growth adjustments are gradual and occur over time. If fatness is the result of unstable weight with abrupt or acute gains, then it is more likely to be abnormal, she says.

Children who are grounded in their internal regulatory processes are more likely to avoid eating errors and to sustain their natural and appropriate body weight regulation throughout life, Satter points out in her book, *How to Get Your Kid to Eat — But Not Too Much.*[4]

Shifting to Health at Any Size

How can we shift to Health at Any Size? Health Canada offers a model through its Vitality public awareness campaign, which gives this simple, eloquent advice: "Eat well, live actively, and feel good about yourself." To this I like to add "and others."

Vitality is an integrated approach to healthy living that shifts the focus away from rigid dieting and prescriptive exercise goals and toward acceptance of a range of body sizes. It emphasizes healthy eating, active living and positive self and body image. Vitality encourages us to be healthy at the weight we are, to get on with life, and to stop obsessing about weight. It's a message of preventing problems before they happen. It is also the basis for new treatment programs.

The Vitality chart on the next page demonstrates this health-centered approach. Other programs advocate similar attitude and behavioral shifts.

Many health leaders, teachers and parents are enthusiastically using this new approach. They say, "Of course, that's right. I'm fed up with all this dieting, fussing about weight. I'm ready to move on."

For others, the shift comes gradually. They may fear change: "If I don't diet, count calories, keep track of fat grams, I'll gain weight and go completely out of control." Or they may accept it professionally, but for themselves, "first need to lose 10 more pounds." Yet the seeds are planted. They think about it, and slowly the process of change begins. I've watched this happen many times among health professionals in the past seven or eight years. The seeds sprout, take root, unexpectedly burst into life, blossom, and bear the fruit of leadership. So I'm happy to plant seeds.

We can help teenage girls and boys shift out of the diet mentality, develop mutual respect, assertiveness, healthy coping skills and self-trust. We can help them find their unique potential as lovable, capable, valuable individuals, so they take pride in themselves and their bodies at whatever size they are.

Vitality puts it this way: "To overcome the influence of a media-dominated culture that judges women on how they look, we must encourage women to accept a wide range of healthy body weights

The shift to *Vitality* from a weight-centered approach

Weight centered approach	VITALITY
DIETING	**HEALTHY EATING**
• Restrictive eating • Counting calories, prescriptive diets • Weight cycling (yo-yo diets) • Eating disorders	• Take pleasure in eating a variety of foods • Enjoy lower-fat, complex-carbohydrate foods more often • Meet the body's energy and nutrient needs through a lifetime of healthy, enjoyable eating • Take control of how you eat by listening to your hunger cues
EXERCISE	**ACTIVE LIVING**
• No pain, no gain • Prescriptions such as three times a week in your target heart-rate zone • Burn calories • High attrition rates for exercise programs	• Value and practice activities that are moderate and fun • Be active your way, every day • Participate for the joy of feeling your body move • Enjoy physical activities as part of your daily lifestyle
DISSATISFACTION WITH SELF	**POSITIVE SELF/BODY IMAGE**
• Unrealistic goals for body size and shape • Obsession and preoccupation with weight • Fat phobia and discrimination against overweight people • Striving to be a perfect "10" and to maintain an impossible "ideal" (thin or muscular) body size • Accepting the fashion, diet and tobacco industries' emphasis on slimness	• Accept and recognize that healthy bodies come in a range of weights, shapes/sizes • Appreciate your strengths and abilities • Be tolerant of a wide range of body sizes and shapes • Relax and enjoy the unique characteristics you have to offer • Be critical of messages that focus on unrealistic thinness (in women) and muscularity (in men) as symbols of success and happiness

The VITALITY approach calls for a shift from negative to positive thinking about how to achieve and maintain healthy weight.[1]

VITALITY/HEALTHY WEIGHT JOURNAL MAY/JUN 1995/AFRAID TO EAT 1997 and shapes, to love their bodies as they are, to value slimness only as it relates to overall health, to refrain from dieting and to reject societal pressures to conform to an unrealistic body size. In doing so, women will improve their self-images and be more realistic in their assessment of body image."[5]

This is no new radical approach to living. The concept of health at any size is natural, nurturing and wholesome. It recalls a time before this debilitating cult of thinness began — perhaps the 1950s, when war-weary parents were happy to nourish their children and didn't have this huge consumer culture to deal with, and into the early 1960s, when health leaders taught that healthy lifestyle means wellness and wholeness, not thinness for its own sake.

Yet, there is an important difference from that earlier time. Both women and men now have a freedom to be themselves that they have never had before. Girls and women are empowered to be at their personal best in any area they choose, without being judged by how they "should" look, or act, or what "their place" should be. They need no longer be regarded as attractive objects or "playthings" — if they are willing to shake loose from narrow appearance constraints.

It's time for our culture to make this shift.

Research supports the health-centered approach

Research confirms the wisdom of the Health at Any Size approach. Good health is associated with positive attitudes, optimism, good relationships, healthy lifestyle, fitness, not with weight loss or added stress or "ideal" weight. People who expect to be well generally are, and they live longer.

Feeling good about ourselves seems to boost our immune systems. There's much evidence that people with more hopeful, positive attitudes recover more quickly from surgery, have less damage after heart attacks, remain cancer-free longer after treatment from advanced breast and skin cancer, and live longer.[6] Optimists expect good things to happen, and they usually do.

On the other hand, negative thinking can be harmful, and research confirms this. What does this suggest for large children who are perfectly healthy, but are continually being warned that they are at severe health risk and will probably die young because of their weight? Will they believe it, live in fear, and possibly make it a self-fulfilling prophecy?

There is no justification for inducing weight fears among children, whether they come from health professionals, teachers, parents, peers or the media. It's false, barbaric, and needs to end.

The research linking overweight and death is controversial and incomplete, and it ignores the fact that there are health advantages as well as disadvantages to being heavy.[7] In fact, research suggests that fitness and activity, not weight, may be the key to good health and longevity.

Steven Blair and his colleagues at the Cooper Institute for Aerobics Research in Dallas studied 25,389 men for more than eight years each and found disease and death rates were related to health behaviors, not fatness. The fit obese men lived just as long as the fit lean men. At every weight, fit men outlived those with lower levels of fitness. Other studies suggest the same for women.[8]

Weight loss may be a deceptive goal. It has been unsuccessful long-term and sometimes dangerous. Treatment, with failure rates of 95 to 97 percent, often ratchets a person's weight up higher than it was before. Even when successful, weight loss treatments have not been shown to improve long-term health. Rather, they may cause the opposite.

There is much evidence that keeping a stable weight through adult life is healthy at any size, that health risk is greatest among weight cyclers (yo-yo dieters), and that large children and adults can be very healthy. Therefore, health professionals are advised to use a wellness approach focused on healthy lifestyle, and skip the weight loss attempts.

People naturally come in a range of sizes. Some are tall, others short, and most are somewhere between. On a graph, this height range makes a nice bell curve. Similarly, some people are naturally thin, some naturally heavy, and most in between. And that's okay. It's not true that thin people are necessarily healthier, even though some of our health leaders seem to think so.

The opposing debate

So, why not Health at Any Size? Opponents say that if people lose their fear of fat and accept size diversity, there'll be tremendous increases in overweight. Others argue that the public needs to keep believing in current obesity treatment because someday there will be drugs that work and people must be kept in a mood to take them. Third, there's fear the weight loss industry may be damaged by a more open approach. Fourth, some obesity specialists say privately that eating disorders can be discounted because they affect so few individuals; therefore, current policy does little damage.

These are weak arguments based on fallacies, not research or reality. The fear of fat has not prevented obesity; instead, it has likely escalated weight gain by promoting dysfunctional eating and weight cycling. Second, the public will recognize and respond to honesty in an area where it has so often been deceived. Health at Any Size does not oppose reliable obesity treatment. Rather, when some future treatment is proven safe and effective, it will fit well into this sound, healthy approach, and size-accepting people will certainly use it when appropriate. Third, yes, there may indeed be loss of profits for diet companies, but those willing to develop worthwhile lifestyle programs can benefit. Fourth, it is past time for obesity specialists to recognize that eating disorders carry a higher incidence and mortality risk than many diseases that get far more attention. Certainly they cause many more deaths among children and teens than obesity.

Moving ahead

We are in the midst of a new movement that will not be stopped. The response is everywhere positive to the nondiet Health at Any Size approach. Diets that don't work, pressures to be thin, and the crisis in disturbed eating — are all reasons why women and men are responding with enthusiasm.

Programs based on this new way of life offer a fresh approach that is flexible, open, accepting, individualized and family-centered. These programs recognize and appreciate local culture and values. Parents are assured they can trust their family traditions, that traditional foods and ways of celebrating with food are valuable to pass down through the generations, shaped and expressed in different ways as they may be. They gain confidence that they and their children can make good decisions.

Leaders in the new programs recognize that parents are confused and shaken by today's conflicting health messages and need to learn to trust themselves again. Their message is: Trust yourself. Trust and empower the child. Support the child in solving his or her own problems, even when that child marches to a different drummer.

These leaders are committed to helping people understand that the body cannot be shaped at will, and that individual differences in body shapes and sizes are natural and desirable, that the weight evolving naturally from healthy lifestyle needs to be accepted as normal.

And yes, the new leaders are willing to accept what has long been unacceptable: that obese youngsters may not lose weight permanently or grow up to be thin. The new guidelines and programs recognize this and deal with it in an honest and straightforward manner.

Changing national policy

By taking the health at any size approach, we put all the issues on the table, recognizing that today's problems are not simple. They include obesity and its risks, the failure of weight loss treatment, pressures to be thin, the high rates of dysfunctional eating, undernutrition and malnutrition, dangerous weight loss methods, eating disorders, the stigmatizing of larger kids, and issues which impact body image for young girls, and increasingly, for young boys. All these factors are in the mix when we consider the complex areas of weight and eating and what they mean in our culture.

Health professionals, educators and parents who are willing to look carefully at all the problems, overcoming the distortion of vested interests, will find positive ways of working together to build strengths in all these areas.

Taking a broader view and recognizing reality is especially important for those who set national health policy. They need to drop the fiction that diet pills and weight loss treatment are working. They need to realize that terrifying people about obesity will not prevent it.

Above all, they need to add eating disorders and the undernourishment of teenage girls to the agenda in Healthy People 2010 and other health initiatives. Only then, when all the issues are on the table, can a comprehensive policy be developed that makes sense and be one that health professionals will support.

Once eating disorders are a recognized concern, I fully expect a major improvement in national health policy. And since this sets the agenda for what happens throughout the country, it will greatly influence how the media reports these issues.

This happened in Canada, where a shift in policy brought a remarkable shift in schools, community and health care.

The origins of Health at Any Size

The health centered approach, Health at Any Size, first found its voice as the nondiet movement. It was led by pioneer nutrition specialists who discovered the harm and futility of putting people on diets, joined by eating disorder specialists who saw dieting's most deadly effects every day, and size activists who have tried everything and know they are worse off for nearly every weight loss attempt.

Nondiet soon became so popular it was co-opted, claimed for the most audacious diet scams: "Diets don't work! This is not a diet!" boast ads for restrictive diets and potentially dangerous pills.

The nondiet movement recently has been rechristened *Health at Any Size*. Credit the Internet. We needed a stronger term for this new paradigm. *Nondiet* was basically negative; it said what it's not, but gave no hint of the many benefits of diet-free living.

Pat Lyons, author of *Great Shape*, has long been talking about the need for doctors to focus on health at any size. Recently the term was picked up by Linda Omichinski, author of the nondiet HUGS program, tossed around and examined by others. At *Healthy Weight Journal* we invited online contacts to consider using it or suggest others. That query generated 55 pages of creative, passionate and thoughtful comments from over 70 people. Not everyone agreed, but there seemed enough consensus to rename the nondiet paradigm "Health at Any Size," with H@AS as a handy acronym. Variations include "healthy," "every" and "for all sizes."

People said Health at Any Size is catchy, easy to remember, simple and tested. It uses conversational English, and stands on its own without explanation. It focuses on an important goal, moving people away from diets and external control. It is compatible with other national and international nutrition messages. And the message to health professionals is clear: Do what you can to help people be healthy, and leave their size alone.[9]

Networking and learning

The Health at Any Size paradigm or philosophy is research based and practical. It unites the work of visionary leaders from many fields.

It has been my privilege to network with many of these leaders through 16 years of writing, editing and publishing *Healthy Weight Journal*. I've been inspired by their vision and insights, and gratified when they are inspired by mine.

There's much to learn from scientists and specialists in the related fields. I feel fortunate that my membership in an eclectic clutch of professional organizations — in the fields of obesity, eating disorders, nutrition, health, size acceptance and health fraud — have enabled me to understand the differing viewpoints. I attend their conferences, listen, present, study research, read journals and newsletters, and talk — by telephone, e-mail and face-to-face — with researchers, specialists, educators, and ordinary people with problems. All have poignant and powerful information to share.

Amazing leadership has come from Canada. Educators and health professionals there have achieved what we in the United States have not yet been able to do: They've changed national policy. Health Canada now encourages a national way of thinking that focuses on health instead of weight, exemplified by the Vitality program. Leaders in the Canadian movement discovered me, back in the mid-1980s, as readers of *Healthy Weight Journal,* and started sending their innovative ideas my way. It's been an awakening experience.

Leaders in the size acceptance movement, who years ago began including me in their communications, have also greatly expanded my awareness. It's been a delight and surprise to have become a

rallying point for size acceptance groups from around the world —
England, Belgium, New Zealand — after we began a regular feature
that showcases their viewpoint in *Healthy Weight Journal*. Their
increasingly articulate views have been important in shaping national
debate.

Women are in the forefront of the Health at Any Size movement,
as they should be. Women know the issues. They are well aware how
disproportionately young girls suffer from eating disorders, dysfunctional eating, undernutrition, and the stigma of overweight. They have
struggled with their own weight and body issues. They are concerned
that boys not suffer as have girls and women. These visionary women,
naturally, are joined by supportive and visionary men who are also
committed to changing the harmful effects of our culture, to speaking
out, challenging, tirelessly presenting the facts, and to reshaping our
national health policy so it is truly health-centered.

A better vision

Working together and supported by a health policy that deals
with weight and eating issues in a sound, comprehensive way, we
can bring about the healthy change needed for our children and our
future.

As we search for answers, it is important to keep a balanced
perspective. We need to remember that weight, eating and health are
only part of what makes life worthwhile. Wellness and wholeness are
not about attaining perfect health or even longevity, necessarily, but
improving our quality of life, so we live well emotionally, intellectually, physically, socially and spiritually.

In the family, caring parents or significant others who understand
the issues set the stage with unconditional love and acceptance, no
matter what, from infancy on. They give reassurance that every child
is okay, just as he or she is, and they model and teach normal eating,
active living and a positive outlook on life.

Schools provide the intellectually stimulating environment needed
for learning when they are safe and accepting — safe from emotional
violence, harassment and bullying, safe from physical violence. And
students, in turn, gain most from the academic process when they are

well nourished, with minds ready to learn, not focused on food, hunger or appearance.

Ways to integrate school and community health programs are being rediscovered. For example, communities across the country are finding new energy by working through a Minneapolis-based program called "Healthy Communities, Healthy Youth," with goals to create an environment in which all young people are valued, problems become manageable, and an attitude of vision, hope and celebration pervades community life.[10]

Programs like this motivate communities to nurture a child-friendly culture through existing organizations and institutions. They emphasize a positive approach, so that instead of looking at problems in a negative way, people shift toward effective preventive action.

As we embrace this new approach, changes will come in five major areas: attitude, lifestyle, prevention, health care and knowledge. Shifting toward a health centered approach in these areas as they relate to eating and weight will further the goal of raising healthy children of all sizes. It will free our children from narrow appearance constraints, and help them live happy, productive, fulfilling lives.

CHAPTER 11

In the family

■

The family is a critical, positive force in defusing this public health crisis. The family is a place for nurturing, sharing feelings, giving reassurance, hugs, a pat on the back, and unconditional love.

Families today take many different structures. Blended or single-parent families are as common as the traditional two-parent household. What's important is that families with healthy attitudes and behavior are at the heart of promoting healthy growth and development for their children.

Parents and other adults can help fearful children restore normal eating, and the sooner, the better. The longer children struggle with eating and weight issues, the more likely it is that they develop severe lifelong problems. If you suspect a child has an eating disorder, it's important to have the problem evaluated by a competent therapist and if needed, get the child into therapy without delay.

Yet it is also important not to overreact. It is all too easy to add to the anxiety, fear and pressure these kids are already feeling. Mothers, fathers or significant others in children's lives who are obsessed or worried over their own weight, continually dieting, restricting fat or calories, and often talking about these concerns, can set children up for eating problems at very young ages. A parent's overconcern about a child's weight further adds to the tension, fear and confusion a child may be feeling. Instead, parents and caring adults can help ease tensions by bringing a flexible, low-key approach to food and weight and focus on supporting the child with love and acceptance.

It's important for the home to be a safe and comfortable place where children are loved and accepted unconditionally. But often parents don't know how to deal with a child who is struggling with dysfunctional eating, an eating disorder, with overweight or size prejudice.

Many children are crying out for help from their families. I receive heartbreaking letters from teenagers who are struggling to cope with weight and eating pressures in their lives. Some write about communicating: *I can't talk to my parents; they're too busy; they won't listen; they don't understand; they want to run my life; they say it's nothing, to forget it.*

What can I tell them? I'm a parent and I've made mistakes. I'm not a therapist. But I tell them "You are lovable, beautiful and capable just as you are. Accept yourself, believe in yourself, find ways to help release the tension that you say is taking over your life and threatening to tear apart your family. And please stop those thoughts of suicide. You said you didn't want to hurt your parents; that's the way to hurt them in the worst way possible."

I tell them to find someone who will listen — your parents, school counselor, pastor or friend. Talking about how you feel will help. It's sad that you, and kids like you, are being made to feel you have to look a certain way to be loved and accepted. Maybe our nation will soon stop this outrageous focus on appearance, and rediscover the richness of diversity. You are okay just as you are. Tall, short, large or small. This is the way we are, all of us, the human race in all its wonderful diversity.

Family communication

It's important that families talk to each other — the small talk about everyday things, the praise and reassurances. Good things to tell kids over and over are: I'm proud of you! You're great! Thanks for helping. I trust you. It's so nice to see you smile! Good work! You did a nice job! You brighten my day! I love you.

Talking about feelings is important, too. Some parents don't know how to express their own feelings or are ashamed of them, or afraid

How to keep communication open

When asked about their problems with parents, teenagers most often cite "not being listened to." Some suggestions for parents:[1]

- **Give your undivided attention** when your teenager wants to talk to you.

- **Listen calmly,** even though you may disagree. Try to understand your teenager's point of view.

- **Use a courteous tone of voice.** A pleasant tone can pay great dividends in improved relationships.

- **Keep the door open** on any subject.

- **Avoid making judgments.** It is not necessary to approve of all your teenager's behavior, but it is important to understand feelings.

- **Allow expression of ideas and feelings.** Listen first and acknowledge your teenager's opinions, even if you are alarmed. Then give your viewpoint, plainly and honestly, recognizing love and mutual respect.

- **Say nice things.** Everyone needs acceptance and appreciation.

- **Encourage positive self-worth.** Help your youngster build confidence by encouraging, but not forcing, participation in sports, music, art, dance or other interests.

- **Be aware of how you treat other children** in the family. Try to be fair and consistent. Showing favoritism can make a child feel rejected, unloved, jealous.

- **Hold family conferences.** Give children the opportunity to participate and work things out together.

NATIONAL INSTITUTE OF MENTAL HEALTH, USDHHS/CHILDREN AND TEENS AFRAID TO EAT 2001 they won't know the right answers. So they discourage their children from talking about feelings. Or they brush them off: "You shouldn't feel that way." Talking about feelings is not always easy, but it helps if moms and dads will ask, "How do you feel about that?" and then listen, without offering advice. In fact, trying to solve problems that should be owned by the child can be controlling and destructive behavior for parents.

Instead, helpful parents will listen quietly when kids want to talk, giving their undivided attention. Acknowledge their feelings in a noncommittal way, "Oh . . . Hmmm . . . I see . . ." Give the feeling a name, "That sounds frustrating." Encourage and trust the child to explore solutions, without taking over.

Use a pleasant tone of voice, and avoid making judgments without hearing it all out. It's a challenge for parents to be clear about important values, yet flexible at the same time. Keep the door open for later discussion of tough subjects.

Communication builds relationships. It lets moms and dads know what their kids are doing and thinking. It helps kids understand their parents. It lays a foundation for positive family life. And it helps kids deal with scary things going on in their lives — transitions to the next school level, separation, divorce, disappointments or grief.

The foundation for free and open expression is laid in childhood. As they get older, kids still want to talk to parents about their problems and freely express their feelings, but don't want them taken over and "solved," or belittled. This is especially important for teenagers, who soon stop sharing if this happens, or if confidences are betrayed.

We don't always know what else is going on in kids' lives: worries about money, not being accepted at school, having trouble with a teacher, not being good at sports, math or reading.

Sometimes a problem seems small to the parent — a favorite shirt torn, a friend's snub, missing out on an event. Enabling them talk it out can help children keep the problem small and let it go. It can help them diffuse anxiety or anger and deal with it in constructive ways. Or it may uncover other, larger factors that need attention.

Sometimes the problem looms so large for the entire family that it seems too terrible to talk about: alcoholism, a financial crisis, marital discord, an unfortunate incident, physical, sexual or mental abuse. It's the "elephant in the living room" that everyone is terribly aware of and steps around, but doesn't talk about. Pretending everything is perfect and conveying the idea that, above all, the family must look perfect in the eyes of neighbors, sets an impossible standard that can cause enormous stress and set children up for emotional problems.

This stress may be expressed in eating disturbances and disorders. Talking about it and expressing feelings diffuses the stress and helps children cope in healthy ways.

Boys need this communication as much as girls, although sometimes it's harder for them to share their feelings. Our cultural code for males makes it difficult for them to share their fears, and this can intensify their distress.

Parents who are too busy to listen and disengaged parents who don't try may want to do some soul-searching about what is really important in their lives. Finding the time and energy to listen at the time it is most needed may be difficult, but it is extremely important in children's lives. On the other hand, some parents are too controlling, too involved. If they will back off, they can empower their children by trusting them to make their own decisions.

It's all part of parenting, of giving our children roots and wings.

Caring neighbors

One of the greatest resources for young people is having ongoing relationships with caring, principled people outside the home, with adults who offer guidance and encouragement, who care about and trust them. They can gain much strength from support across the generations, by hearing consistent messages about boundaries and values from neighbors, relatives, older and younger adults from school, church and community, adults who call them by name and are their friends.

Many children and teens are missing this support network today. In one Minneapolis study, only 29 percent of youth reported having caring neighbors.

Many adults have pulled back from offering their support to neighborhood kids because they feel overwhelmed by frightening youth problems that dominate the headlines. Often neighbors don't get involved in the lives of children on their block, and may not even know their names. Instead of offering support, they defer problems to professionals.

The Search Institute in Minneapolis turns this around by urging people to take action on their own. Through the "Healthy Communities, Healthy Youth" program, adults are encouraged to do simple things: look at and speak to every child or teen you see; talk to youngsters about their interests; send a birthday or congratulatory card; invite a young person to go along to a ballgame; have an open-door policy so neighbor kids feel welcome to come in for conversation, refreshments, or just hang out.[1]

Building assets for children

Search focuses on 40 assets, or building blocks, to help promote the healthy development of children. Surveys by the Search Institute have shown that the more of these assets young people have, the more they engage in positive behaviors, such as volunteering and succeeding in school. The fewer assets they have, the more likely they engage in risk-taking behaviors, such as violence, sexual activity, alcohol and drug use. Each asset is important, and together the benefits are additive.

Communities should strive to increase the number of each child's assets, the Search Institute teaches. Following are examples of these assets:

- Support from three or more non-parent adults
- Caring neighbors
- Active, involved parents
- An attachment to school
- Desire to help other people
- Commitment to serve in your community
- Training in music and the arts
- Religious participation
- Skills to resolve conflict nonviolently
- Optimism about your personal future

Restore normal lifestyles

An emphasis on sound, healthy lifestyles is the best known prevention for weight and eating problems of all kinds. As in the Canadian Vitality healthy weight programs, a healthy family focus will be on eating well, living actively and feeling good.

"Vitality is a shift in thinking about what healthy living really is. It's a lifestyle for everyone. It's throwing a Frisbee with the kids, having friends over for a potluck dinner, curling up enjoying a good book. It's about healthy eating and active living. It's gardening and cycling, laughing and relaxing. It's good for you — body and soul."[2]

Mothers, fathers and children who feel good about themselves and each other make healthy choices easy — not just for a short period of time but for a lifetime.

Restoring normal eating is a priority for those who have restricted their eating, or who habitually overeat. Unfortunately, today many parents are so confused and fearful of their own eating, weight and health, that their fears are multiplied in their children. They need to stop dieting, stop talking about hips and stomachs and thighs, and realize that their own attitudes and behaviors may contribute to their children's eating and weight problems. Giving oneself a year to normalize eating will make a great difference.

Normal eating

Eating well has two aspects — how and what one eats. How children eat is often being ignored today, yet eating behaviors are often at the root of many of their problems.

Normal eating means usually eating at regular times, typically three meals and one or two snacks to satisfy hunger. It is regulated by internal signals of hunger, appetite and satiety — we eat when hungry and stop when satisfied. If kids will do this they may avoid many of the eating and weight problems that plague our society today.

Normal eating enhances feelings of well-being. It nurtures good health, vibrant energy, and the healthy growth and development of children. Normal eating furthers clear thinking, the ability to concentrate, mood stability and healthy relationships with family, friends and community. Normal eating promotes natural weight and stable weights as young people mature.

In normal eating, kids take pleasure in taking meals with family and friends, sometimes eating for fun and social reasons. After eating, they feel good. Thoughts of food, hunger, weight and body image are relegated to the "back burner," and take up only a small part of the day. Normal eating is natural and simple. It is trusting yourself.

"Normal eating is three meals a day, most of the time, but it can also be choosing to munch along. Normal eating is flexible . . . giving yourself permission to eat sometimes because you are happy, sad or bored, or just because it feels good. . . . Normal eating is trusting your body to make up for your mistakes in eating," writes Ellyn Satter in *How to Get Your Kid to Eat . . . But Not Too Much.*[3] In normal eating, people go to the table hungry, and eat until they are satisfied.

When children and teens eat normally, at mealtimes, they are more likely to make good food choices, enjoying balance, variety and moderation. Normal eating means choosing foods they like, foods that satisfy and taste good, and eating that food in moderate, relaxed ways. It means they can eat their favorite foods now — or later. In normalized eating, there are no good foods or bad foods. All foods can fit. Eating is a natural part of our lives; however, it is only one small part, and should not dominate.

Normal eating is not about rules, but developing reasonable habits that allow us to put eating in a comfortable groove and get on with life. It will differ for different individuals — we each need to find what works, trusting ourselves, and make it a habit. When families eat normally, children are less likely to gain excessive weight. They grow normally, and their weight tends to stabilize at appropriate levels.

Both restricting food and habitually eating past the point of satiety can cause excess weight gain. Sometimes moms and dads need to remind themselves and their children that we feel better if we stop eating when satisfied. Yet, we can trust our bodies to balance out an episode of overeating, such as a big holiday meal, over a few days.

Parents can help de-emphasize food in the home by keeping

snacks and food reminders out of sight, by not talking excessively about food or recipes, and by avoiding food symbolism — not using food as an important way of expressing love, or to reward, punish, or comfort (a kiss is better than a cookie for a hurt finger).

Kids who eat normally will not all be thin. They will be in a range of sizes, as their natural weight is expressed through a variety of inherited and environmental factors. All this is part of normal living.

Normal eating

What is normal eating?
- Normal eating is usually eating at regular times, typically three meals and one or two snacks to satisfy hunger. It is regulated mostly by internal signals of hunger, appetite, satiety — we eat when hungry and stop when satisfied.

How does it promote health and well-being?
- Normal eating enhances feelings of well-being. We eat for health and energy, also for pleasure and social reasons, and afterward, we feel good.
- Normal eating promotes clear thinking and mood stability. It fosters healthy relationships in family, work, school, and community. Thoughts of food, hunger, and weight take up only a small part of the day.
- Normal eating nurtures good health, vibrant energy, and the healthy growth and development of children. It promotes stable weights, within a wide range, expressing both genetic and environmental factors.
- Normal eating — eating meals — means that food choices will likely provide variety, moderation and balance.

How can parents encourage normal eating?
- Offer a variety of nutritious food at regular, planned intervals.
- Help the child identify hunger and fullness.
- Set a good example of normal, healthy eating and lifestyle.
- Let your child decide how much and whether to eat.

CHILDREN AND TEENS AFRAID TO EAT 2001

Eating well means combining all this with active living, which ensures that appetite mechanisms and other body functions are activated into a natural body rhythm.

Let's look at how to eat in normal, healthy ways.

Positive feeding

Learning how to eat well — for those who have restricted their eating or who habitually overeat — begins by stopping all diets, stopping skipping meals, stopping mindless, chaotic eating, and restoring normal eating as a priority.

Once it came naturally. As babies, when our stomachs were hungry, we cried. We ate. It felt good, and when full, we stopped eating. Simple as that. Unfortunately, in our society many kids and adults override this natural regulation system. They learn to ignore their internal signals when told by overanxious or controlling parents that they must eat more — or less — than their bodies really want.

Satter says it is essential for parents to maintain a positive feeding relationship through the growing up years that will allow kids to feel relaxed and comfortable about eating and in touch with their internal cues of hunger, appetite and satiety. Underfeeding interferes with this, as surely as does urging a child to eat more than he wants.

Feeding disruption often begins with the bottle. It's easy to get in the habit of expecting baby to drink those 4 ounces of formula, or 6 or 8 each time. It's easy to coax and urge, or stop too soon. Thus, the parent wielding a bottle needs to be especially attentive to the baby's response. One reason breast-feeding is preferable, is that mom is likely to accept that her baby wants to self-regulate, and can naturally do this well.

Satter teaches a *Golden Rule for Parenting with Food.* "Parents are responsible for what is presented to eat and the manner in which it is presented. Children are responsible for how much and even whether they eat." This means parents are responsible for the purchase of food, preparing and serving meals, and getting everyone to the table. Then they need to stop, and trust that the child will eat what is needed. It is the child's responsibility to decide which foods and how much to eat, and even whether or not to eat.

Satter explains that parents should not interfere with the natural eating and regulation process by urging, bribing, scolding or praising for eating. Let children eat as much or as little as they want. Allowing them to make their own decisions lets them respond appropriately to their internal cues of hunger and satiety.

Unfortunately, this natural division of responsibility is often violated by parents with rigid or restricting eating styles of their own, who try to take over their children's eating, who urge them to eat more, to clean their plates — or to stop eating before they are satisfied. This sets the stage for disruptive and disturbed eating patterns.

Satter says it is sometimes hard to convince parents that "Even

Developing positive eating habits

Instead of . . .	Try this
Using food as reward or bribe	Give hugs instead of food
Letting child drink from a bottle	Have your child use a cup
Letting your child eat whenever he/she wants	Set regular meal and snack times
Letting your child eat whatever he/she wants	Offer a choice of healthful foods
Quieting your child with food	Comfort your child with attention and affection
Setting stricter limits for larger child than rest of the family	Use the same limits and foods for all members of family
Letting your child help himself/herself to food	Store food out of sight and out of reach
Letting your child watch TV or play with toys during mealtime	Take away distractions during mealtime

Wisconsin Department of Health and Social Services, adapted from Child of Mine, *by Ellyn Satter, and* Your Growing Child, *by the California Department of Health Services.*[2]

CHILDREN AND TEENS AFRAID TO EAT 2001, 1997

the fat child is entitled to regulate the amount of food he eats."

Mothers and fathers have three responsibilities in feeding children, advise Iowa State University Extension specialists, Carol Hans, RD, and Diane Nelson.[4]

1. Offer the child a variety of nutritious foods at regular intervals. Planned meals and snacks give the child regular sources of energy, help the child develop sensible eating patterns, and encourage positive food behavior in social situations.

2. Help the child identify and pay attention to feelings of hunger and fullness. This starts by learning to distinguish a baby's hungry cry from other cries. It means not urging a toddler to eat more. It means allowing second or third helpings.

3. Model a healthy lifestyle. Children learn by example and are likely to do what parents do, whether it is eating chips while watching television or bicycling after supper.

Eating meals together

Family meals eaten at home help to structure children's eating in healthy ways. In eating together, families gain a better sense of unity. Family traditions, values and humor are shared in a pleasant, relaxed setting. All this, yes, with the television turned off (please!) so family members can talk about the good things, and not so good, that happen and how everyone feels about them.

"Family meals establish traditions and create pleasant memories as members discuss events of the day. Teens benefit greatly from this time together," says Kathy Walsh, Family Consumer Science teacher in Harvey, N.D., and mother of three. "Meals promote communication skills, cooperation, cooking skills and table manners. (And) children who eat meals with their parents and siblings tend to eat a more varied and nutritious diet. Let the kids help prepare the meal and they are more likely to eat it. If this is a new idea to your family, give it a try . . . it could surprise you and provide some great memories."[5]

For families on the run, Walsh suggests being creative and flexible. "Bring the family together for a late dessert or eat breakfast together. Make weekend meals the family focus."

Satter, also, is adamant about having family meals. "Meals are as essential for nurturing as they are for nutrition . . . Without meals, a home is just a place to stay," she insists in her 1999 book, *Secrets of Feeding a Healthy Family.*[6]

Eating breakfast gives children a healthy start to their day. Young people who eat breakfast perform better in school through increased problem-solving ability, memory, verbal fluency and creativity and are less likely to be absent, says the American Dietetic Association in a review of the scientific literature.[7]

The dieting child

What can parents do when a teenager is determined to lose weight in unhealthy ways?

As a parent of wrestlers, I understand this all too well. Our two sons were champion wrestlers in the lower weights and they believed that to be champions they had to lose a lot of weight. High school wrestling is a great sport and I enjoy it. But losing too much weight is a major problem that needs fixing in many schools.

With our older son Rick, I did everything wrong. His single-minded purpose was so devastating, his level of nutrition so low, and his eating so chaotic, that I felt helpless. I was a nutrition teacher, but didn't know what to do. At the gym after a match Rick stuffed himself with hot dogs and candy bars, and next day ate big meals, cookies and snacks. Then back to almost nothing, even restricting water the day or two before a match.

The rest of our family ate as usual. We'd try to coax him to meals, but mostly we tiptoed around and tried not to notice his irritability. Now, I understand that being irritable and moody is a classic, textbook reaction to hunger and malnutrition.

One day, I had just taken brownies out of the oven when Rick came home from a hard workout. The house was full of good baking smells. He walked into the kitchen with an expression of anger, frustration and despair in his face. "You baked brownies! How can you do this to me?" That really hurt. I was trying to be a good mother and keep goodies in the house for the rest of the family. But he was right. Instead of helping him, I was tempting him with just the kind of high-calorie food he didn't need.

With our younger son Mike it was easier. I fixed the same small nutrient-dense meals for all of us, no frills, with limited fat and sugars. He still ate almost nothing those two days before matches, but otherwise ate quite well.

One of the tough things about high school wrestling season is that it comes during both Thanksgiving and Christmas holidays. One mother whose three sons were also wrestlers told me their family hadn't had a Christmas dinner in 10 years where one of the boys hadn't rushed from the table in tears, run upstairs and slammed his bedroom door.

At our house, we tried to solve the problem this way. We normally celebrate holidays with the traditional bountiful table, but when Mike was wrestling, I'd fill everyone's plate in the kitchen, spreading out the food so it looked like more, adding big no-calorie gelatin salads. They weren't great meals and I knew Mike's thoughts were on the turkey in the kitchen, but we tried to make them fun.

Yet the night Mike won the state championship at 105 pounds, as a junior, he probably needed another 15 or 20 pounds just for endurance — and his opponent was in much the same shape. It still hurts to see that photo of Mike with his championship trophy, gaunt-faced, with sunken eyes and cheeks.

Sometimes all parents can do with a dieting teenager is to ease the stress as best they can. They can encourage full nutrition, but decisions on how much and what to eating belong to the child, and this cannot be infringed.

Reassurance on size

It's natural for parents to want their children to be as perfect as possible, but when it comes to weight, "perfect" must be broadly and individually defined, advise Carol Hans and Diane Nelson. In their brochure, *A Parent's Guide to Children's Weight*, they remind parents that children grow at different rates and may have very different body structures from their own brothers and sisters. They advise parents that a child who is too thin needs the same emotional support as one who is too heavy.

"Parents can help the child learn to see food as only one of many possible ways to celebrate a happy event, to ease disappointment, or to erase boredom." And parents can refrain from comments about their children's size or shape, except in a reassuring way.

Moms and dads need to examine closely their dreams and goals for their children. Are they emphasizing beauty and body shape, especially for daughters? A visit to a compassionate pediatrician can help put size in perspective and provide the basis for reminding a child that individuals grow at different rates. When a child shows a sudden weight drop, medical or emotional problems may be suspected. Professional help from a pediatrician, dietitian or child psychologist may be necessary.

Family coping with eating disorders

Parents who are concerned that a child may have an eating dis-

Preventing eating disorders

10 things parents can do

by Linda Smolak and Michael P. Levine

1. **Avoid conveying an attitude** about yourself or your children that "I will like you more if you lose weight, eat less, wear a smaller size, eat only 'good' foods." Avoid negative statements about your own body and your own eating.

2. **Educate yourself and your children** about (a) the genetic basis of differences in body shapes and body weight; and (b) the nature and ugliness of prejudice. Be certain your child understands that weight gain is a normal and necessary part of development, especially during puberty.

3. **Take people, especially females, seriously** for what they say, feel, and do, not for how they look.

4. **Scrutinize your child's school** for posters, books, contests, which endorse the cultural ideal of thinness. Make sure the school includes images of successful females in the curriculum.

5. **Encourage children to ignore body shape** as an indicator of

order or severe eating problem should see their family doctor, dietitian or an eating disorder specialist.

A teenager may feel uncomfortable talking about her eating with anyone, and refuse to see a professional. Try negotiating, suggests Stephanie Fortin, MA, a Canadian eating disorder specialist in the *National Eating Disorder Information Centre Bulletin.*[8] Rather than demanding she enter treatment, she says, negotiate slowly, one step at a time, while reassuring her of your concern for her health and well-being.

The National Eating Disorders Organization advises choosing a therapist with care: "You have the right to choose the gender of your therapist; you have the right to ask to talk with the therapist ahead of time to clarify his or her experience in this area and treatment approach. Listen to your feelings . . . If you feel you can work well with

anything about personality or value. Phrases like "fat slob," "pig out," and "thunder thighs" should be discouraged. Being teased about body shape is associated with disturbed attitudes about eating.

6. **Help your child develop interests and skills** which lead to success, personal expression, and fulfillment without emphasis on appearance.

7. **Teach children** (a) the dangers of trying to alter body shape through dieting; (b) the value of moderate exercise for health, strength, and stamina; and (c) the importance of eating a variety of nutritious foods. Avoid dichotomizing foods into good/safe/lowfat vs bad/dangerous/fattening.

8. **Encourage your children to be active** and to enjoy what their bodies can do and feel like.

9. **Limit how much television children watch.** Watch with them and discuss the images of females presented. Do the same with fashion magazines.

10. **Make family meals relaxed and friendly.** Refrain from commenting on children's eating, resolving family conflicts at the table, or using food as either punishment or reward.[1]

Reprinted with permission from the National Eating Disorders Organization.

this person, then make a commitment to treatment."

NEDO cautions parents that recovery can take time. "Working through an eating disorder is very difficult, an 'up and down' process." Relapse back to baseline or worse is a recognized pattern, even after seemingly successful treatment.

Once the child is in treatment, the helpful parent will be there to listen, keep communication open, and share in supportive ways, says Fortin. Parents may wonder whether they are too involved or not involved enough. They need to allow their eating-disordered teen to grow up, to do the things others her age are doing. Giving advice and opinions in a respectful manner, as with another adult, will help.

Parents may want to examine their own feelings about weight and food, and work toward self-acceptance and size-acceptance. Modeling healthy behavior means having ordinary nondiet foods and meals in the home, and exercising for fun and fitness, not appearance.

But parents are not responsible for making the eating disordered patient well, she cautions. "The therapist will be responsible for that portion of the recovery process. This does not mean that you ignore the eating disorder altogether: Your support is important."

The therapist can help parents with coping strategies. Don't let the eating disorder take over all of family life, Fortin advises. Focus on other interests you share. If family communication has broken down, family therapy may be advised. Recovery may be slow, and parents should not be discouraged by good progress followed by a plateau or setback. This is part of normal recovery. This is hard work, so families can celebrate small improvements.

Fortin offers these tips for parents of eating disordered youth:

- Learn as much as you can about eating disorders. You can be supportive by just learning the issues your teen will be facing in therapy.
- Focus on health and well-being. Avoid commenting on weight or appearance. She/he is already overly focused on it.
- Understand the eating behavior as a coping strategy for dealing with painful emotions and conflicts. Do not blame or shame.
- Encourage discussion of conflicts and concerns. Be ready to help problem-solve and find supportive professional help.

- Be prepared to seek help and support for the entire family. This is a good way to develop mutually respectful coping strategies.
- Youth with eating disorders may benefit from structure in meals. Regard meals as a relaxed time when family members can catch up with each other's interests. Do not focus on food, or force or withhold food.
- Avoid power struggles over food. Do not prepare or buy food for the adolescent and other food for the rest of the family.
- When the eating disordered person's behavior affects others, she/he is responsible. Bathrooms and kitchens should be left clean by everyone. Household or shared foods depleted by bingeing should be replaced by the person who binged.
- Take your child to your doctor if you are at all worried about her health. Signs of medical instability can be subtle, and might include dizziness, tingling sensations and blacking out.

One new approach to eating disorder treatment enlists parents in therapy. It doesn't work for all families, particularly if there are other disruptive forces, but when properly trained, parents can monitor and guide the eating process, says Amy Baker Dennis, PhD, an assistant professor at Wayne State University Medical School in Detroit. Parents are with their daughter for hours each day; they intimately know their daughter and her social life. When a truce is called in the battle for control, they can help her solve problems and surmount the hurdles she faces.[9]

The most effective and long-lasting treatment includes some form of psychotherapy or psychological counseling integrated with nutritional and medical care. Many patients respond well to outpatient therapy; for others, inpatient care at a hospital or residential center is needed. The newly revised Practice Guidelines for Treatment of Eating Disorders are available in the January 2000 edition of the *American Journal of Psychiatry*.

A wealth of information for parents, coaches and friends in how to help and how to prevent eating disorders is available from Eating Disorders Awareness and Prevention in Seattle (www.edap.org).

Dads and Daughters is a campaign to help fathers understand

10 Tips for Dads with Daughters

1. Listen to girls. Focus on what is really important — what your daughter thinks, believes, feels, dreams and does — rather than how she looks. You have a profound influence on how your daughter views herself. When we value our daughters for their true selves, we give them confidence to use their talents in the world.

2. Encourage her strength and celebrate her savvy. Help your daughter learn to recognize, resist and overcome barriers. Help her develop her strengths to achieve her goals. Help her be strong, smart and bold!

3. Respect her uniqueness. Urge her to love her body and discourage dieting. Make sure your daughter knows that you love her for who she is and see her as a whole person, capable of anything. Your daughter is likely to choose a life partner who acts like you and has your values. So, treat her and those she loves with respect. Remember 1) growing girls need to eat often and healthy; 2) dieting increases the risk of eating disorders; and 3) she has her body for what it can do, not how it looks. Advertisers spend billions to convince our daughters they don't look "right." Don't buy into it.

4. Get physically active with her. Play catch, tag, jump rope, basketball, frisbee, hockey, soccer, or just take walks . . . you name it! Help her learn all the great things her body can do. Physically active girls are less likely to get pregnant, drop out of school, or put up with an abusive partner. Studies show that the most physically active girls have *fathers* who are active with them. Being physically active with her is a great investment!

5. Get involved in your daughter's school. Volunteer, chaperone, read to her class. Ask tough questions, like: Does the school have and use an eating disorder prevention or body image awareness program? Does it tolerate sexual harassment of boys or girls? Do more boys take advanced math and science classes and if so, why?

Are at least half the student leaders girls?

6. Get involved in your daughter's activities. Volunteer to drive, coach, direct a play, teach a class — anything! Demand equality. Texas mortgage officer and volunteer basketball coach Dave Chapman was so appalled by the gym his 9-year-old daughter's team had to use, he fought to open the modern boy's gym to the girls' team. He succeeded. Dads make a difference!

7. Help make the world better for girls. This world holds dangers for our daughters. But over-protection doesn't work, and it tells your daughter that you don't trust her! Instead, work with other parents to demand an end to violence against females, media sexualization of girls, pornography, advertisers feeding on our daughters' insecurities, and all boys are more important than girls attitudes.

8. Take your daughter to work with you. Participate in every April's Take Our Daughters to Work Day and make sure your business participates. Show her how you pay the bills and manage your money. Your daughter will have a job and pay rent some day, so you need to introduce her to the world of work and finances!

9. Support positive alternative media for girls. Join with your family to watch programs that portray smart savvy girls. Subscribe to healthy magazines like *New Moon* and visit online girl-run 'zines and websites. It's not enough to condemn what's bad, we must support and use media that support our daughters!

10. Talk to other fathers. Together, we fathers have reams of experience, expertise and encouragement to share. There's a lot we can learn from each other. And we can have a lot of influence – for example, Dads and Daughters protests stop negative ads. We can make the world better for girls when we work together![4]

Reprinted with permission. Copyright by Dads and Daughters. *To learn more about the nonprofit group Dads and Daughters, call 1-888-824-DADS or visit www.dadsanddaughters.org*

and become more involved in their daughters' lives in an effort to prevent body image problems and eating disorders. From Duluth, Minn., it urges fathers to listen to their daughters, focus on what's important (not appearance), to give them confidence in valuing their true selves, and to get involved with their activities, their schools, to know and respect their friends. It urges men to "help make the world a better place for girls by demanding an end to violence against females, media sexualization of girls, advertisers making billions feeding on our daughters' insecurities, pornography, and all 'boys are more important than girls' attitudes." (www.dadsanddaughters.org)

Helping the large child

The large child needs lots of love and attention, as do all children, and to be reassured of parental love regardless of weight.

Diets and weight loss programs are not an option, since they disrupt normal eating, will likely fail, and may set up a lifelong pattern of excessive weight gain following weight loss. Putting children on diets is a form of punishment that asks them to ignore feelings of hunger and may lead them to believe there is truly something wrong for wanting to eat more than their parents want to give them.

The best course is for parents to expect the child to grow into his or her weight, while taking appropriate action to improve communication and habits, and reduce stress levels. The family can work together to plan and initiate changes for everyone's benefit.

Parents should not treat the overweight child differently, such as giving one child different meals, desserts or snacks from the rest of the family, say Hans and Nelson. "Since a parent's primary role is to give support, any action that denies support should be avoided. For example, when a child is upset by playmates' teasing, a parent who responds with, 'When you get thinner they won't tease you anymore,' only reinforces the child's suspicion that there is indeed something wrong with him or her. A more positive response is to listen to the child express his or her feelings about that teasing, and then perhaps, ask if other children are getting teased and for what reason. This can lead to a discussion of: 'What do you think you can do about this situation?'"

Thus, it is time to look at childhood obesity in a different way. New research suggests that genes may account for 75 to 80 percent of the body fat children carry. Instead of fighting against this, parents need to work with the child's natural tendencies. Most parents are very aware of the social stigma associated with being fat. Many have experienced size discrimination first hand, and all have witnessed it. They are determined not to let this happen to their children. But the steps they take to prevent obesity may backfire.

When parents are afraid that a child is becoming fat, they often restrict food, says dietitian Joanne Ikeda. But recent research shows this can make it worse. Children whose parents control their food intake are less able to self-regulate their energy intake. Thus, they may be at higher risk of obesity than kids who are allowed to choose how much food they eat.[10]

Therapists often find these children develop a fear of hunger, expressed by begging, scavenging, and even stealing food. Some parents act more like prison guards than nurturers and caregivers, Ikeda suggests. She tells health professionals they must assure parents that infants are born with the ability to regulate their energy intake and this ability needs to be fostered throughout childhood, not interfered with.

Even if we don't actively discriminate against people who deviate too greatly from our standards for beauty, our silence condones it. Our children watch us and model their behavior after ours.

"Fat has become the bogeyman, the monster that terrorizes our children," Ikeda says. "Overdramatic? Only as dramatic as the newspaper headlines, 'Too Fat Boy Murders Classmates who Teased him, Then Kills Self,' 'Girl drops Dead of Starvation — Afraid of Becoming too Fat,' and 'Girl Commits Suicide because Mom nagged her to Lose Weight.' These are not from the *National Enquirer*. They are all articles I have clipped from California newspapers over the past couple of years."

Ellyn Satter charges that our current attitudes and approaches blame children and parents for a child's fatness and promise cures that health professionals can't deliver. "We have led parents to believe that children are too fat because they eat too much and that children can become slim if they eat less. In so doing, we set parents and children up for disappointment and unnecessary self blame. In encouraging patients to try for weight loss, we find ourselves administering programs we don't totally believe in and accepting outcomes that leave us feeling discouraged and dishonest. It's time to define the problem of juvenile obesity in a way it can be solved."

She says we have overreacted to normal fatness and the growth process — often children will slim down naturally. However, some children are genetically fat. "It is possible that our interventions — restriction of food intake and subsequent struggles and preoccupation with eating — have exacerbated tendencies to fatness and interfered with a child's normal inclination to slim down. Even when obesity does exist, we don't know what causes it. Fat children eat no more, or no differently, than thin children. Nor do we know how to cure it."

Satter cites research that shows children are less able to regulate intake when parents are preoccupied with keeping them from being fat.[11] She says when parents restrain food and fail to gratify children's appetites, they can lose their ability to regulate food, and when controls are relaxed are prone to overeat. She reports children can get too fat when they are systematically overfed, although normally if they overeat, they will compensate by eating less the next day.[12]

Kids can get too fat when their emotional needs are not met, when they don't feel safe, when there is family or social stress. In response to these situations, children may demand food too often as a way of attracting the parents' attention, or become underactive because they are despondent. A child may also overeat because she is depressed or anxious and has learned to use food for comfort. A child may underexercise because someone is overprotective, is intolerant of her noise and mess, or because she is depressed and lacks energy.[13]

Satter warns, "In all cases, rather than attempting to shift calorie balance with diet and exercise, it is essential to identify and resolve underlying causes to restore the child's normal regulatory and growth patterns. That outcome goal is achievement of the child's weight, not some externally defined (even modest) standard of weight. Striving for a particular body weight creates distortions with eating and feeding and interferes markedly with nurturing the child."

In treatment programs, Satter suggests setting aside weight loss as a goal and focusing instead on achievable goals: improving the attitudes and behaviors that accompany the overweight. "We can help our patients learn to eat and exercise in a healthful and positive way, feel better about themselves, and feel good about their bodies. If we — and they — institute these changes, they might be thinner.

Guidelines for parents of large kids

- **Provide the child with lots of love and attention.** Don't pressure the child to lose weight.

- **Have regular meals and snacks.** Try to discourage eating at other times.

- **Let the child decide how much to eat.** Don't limit the amount of food a child can eat, or make a child clean the plate.

- **Serve the same healthy food to all family members.** Don't put the child on a special low calorie diet.

- **Have appealing snack foods available** . . . like popcorn, frozen fruit juice bars, string cheese, and frozen low-fat yogurt. Don't have lots of high fat snack foods like chips, cake, pie, ice cream, cupcakes and doughnuts.

- **Expect the child to grow into his/her weight.** Don't expect the child to lose weight.

- **Encourage the child to be more active** by playing with toys like balls, frisbees, jump ropes, and bicycles, by joining a sports team, by taking gymnastics, swimming, tennis or other lessons, by walking the family dog, or by joining a 4-H club, Girl Scout, or Boy Scout troop . . . don't let the child spend a lot of time watching TV or playing video games.

- **Go on family outings that include hiking,** swimming, and going to parks and playgrounds where everyone can play actively. Don't let your family become "couch potatoes"![5]

California Guidelines for Parents of Large Kids. Reprinted with permission from If My Child Is Too Fat, What Should I Do About It? *Joanne P. Ikeda, University of California/ Afraid to Eat 2001, 1997*

But we can't count on it, and we must not promise it."

Thus, rather than requiring the child to eat less or exercise more, Satter advises indentifying and correcting the destabilizing influence, which in turn restores the normal regulatory and growth processes.

Helping parents understand feeding management may correct the underlying cause of a child's energy imbalance, but it must be focused on parents' feeding practices rather than on what and how much children eat, she says. Parents must respect the division of responsibility, which allows children the freedom to pick and choose from food that the parent has made available.

It is when parents don't live up to their feeding responsibilities or intrude on the child's prerogatives that feeding difficulties and disturbances of food regulation occur. Parents may fail to get a meal on the table, then try to control what and how much their child eats."

However, Satter finds that some parents are so rigid and controlling, or so fearful of the child's fatness, that they can't trust the child's eating. Other parents are so chaotic, both internally and externally, they can't bring order to feeding. At both extremes, families may need mental health professionals to help them correct the rigidity or chaos.

Frequently, such families will not participate in treatment and only want the child put on a diet. But, "It is absolutely unrealistic to expect the child to lose weight when the whole family system is set up to promote the opposite."

Putting a child on a weight loss diet or restricting food even in indirect ways — such as specifying free and limited foods — profoundly distorts the developmental needs of both parents and children. Children need to be nurtured. Parents need to nurture them. Children need to be able to trust their internal processes. Parents need to be able to relax and trust their children and those processes — not be police officers.

Sometimes it is the health provider who urges weight loss. It's important for parents to stand firm in their refusal. They might refer to their own experience. "Dr. Johnson, I've tried many times to lose weight, and always lost weight, but regained it quickly, and sometimes more. I don't believe that yo-yoing weight up and down is healthy, or that it would be healthy for Jimmy. So we will wait until there is a safe method that works long term."

If the health provider persists, and claims he or she already has used that method, it is appropriate to say. "All right, we're willing to consider it. We'll wait two years. Then if you can show us proof that your patients have safely kept off all lost weight for two years, we'll talk about it again."

For the child who naturally has high fat levels, or who remains fat despite restoration of positive feeding and family dynamics, the goal is to allow him to grow up to achieve a healthy body and feel good about his body and himself. Large children can be physically active and successful in sports. They can feel good about their eating, and have varied diets of high nutritional quality. And they can have good social and emotional skills. In fact, to be successful, fat children must acquire better-than-average social and emotional skills, says Satter.

Overweight is a stigmatizing condition. Larger children and their parents may need help learning to deal with prejudice and social and emotional challenges. They grow up thinking less of themselves only if their parents think less of them. Some parents are unaccepting and insist on changing their children. Others blame themselves and are overprotective. Children grow up to feel good about themselves if their families value them for their considerable worth, expect them to be capable, and see their size as only one of their characteristics.[14]

Prevention starts at birth

To the extent that it is an abnormal and unnecessary condition for the child, obesity can be prevented, Satter explains. This process starts at birth, with a positive feeding relationship between parent and child. Infants know how much they need to eat. They give cues to guide the feeding process, and to grow properly they must be supported in eating according to their internal regulatory processes of hunger, appetite and satiety.

For the parents of the large child, an important part of prevention is helping them resist pressure to put their child on a diet. Parents feel guilty and responsible. Their guilt is reinforced by health professionals, school, media, family and friends who think parents have "done something wrong" and expect them to remedy it. Parents need support in pursuing a moderate approach, and help with their feelings. They don't benefit from criticism.

Weight may level off and allow the child to grow into his or her weight. But trying to manage this amounts to an attempt at weight loss that distorts the feeding relationship, Satter warns. Instead, health providers must measure outcome by the degree to which they have helped the parents and child establish positive eating and exercise behavior and functional social and emotional skills. Then they must

Intervening with childhood obesity

Maintain structured meals and snacks

- Have meals and snacks at reliable times

- Limit *random* eating and (caloric) drinking between times

Keep the caloric density of food moderate

- Make moderate use of high-fat, high-sugar foods

- Don't deprive the child of "treat" foods; it only makes them more appealing

Maintain a division of responsibility in feeding

- Parents take primary responsibility for planning, procuring, preparing

- Let *even the fat child* decide what and how much to eat from what has been provided

- Don't criticize how much the child eats or give the child "looks."

Help the child to detect and trust hunger, appetite and satiety

- Have pleasant eating times where the child can be relaxed

- Teach and model focused, mindful eating

- Expect reasonably civilized table manners — be realistic

- Don't promote "stocking up" sometimes by restricting food other times

- Don't reward with food or use it for comfort — but do be supportive

Cut down on feeding cues (reminders)

- Confine most eating to the

let weight find its own level.

Of course, we can continue to hope that if families achieve these goals, children will grow up to be slim — or at least slimmer than they would be otherwise. The odds are good: Longitudinal studies show that more children slim down than stay fat. We can help children institute positive lifelong eating and exercise patterns and attitudes toward self and others. We can let them grow up to get the bodies that are right for them. But we can't make them lose weight. We can only do all we can — then we need to let go of it.[15]

Joanne Ikeda conducted weight management programs in the

---

table
- Make most eating at either meal or snack time
- Put food out of sight to limit absent-minded eating
- Turn off the TV at eating times.

Think of the child as "normal" when making food decisions
- Plan and provide nutritious meals and snacks
- Make food selection decisions as you would for any child
- Trust your child's food regulation — don't fake it by serving low-calorie food

Use your own good judgment in setting feeding limits
- It is helpful to teach orderly,

deliberate and satisfying eating
- It is helpful to be firm about structure with eating
- It is not helpful to deprive

Goals in treatment programs
- Be realistic about outcome
- Allow the child to develop the weight that's right for him/her
- Prevent overeating; don't promote undereating
- Develop regular and reasonable exercise
- Support/enhance social functioning, including coping with a "handicapping condition"[6]

Copyright 1995 by Ellyn Satter. All rights reserved. From *Feeding with Love and Good Sense: Training Manual*. Ellyn Satter Associates, 4226 Mandan Crescent, Madison, WI 53711.

early 1980s for teens using a behavior modification approach.[16] [17]

"Some of the youngsters I worked with lost weight, some maintained, and some gained," she reports. "All needed more love and acceptance. There was the large boned, aristocratic looking girl accompanied by a mother who wore a size four petite. 'I hope you can do something with her, because I can't,' said the mother haughtily. I felt like saying, 'Sure, I'll just touch her with my magic wand and make her look just like you,' but of course, I didn't.

"There were two bosom buddies; one looked fatter than the other. The larger girl kept worrying that her friend would lose weight, and thus have no need of their friendship. She made sure they visited the candy machine before and after every meeting.

"The only adolescent who appeared to have escaped serious damage to his self-esteem was a big kid whose mother brought him in, saying, 'Everyone in our family is big, so I don't expect him to lose weight. I just want him to learn some healthy habits.'

"'Yes, yes, yes!' was my enthusiastic response. She was right, this boy was big. Big enough to intimidate any peers who wanted to make his size an issue. Plus he was good at using humor to help our group 'lighten up,' and even I was vulnerable to his charm. We needed his levity to ease the pain — the pain of knowing that your parents would love you more, your teachers would like you more, and your life would be wonderful if you could just look like the kids featured in *Sassy* or *Seventeen*.

"I stopped working with fat youngsters when I realized that I was contributing to their distress by reinforcing the idea that there was something 'wrong' with their bodies. But their pain remains with me. It sustains me and provides the motivation for my efforts to promote size acceptance in some very concrete ways," says Ikeda.

Children have no control over their genetic makeup, and health professionals need to help parents be realistic, Ikeda points out. "When a tall, large man and a short, fragile-looking woman have children, they may expect their daughters to resemble the mother, and sons, the father. But this may not be the case."

Parents who try to pressure children by making their love conditional on weight loss need to be told that they are harming, not

helping, their children, she says. Size discrimination is often practiced under the guise that it will motivate large children to change
their eating and exercise habits so their bodies will become "normal."

Health providers and educators are in a unique position to influence attitudes and opinions, and point out flaws in this thinking, she
says. "Our children did not create this world where an overabundance of appealing, low-cost, high-fat foods is widely available at a
moment's notice. A world where machines perform most of the tasks
that used to require human energy expenditure. As adults, we must
assume the responsibility for this situation and make every effort to
change it . . . in ways that help, not punish our children."[18] [19]

"There is no reason your child cannot lead a happy, productive,
full life at whatever size she turns out to be," explains Ikeda. In the
brochure, *If My Child is Overweight, What should I do about it?*, she
tells parents, "Being overweight may seem like the worst possible
fate. However, it isn't. A worse fate is feeling rejected and unloved
because one is overweight. You can make sure this does not happen
to your child. Reassure your child she will be loved by you always,
whether she is thin or fat. Help your child to feel good about herself
so that overweight is not compounded by low self-esteem."

Raising largely positive kids

Big kids have a hard time in our thin-obsessed society.

Carol Johnson, author of *Self-Esteem Comes in All Sizes,* and
founder of Largely Positive support groups, says adults must send
them enough positive, loving messages to counteract the negative
ones they will hear at school, the beach, at parties, and from the
media.[20] "As hard as it is to be a fat adult in America, it's even
harder for fat kids. Kids long to fit in and be accepted by their peers.
Damage to self-esteem can begin at a very young age. If it's not
mended, the scars can last a lifetime.

"I'm not opposed to weight loss. What troubles me is our inability to separate weight loss from self-esteem. Large kids should not be
led to believe losing weight will make them better people. Because
despite their best efforts, not all kids will lose weight permanently.
It's imperative that parents and supportive adults provide larger kids

with the tools to realize they're just as good as thinner kids, that weight is not a measure of their self-worth."

Johnson's suggestions for raising largely positive kids are:

• Be sure your understanding of obesity is accurate and that you can separate myths from facts. This will help you to view a child's chubbiness as physiology, rather than defect.

• Do *not* put a larger child on a diet. Most experts now agree this is one of the worst things done to overweight children.

• Teach larger children that their self-worth has nothing to do with their weight. Emphasize positive attributes and talents, and teach them that these are the things that have lasting value. Give frequent praise for talents, accomplishments and for just being who they are.

• Be honest with larger children about remarks they are apt to encounter about their weight. Help them decide how they will respond. Tell them that many groups of people have suffered discrimination, and that larger people are one of those groups. Teach them that diversity of size is no different from diversity of culture — we must learn to respect both.

• Be a good role model. Don't criticize your own body. If children see you appreciate your own body, they'll find it easier to like themselves.

• Don't *ever* suggest that a larger child's weight makes him/her less attractive or that no one will want to date them. This can cause lifelong damage to self-esteem. A larger young girl may be thankful for any attention a boy gives her. Teach her that she deserves respect and affection and that anything less should not be tolerated.

• Make an extra effort to help your larger child find clothes that are in style.

• Encourage physical activity. But let the child decide what activities he or she prefers. Don't force a larger little girl into a ballet class if she doesn't feel comfortable there. On the other hand, if she wants to twirl a baton, don't discourage her because of her size. Physical activity can be a family affair. Take a family walk every evening or set up a badminton game.[21]

Children need reassurance that every body is a good body, and that they can be healthy at the size they are.

CHAPTER 12

Prevention in schools

■

Schools reflect society's obsession with thinness and scorn for large people. The pressure, the harassment is all there — between students, between teachers, between students and teachers, in the classrooms and in the halls.

Teachers tell me that they see girl after girl in the lunchroom choosing the salad bar over main-course meals, and coming out with only a small plate of lettuce. "I hope they are making up for it with healthy meals at home," one teacher said. Then she sighed — we both knew it wasn't happening at home, either.

The mini-world of the school is an important and natural player in the effort for change. But a greater awareness is needed so parents and educators will recognize eating and weight problems, and decide to approach them in a comprehensive way, using health at any size concepts which benefit all children and harm none.

Schools have long recognized the problems of hungry children. Many provide both breakfast and lunch for kids who are neglected, of low income, or whose parents both work.

This is just one step. It does not begin to touch the problems of girls and boys hungry from self-starvation. Schools could do far more to address the role they play in children's lives when it comes to eating, socializing and developing self respect — qualities that aren't part of the curriculum but nonetheless are critical in the learning process.

"A student who is not healthy, who suffers from an undetected vision or hearing defect, who is hungry, or who is impaired by drugs or alcohol, is not a student who will profit from the educational process," says Michael McGinnis, director of the Office of School Health, Centers of Disease Prevention and Health Promotion, Atlanta.[1]

Today one in four children lives with a single parent; one in five lives in poverty; one in five is of a minority race; and one in 10 has a physical or mental disability, factors which may increase the risk of health problems and educational failure, says Lloyd J. Kolbe, PhD, chief and researcher at School Health, CDC. The major health problems our society faces are caused in large part by behaviors begun during youth, he notes.

Given these challenges, school health programs can become one of the most efficient means the nation could employ to prevent the major health problems that confront us, he says. Comprehensive school health programs can prevent future health problems, improve economic productivity, reduce the spiraling costs of health care, and improve educational outcomes. Schools can prevent many health problems from happening, detect others at early stages, and treat those that have not been prevented, thus avoiding the worst effects. Kolbe calls for a regeneration of school health programs to bring about these changes.[2]

An awareness of the severity of the weight and eating crisis for youth today and effective preventive measures fit well into this scenario. This is a major health crisis, and school administrators, boards and parents need to take effective steps to address these problems.

Integrating the approach

Most schools use the Comprehensive School Health Program, developed by Kolbe and the Centers for Disease Control and Prevention Division of Adolescent School Health. This program recognizes that education and health are interrelated and that healthy children who feel safe and accepted in their environment can learn better and achieve more academically.

Comprehensive school health programs provide unique opportunities throughout the school experience for health promotion and preventive health measures. They make important changes in the health and lives of the 45 million American school children, and for their families, school staff and community.

The CDC program includes the following eight interdependent components, all important in a comprehensive school program that addresses eating and weight issues:
1. Health education
2. Physical education and activity
3. Counseling services
4. Food service
5. Healthy school environment
6. Health programs for faculty and staff
7. Health services
8. Parent and community involvement

In each of these components, schools address six high risk behaviors: injuries from accidents, violence or suicide; tobacco use; alcohol and other drug use; poor nutrition; lack of physical activity; sexual behavior, sexually transmitted diseases and unwanted pregnancies.

Many of these risky behaviors are also involved with body image, weight and eating. Poor nutrition and lack of physical activity are closely related to a wide range of problems. Violence, harassment and suicide are linked to dysfunctional eating, eating disorders, size prejudice, low self-esteem and depression. Sexual or physical abuse may trigger eating disorders. Teenage girls smoke to lose weight and won't quit for fear of weight regain. And the risk of preteen pregnancies increases with early puberty, apparently related to higher levels of body fat and sedentary living.

The challenge is to develop and integrate into the school's health program the components that can prevent eating and weight problems Such a program can do much to stimulate students' intellectual growth and their ability to learn.

1. Health education in the classroom

Health education can help youngsters integrate normal eating, healthy food choices, and balanced, active living from kindergarten through high school. Classroom curriculums can expand to deal with the level of dysfunctional eating, undernutrition, hazardous weight loss, eating disorders, size prejudice and overweight that are real issues for students today. Creating awareness is a first step in helping teachers recognize these problems so they can be dealt with at early stages.

At junior high and high school levels, required classes in nutrition, child development and family living give students a solid foundation to incorporate healthy living concepts into their lives. Unfortunately, when budgets are tight many schools cut back on these essential classes. Concerned parents can make a big difference in influencing these decisions. Recognizing how fundamental these subjects are to healthy living, they can insist their schools offer and require these classes. The eating and weight crisis is truly a high-cost health emergency and we must regard it this way.

Everywhere I go now people tell their terrible stories with haunted eyes: a sister who doesn't eat; a beloved 16-year-old granddaughter, hospitalized in long-term care for her anorexia; a daughter with bulimia who quit college because she couldn't focus; a nephew's suicide related to his body shame and being picked on in school; a stepdaughter who "lives on coffee and cigarettes."

Teachers are hearing these same stories and watching them being played out every day in their classrooms.

2. Physical education and activity

Healthy kids need daily opportunities to exercise, play and learn new skills in school, to help them maintain strong and healthy bodies.

Many schools are well on their way to shifting physical education emphasis toward keeping all youngsters active in ways that last a lifetime. These schools focus on getting all kids involved, less on winning games, grooming star athletes, and showcasing spectator sports. They don't excuse youngsters with special needs from PE, but broaden programs to include them.

Good things are happening for girls in sports and athletics. In the more than two decades since Title IX mandated equality for female athletics in schools, the percent of girls in sports has grown from 4 to 42 percent, and 27 percent of high school girls play on sports teams run outside of school. Most schools strive to improve the quality of physical education and increase class time so they are providing both training in lifetime skills and the daily exercise needed by today's youngsters — who are often sadly inactive outside of school.

Healthy People 2010, which sets the nation's health goals, calls for daily physical education for all students and that 50 percent of class time be spent actively by every child. It also calls for kids to engage in moderate activity for at least 30 minutes on five or more days a week, and vigorous activity of 20 or more minutes on three or more days a week.

Focusing on fun and creativity, not competition, is important to all students, but particularly to kids who are physically underdeveloped. These are the students most likely to lead sedentary lives. Competition isolates and discourages them from being active. With special help they can keep motivated and find pleasure and success in physical activity. The President's Council on Physical Fitness and Sports identifies this as "the most urgent task facing physical education and other youth programs." The Council recommends fitness testing and remedial programs for students who don't meet standards. But sensitivity is important to avoid stigmatizing or humiliating the less fit or larger youngsters.

Many experts are calling for more after school intramural sports, and less focus on fielding winning teams. Communities that support intramural sports find it can be difficult to compete for time, gymnasiums and coaching staff, but that more children get to play, they often have more fun, and it lessens the sometimes-bitter competition between schools. Dedicated athletes, too, can benefit from a more open system that frees up their training time for other interests.

Assigning a sports nutritionist to work with school athletic teams helps prevent problems of undernutriton, and the dangerous weight loss practices common in sports like wrestling, gymnastics and running. The sports nutritionist consults with athletes, coaches and parents at the beginning of each season. She helps them identify and alleviate obsessive exercise behaviors and disturbed eating patterns.

Fitness testing is a valid part of many physical education programs. Four measures — aerobic capacity, flexibility, strength and endurance — help individuals and their coaches develop reasonable goals and evaluate improvement. But unnecessary problems arise when weight (or body composition) is included as a fifth measure of fitness, as in some testing programs. Such scoring is unfair to the larger child who improves in fitness, but receives a low score because of weight. It robs that child of the sense of accomplishment and pride that should be earned from working hard, and it adds to the stigma and shame that heavy children suffer, warns Karen Petersmarck, PhD, RD, a Michigan public health consultant with the Department of Community Health.[3]

Weighing and body fat testing also frequently misclassify children. Kids go through several growth spurts in a year, and each time fat may be depleted or deposited. This is entirely normal, yet focusing on it can set off a destructive cycle of dieting and weight obsession.

Petersmarck advises separating the concepts of fatness and fitness when evaluating progress. Fatness is not a measure of fitness, and teachers need to understand and assure students that good physical health is possible at higher body weights. Two fitness tests not dependant on weight in scoring are the Presidential Physical Fitness Award Program and Chrysler Fund AAU Physical Fitness Program.

3. Counseling services

School counselors and school nurses play key roles in identifying factors that hinder optimum school performance and adjustment, provide broad-based intervention programs, and connect students to appropriate services. Integration of weight and eating issues into the counseling program is important in helping schools deal effectively with these problems. Special training in nutrition, weight and eating issues is needed, or the assistance of someone who has this training.

What perhaps would be most effective is a nutrition coordinator or designated point person in each school committed to the health at any size philosophy and trained in eating and weight issues. These individuals would be team leaders working with teachers, coaches, counselors and administrators to identify and prevent eating and weight problems. They could also train staff in health at any size attitudes, and help them probe their own biases and concerns.

Ideally, these individuals would coordinate healthy body image and lifestyle curricula into all grade levels, including eating disorder prevention programs. They would work with individual students and parents as needed, develop support groups, refer students to specialists when needed, and extend team efforts into the community. They would promote zero tolerance policies for size prejudice, sexual harassment and bullying.

Antismoking programs also need to move ahead with the issue they have feared to address: smoking and weight. Girls need to hear messages that minimize weight concerns and emphasize the relatively small effect smoking has on weight-suppression.

4. Food service

Nutritious and appealing meals that coordinate with health education help students develop strong healthy bodies and good eating habits. Having a staff nutritionist means she can assist with lunch and breakfast menus, vending machine food and drink choices, and ways to encourage healthy food choices.

Scheduling adequate time for eating is being sadly neglected in many schools. A new study shows it takes the average child about 25 minutes to eat, and longer for younger children. Yet, typically after being served, a child has only about eight to 12 minutes. Meals need to be pleasurable, with enough time to eat and socialize. When time is short some don't get enough food, and it adds to plate waste.[4]

Timing of school lunch makes a difference, too. One study in grades one to three found that when recess comes before lunch, children eat more vegetables and meat or meat alternate and drink more milk. They come to lunch ready to eat and are less rushed or distracted by wanting to go out and play with friends. They have less stomach discomfort and dizziness, and less food is wasted.[5]

Vending machines are another urgent concern. Sadly, many schools are now signing the aggressive "Exclusive Pouring Rights" contracts that include a financial trade-off for vending and giveaways of soft drinks and advertising for companies such as Pepsi and Coke. It's a form of corporate sponsorship that feeds school revenue at the expense of children's health habits, particularly since many are already drinking so much soda that it has displaced milk altogether. Some nutrition, health and parent groups propose a ban on these contracts.

5. Healthy school environment

Children will perform according to the expectations their teachers have for them. Schools are responsible for supervising conduct and protecting students, and for giving guidance in how to get along in society. Keeping the school environment free of bullying and harassment is an important and challenging goal.

Physical, emotional and social surroundings that are safe, secure and accepting of each individual will enhance the well being, intellectual development, and productivity of students and staff. Kids who feel safe are free to direct energies to learning and can develop in natural, healthful ways. Victims are liberated.

Many schools now integrate the Character Counts' six pillars of character into every classroom and through the school. These are:

- Trustworthiness (honesty, integrity, loyalty)
- Respect (consideration, tolerance, dignity, courtesy)
- Responsibility (accountability, perseverance, discipline)
- Fairness (equality, consistency)
- Caring (kindness, gratitude, forgiveness)
- Citizenship (service, cooperation, environment)

When values like these are held by students and staff, our schools and communities become better places for everyone.

Insisting on respect for each individual *does* work. In the same way schools have "zero tolerance" for drugs and weapons, I would challenge them to establish policies of *zero tolerance for size bias,* to apply in classrooms, halls and grounds. This would refuse to allow size discrimination, harassment, bullying, or the singling out of any student for special torment.

Size prejudice not only hurts large kids but all kids, because they fear not being thin enough to be safe. It keeps them all striving to be thinner. Awareness programs on size acceptance for teachers and staff can be a first step. They may need to assess their attitudes and behaviors so they don't inadvertently model body dissatisfaction or size prejudice. Other schools may begin by surveying potential problems and developing focus groups to study them.

A program to teach students about size bias and reduce the stigmatization of large students has been developed by the Council on Size and Weight Discrimination, led by Nancy Summer and Cathi Rodgveller.[6] In workshops for sixth to ninth grade girls, Summer begins by inviting students to "get all the negative things out of their systems" that they think and say about large people.

"We cover a lot of ground: everything from discrimination to health to sports to fashion magazines. But always I stress my basic message: bias against fat hurts people of all sizes . . . because as long as fat is hated, everyone will be afraid of becoming fat . . . I share a lot of personal stories and listen to theirs. Some of the stories I hear are sad and frightening."

An important part of her workshops is looking at models and classic art, discussing differences between glamour and thinness. Summer says the girls tell her the larger models are the prettiest, "And I have to remind them that girls and women of all sizes are beautiful."

She encourages kids of all sizes to fight size bias by speaking up every time they see it, explaining that large kids need allies when they are being picked on. They discuss ways of doing this. "It isn't enough to just not laugh along with a joke. It's important that you say something, whether it's privately to the person being picked on, or publicly to the mean kids that what they are doing isn't okay."

The bully needs to be stopped so that all kids feel free to be themselves. How to defend themselves and others against prejudiced attitudes are explored. By the end of the workshop, they really understand this concept, she says. What matters most to larger girls is often what they hear their classmates say about size bias, such as, "I learned that it's not okay to pick on fat kids."

An improvisational theater team of high school students in Spearfish, S.D., tackles size prejudice in another way through elementary classrooms. They set the scene in a hallway lined with students, through which sixth-grader Josh must walk as classmates point, laugh and ridicule his size. Josh mutters, "I hate this place!" The actors freeze and processing begins, led by advisor Sandy Klarenbeek: *Who are the these kids? What did you see happen? How does it make you feel? Could this happen in your school?* "It is important for them to realize there is more to Josh than his size. He has feelings, is an individual," says Klarenbeek. "This kind of peer teaching is very effective."

6. Health programs for faculty and staff

Teachers and staff with healthy lifestyles and attitudes are powerful role models for kids. And since teachers reflect the problems and biases of our society, many need help with their own weight and eating issues. Thus, there is an urgent need for in-service training and attitudes of acceptance among school staff.

7. Health services

The school nurse, public health nurse, and other school resources provide support and a consistent approach with weight and eating issues. They may be involved in testing, identifying students with special needs, and making referrals to health professionals. Screening for disordered eating in all students, or for students considered at risk, may be advisable.

Whether schools need to measure height, weight or body fat is controversial, however. When done, it is important to avoid shaming or stigmatizing the larger child. Weighing needs to be done in private with no other children present. Comments should be neutral.

Joanne Ikeda, California nutrition specialist, suggests that if a child makes a negative comment about his or her body, it is appropriate to ask, "Why do you feel that way?" and, "I wish you felt more positive about your body. Your body is a good body. I hope you will take good care of it."

8. Parent and community involvement

Successful programs integrate parents and other community members into school planning and programs, so that school efforts will be supported and reinforced in the home and community. Moving ahead to integrate school and community efforts, a network of administrators, teachers, counselors, parents and others, can find ways of extending healthy weight and eating programs. These people serve on teams, committees and advisory committees and are involved in health conferences, training sessions, and as classroom volunteers.

Team conferences

Training conferences and in-service workshops for school staff and community health teams offer excellent opportunities to integrate preventive programs for weight and eating problems. Many states bring health teams together for annual training and program planning.

Recently I've had the privilege of presenting seminars at the North Dakota Roughrider Health Conference and the Wisconsin Wellness Conference. These groups value personal wellness skills for each team member, along with building strong coalition teams and giving them the training and motivation needed to develop meaningful school and community health programs. Here and elsewhere, I've found teachers deeply concerned about these issues.

"We in North Dakota consider every teacher a health teacher, both because each is a personal role model and because anyone who reaches into the lives of children has the opportunity to integrate education into all subject areas," explains Linda Johnson, MS, director of School Health Programs, N.D. Dept. of Public Instruction

Promoting active lifestyles

Sports Play and Active Recreation for Kids (SPARK) is an ongoing federally-funded program to research ways of restructuring elementary school PE so it promotes more activity. SPARK emphasizes fitness activities that can be enjoyed over a lifetime such as swimming, biking, walking and aerobic activities. Kids play frisbee games, jump rope, and learn aerobic dances.

Fifth grade teacher Julie Harris of the Turtleback Elementary School in Rancho Bernardo, Calif., is enthusiastic about her five years teaching the SPARK program. "More kids are more active and even nonathletic students learn skills and achieve a measure of success."[7]

Important features are:

- Training and follow-up for teachers. During the first year, SPARK trainers take a half-day refresher course every four months and are visited weekly by a consultant.
- A detailed curriculum of four-week units, each centered around a specific sport. Skills transfer from one sport to the next.

"We want to create a model grade school PE program that will help instill lifelong exercise habits," says Sallis. "Because we want to connect physical activity to the rest of children's lives, there is a weekly class on how to develop activity routines outside the classroom. And it includes homework — just as in math classes."

In 12 schools on the Navajo reservation near Window Rock, Ariz., the SPARK program has helped 1,250 children in third through sixth grade integrate activity with their tribal culture, while spending 30 minutes, three times a week in moderate to vigorous activity. The first 15 minutes is spent on teaching aerobic skills, the second 15 minutes on sports skills. Native dances are taught in the aerobics unit.

Project leaders hope this program will make a difference in the high prevalence of overweight among these children. The aim is to turn kids on to movement, so they find activity fun and exciting. Teachers say it works.

But while special programs work in school, Sallis says that getting children to continue to be active outside school hours has been more difficult than expected.

Curbing abuses

For sports in which weight is important for peak performance, it is essential that coaches, parents and athletes keep a healthy perspective. Full nutrition and healthy growth and development for the athlete cannot be compromised.

Every sport has athletes with eating disorders. Athletes may be asked or encouraged to lose weight quickly — requests that often lead to restrictive dieting and, in some cases, eating disorders. Weight loss may help their performance temporarily, but can lead to serious health problems and even death.

The U.S. Olympic Committee states that the average and healthy range of body fat for young women is 20 to 22 percent. But many female athletes and dancers and their coaches strive for 10 to 14 percent or even lower.

Barbara Bickford, a lawyer and assistant professor of exercise and sport science at the University of North Carolina, says schools could be held liable if they allow students with eating disorders to participate in sports. "What's right for the athlete is often in conflict with what's right for the team or the coach's career advancement," she says.[8]

It may take lawsuits and deaths to get this problem the attention it deserves, she suggests. At Southern Methodist University, a formal eating disorders prevention program was put in place in the aftermath of the death of a 20-year-old student with an eating disorder.

Wisconsin, a leader in working to resolve wrestling's inherent weight problems, raised the requirement to 7 percent body fat for males, and an athlete cannot wrestle in a weight class for which he would need to lose more than three pounds a week. A sports nutritionist works with wrestlers, coaches and parents; healthy eating practices are expected and actively integrated into the training program.

Coaches now overwhelmingly support the new program, and have many more students participating in the program, although many were reluctant at first, says Don Herrmann, associate director of the Wisconsin Interscholastic Athletic Association. "Probably 60 percent of wrestling coaches openly opposed this in the early stages. They said we didn't need it, that skinfold measures aren't accurate enough, and it would bring too much attention to wrestling weight concerns." But he says there was a dramatic swing in acceptance and after only a short time, 97 to 98 percent of coaches favored the new program. Coaches in other sports soon asked to be included.[9]

Planning prevention programs

Efforts to prevent eating and weight problems have proceeded slowly, with mixed results. Most have proven more effective at increasing knowledge than changing attitudes and behavior. Meanwhile problems have worsened.

A major concern — in the current climate of emphasing obesity risks — is that obesity prevention will forge ahead without integrating eating disorder prevention. This could do great harm.

It is important that prevention of eating and weight problems be addressed together in integrated, comprehensive ways. The Health at Any Size paradigm addresses the needs at either end of the weight scale, and any extreme of eating behavior. It bridges the barrier of contradictions that some have seen between eating disorder prevention and obesity prevention.[10]

10 things coaches can do to help prevent eating disorders in athletes

1. **Educate your coaches and trainers** about the signs and symptoms of eating disorders and your staff's role in helping prevent unhealthy behavior.

2. **Provide athletes with accurate information** about weight, weight loss, body composition, nutrition, and sports performance to reduce misinformation and to challenge practices that are unhealthy.

3. **Emphasize the health risks of low weight,** especially for females with menstrual irregularities. Refer athletes for a medical assessment in these cases.

4. **Refer to a therapist or sports psychologist** skilled at treating eating disorders if an athlete is chronically dieting or practicing mildly abnormal eating. Early detection increases the likelihood of successful recovery.

5. **De-emphasize weight** by not weighing athletes and by minimizing or eliminating comments about weight. Instead focus on other areas to improve performance such as strength,

"Prevention is neither a luxury nor a fantasy, but a necessity," says Michael Levine, PhD, Professor of psychology, Kenyon College, and president of the board of directors of Eating Disorders Awareness and Prevention (EDAP). He says preventing eating disorders is challenging and controversial, because it promotes change in education, mass media, public health and politics.[11] It is now clear that prevention efforts must start early, focus on changing behavior rather than attitudes and knowledge, and must be a sustained effort.

"Prevention is a marathon, not a sprint," says Linda Johnson. "Many prevention programs have fallen short because our approach

---

conditioning, and mental preparation.

6. **Do not assume** that reducing body fat or weight will enhance performance. Many individuals respond to weight loss attempts with eating disorder symptoms.

7. **Understand why weight is such a sensitive** and personal issue. Eliminate comments or behaviors about weight and body image. If an athlete's weight becomes a concern, refer the athlete to a skilled health professional.

8. **Do not automatically curtail athletic participation** if an athlete is found to have eating problems, unless warranted by a medical condition.

9. **Sports personnel should explore their own values** and attitudes about weight, dieting, and body image, and how these values may inadvertently affect their athletes. Recognize your role in promoting a positive self-image in your athletes.

10. **Take warning signs and eating disorder behaviors seriously.** Eating disorders have high mortality and suicide rates.[1]

Reprinted with permission from Eating Disorders Awareness and Prevention, Inc. (EDAP). For more information, contact EDAP (800-931-2237) www.edap.org

262 CHILDREN AND TEENS AFRAID TO EAT

has been single-pronged and of short duration. Often what is convenient, easy and cheap does not benefit youth."

She says a successful prevention program will:

- Develop a needs assessment
- Build in measurable goals and objectives
- Use researched, theory based, proven effective programs
- Deal with problems in a comprehensive way
- Work with an active advisory council
- Include ongoing evaluations[12]

A comprehensive effort that includes school, community and families is most likely to bring about real change, says Johnson. Prevention programs also must do no harm to vulnerable individuals. It's clear the wrong kind of prevention is useless and can make matters worse.

What does not work are one-shot programs or prepackaged events used in isolation, with no long-term effort. Information-only programs that change knowledge, but do not teach skills or change behavior, do not make people healthier. Scare tactics don't make them safer. It is illogical to spend time, money, and energy on untested programs or efforts that will not be sustained over time, experts say.

Unfortunately, most eating disorder prevention efforts have been of this nature. They have come too late and offered too little. Much time has been wasted. Too often prevention has missed its mark with efforts that began in high school, or showcased speakers who inadvertently glamorized their eating disorder experience, or even gave disordered behavior details that listeners put to use.

Obesity prevention efforts, too, have mostly been sporadic and unhelpful, sometimes singling out and stigmatizing certain students, promoting useless weight loss plans, and stirring up size prejudice.

Prevention at three levels

Prevention involves intervention at three levels:

1. Primary, aimed at preventing eating and weight problems in the general population
2. Secondary, focused on early stage problems or high-risk individuals

3. Tertiary, treatment of eating disorders or weight problems[13]

Currently, both eating disorder and overweight prevention are focused at the third level — on treatment. Treatment results in improvement or recovery for most eating disorder patients. However, success is not easy, and advanced cases end in death in alarmingly high numbers. Overweight has been treated without success for many decades as described elsewhere in this book. Primary and secondary prevention is in its infancy.

A remarkable example of a comprehensive program that addresses all three levels, prevention and treatment, and includes both eating disorders and obesity comes from a kibbutz in northern Israel. Launched through the community clinic, the program shows two-year success in reducing disturbed eating and eating disorders in a population of 680 persons.

Targeted for individual attention were all 38 teenage girls and their parents, teachers and significant other adults. Three girls were diagnosed with anorexia nervosa and another one at high risk, and were referred to a specialist. Twelve were referred with eating problems and received individual counseling in a non-judgmental, supportive, empathetic approach for both teenagers and parents. Six girls with weight problems, who said they wanted to lose weight, were assessed as to eating issues, and followed a program of individualized nondiet counseling. In all, 23 girls and women and five boys and men received help. Expenses were kept low, using resources already in place.

At the end of two years, two girls with anorexia had recovered and the third was much improved. The high-risk girl developed anorexia nervosa, was diagnosed early and recovered within a year. The others recorded marked improvement in condition and behavior, and had a greater sense of well-being.

Interestingly, attitudes of clinic team members changed dramatically as the intervention progressed. In two years, they made a paradigm shift from being focused on calories and weight to valuing the broader aspects of eating behavior, internal regulation, feelings, self-image and coping with social pressures. Through all this, the highly committed team gave strong support to both youth and parents, and now helps train teams in other communities.[14]

Primary prevention

Because treating eating disorders and obesity is so difficult, primary prevention is urgent. The sooner good programs can be put in place, along with strong secondary care, the less need for treatment.

Preventive programs are most promising when they have first assessed the need and timing for prevention, then deliver the program about one year before the age when the behavior starts, experts say. Research-based, theory driven curricula are most effective (such as social learning theory or behavior change theory). Comprehensive programs are integrated throughout the school and involve the home.

Two major models of primary prevention are identified by Michael Levine and Niva Piran, of the University of Toronto. The first is what they call *Top-Down* or leader driven. Patterned after drug and smoking prevention programs, this model aims to give students the knowledge, skills and encouragement needed to reduce their risks and increase their strengths. It decreases negative body image, dieting and other stresses, and improves communication, problem-solving, decision-making, healthy lifestyle and other competencies.[15]

The second method is the *Feminist-Empowerment-Relational* model, developed by Piran when she was asked to help curb the high rate of disturbed eating and eating disorders at an elite Toronto ballet school. The school was recording nearly two new cases of anorexia or bulimia nervosa every year, or about 10 percent of the girls (age 10 to 18). Piran met with all students two to six times in small focus groups and used their knowledge and experience to guide action and changes in the system. All staff were included in exploration.

Her method empowers girls and women to change themselves and their environments through group dialogue, similar to that in a consciousness-raising group, fostering respectful discussion about issues that are often silenced or felt to be shameful, and working with the system to bring about favorable changes. It encourages girls and women to work individually and together to change what they as a group identify as unhealthy and unfair influences in their lives.

Students began strongly demanding safe and respectful treatment of their bodies by school staff and peers.[16]

During Piran's 10 years of intervention, no cases of bulimia and only one of anorexia developed at the school. Eating disorder test scores dropped from 50 percent in 1987 to about 15 percent. Surveys revealed similar decreases in body dissatisfaction and the number of students who binged, vomited, used laxatives, went on diets or skipped meals.

Levine and Piran advocate combining these two models into pre-

Basic principles for eating disorder prevention programs

1. **Eating disorders are serious and complex problems.** One should avoid thinking of them in simplistic terms.

2. **Prevention programs need to involve both girls and boys.** They have interrelated problems, and both are at risk.

3. **Prevention efforts must address:**
   - Our cultural obsession with slenderness;
   - The distortion of femininity and masculinity in today's society;
   - Self-esteem and self-respect.

4. **Programs should include opportunities** for students and adults to speak confidentially with a trained professional, if at all possible, and be referred for competent, specialized care when appropriate.

5. **Systems should be developed** to make it easier to reach out and help students who may be having eating problems. Such systems must be able to provide referrals to competent treatment resources while being sensitive to the needs and rights of the family and child.[2]

Adapted from Eating Disorders Awareness and Prevention materials. For more information, contact EDAP (800-931-2237) www.edap.org

CHILDREN AND TEENS AFRAID TO EAT 2001

vention programs that include these components:

- Media literacy and ways of analyzing the culture
- Student discussion of the impact of culture
- Nutrition education that promotes healthy eating and challenges dieting
- Techniques for developing personal competencies[17]

There is a great need to support teen girls by increasing social support and mentoring, reducing environmental stressors like sexual harassment and teasing, transforming girls' lives by reducing the importance of appearance, and changing institutions such as the mass media that disempower them. A variety of techniques for resisting these negative influences is included in successful prevention efforts.

In addition, experts say that comprehensive preventive programs need somehow to address boys and men, their power, their fears, their dreams, and their capacity to care for themselves and others.

Media literacy

Training in media literacy develops the ability to question, evaluate, understand and respond thoughtfully. It helps students insulate themselves against thinness messages in advertising and the media. It helps them ask needed questions: Is this a realistic portrayal? Am I or my experience similar? Do I want to act or be like this person?

Media literacy also helps students learn how to use the media for positive change. They can become proactive in contacting advertisers and organize boycotts of products which are offensively advertised.

GO GIRLS! (Giving Our Girls Inspiration and Resources for Lasting Self-esteem!) from EDAP is an action oriented prevention program that follows through with activism and advocacy projects.

Teenage girls develop critical thinking skills, learn how to be critical viewers of the media, and use the media to communicate their own messages in their own words with the goal of changing important aspects of their environment in regard to marketers' images of women.

The Internet plays an increasingly important role in how people respond to these issues. It offers many opportunities for communication, new forms of multimedia and interactive educational opportunities. It provides a wealth of health information, and ways of exchanging prevention and treatment information around the world. Increasingly, it will be an important resource for engaging students in both the analysis of media and preventive education and action.

At the same time, the world wide web clearly has destructive elements. Young people need training in how to deal with the explosion of exploitive marketing and false information on the web.

Teacher training needed

Teachers are telling me they get little or no training on eating disorders or their risks, even though they are seeing enormous problems that look like eating disorders at every grade level. Their students are truly afraid to eat, afraid to gain weight, afraid their bodies are wrong, and they often talk about their fears.

This training is urgently needed and teachers are asking for it. It is also important for teachers to understand and evaluate the process of referral and parent notification in their schools. Many need improvement; currently, it can be difficult to get effective help for students at early stages of disturbed eating.

Teachers also need to assess their own attitudes and eating behavior. It is urgent that colleges soon address the problem of sending out young teachers, coaches and other professionals in health, nutrition and education fields who have not resolved their own severe eating issues.

Stanford University offers a class that shows promise of changing behaviors for such young professionals-to-be, called *Body Traps: Perspectives on Body Image*. While the focus is on objectively evaluating the issues, results show significant personal change: improvement in body image, eating attitudes and eating behaviors for class members as compared with a control group. The class includes multimedia presentations and discussions on body image, media and advertising, history of beauty, and disturbed eating. Students are required each week to write a two to three page reaction paper expressing their thoughts, feelings and criticisms from assigned readings.[18]

Issues strong by fifth grade

Evaluation of eating disorder prevention programs in schools show they need to begin early, by fifth or sixth grade. By this time, up to half of girls already "feel too fat" and 20 to 40 percent are dieting. By eighth grade, over half say they have dieted during the past year. These figures do not reflect the immense pressure felt for body dissatisfaction by other girls who are not dieting.[19]

In lower grades these attitudes and behaviors are measurable, but the girls lack dieting commitment, and their beliefs about the importance of thinness have not yet crystallized. Therefore, until about fifth grade the focus should be on learning about healthy nutrition, positive eating habits and body acceptance, not eating disorders, experts say.

But by fifth grade, body shape is much more important. Children who are already dieting at this age may be at increased risk for developing eating disorders because of the effects of calorie restriction and weight loss failures. Yet their susceptibility to thinness messages may be modifiable at this point. This is a time when children's social attitudes and beliefs can be changed, their thinness attitudes are still evolving, and a time when it is likely that parents will prohibit extreme dieting.

Discussion of eating disorders should begin between fourth and sixth grade when puberty development becomes obvious, says eating disorder specialist Paula Levine. For girls, this is younger than age eleven, and certainly before junior high, "before their self-esteem begins to plummet for other reasons."[20] Yet, eating disorder specialists warn there is risk that explaining eating disorder behaviors too plainly, such as by vomiting and laxative use, can promote these behaviors.

While fifth grade may be early enough for discussion of eating disorders in school, it may not be early enough for parents. Paula Levine speaks to new parents in newborn classes about eating disorders, and believes this may have an important impact.

Eating disorder prevention programs should have the following goals and principles, say Smolak and Michael Levine.

Goals:

• Acceptance of diverse body shapes, including causes of body size and prejudice; body changes in puberty.

- Understanding that body shape is not infinitely mutable.
- Understanding proper nutrition, including the importance of dietary fat and risks of malnutrition.
- Discussion of the negative effects of dieting.
- Information on the positive effects of moderate exercise and the negative effects of excessive exercise.
- Development of strategies to resist teasing, pressure to diet, and propaganda about the importance of slenderness.

Principles:

- Involve parents. Cooperation is needed, and possible family problems may be averted or improved (parents who diet or encourage dieting, concern over their own or daughter's weight, teasing, detrimental control over family eating). Parents need to know the indicators of eating problems and that such disorders can occur in younger children.
- Tailor materials to the child's level. Simple rules might be provided, such as "children should play outside for an hour or more daily, and limit television watching." Discussion on dieting might focus on the short-term effects such as hunger, crankiness, poor concentration and fatigue.
- Provide new ways to classify, evaluate and interact with people. Characteristics ranging from reliability to kindness might assess a person's value. Girls need to find attributes other than attractiveness or body shape by which to judge themselves and their success, such as academic, personal or social labels.
- Focus on healthy nutrition and body acceptance.

Highly recommended classroom curricula, both from EDAP, are:

- *Healthy Body Image — Teaching Kids to Eat and Love Their Bodies Too,* by Kathy Kater; grades 4 to 6.
- *A Five-Day Lesson Plan on Eating Disorders: Grades 7 to 12,* by Michael Levine and Laura Hill.

Appropriate to use as either 10 to 12 week classroom curricula or in outside programs are:

- *Teens and Diets — No Weigh,* by Linda Omichinski, ages 12 to 17 (www.hugs.com).

- GO GIRLS, middle and high school girls (www.edap.org).

In the Seattle area, an eating disorders prevention puppet show is making a big hit in elementary schools. Developed by EDAP with professional puppeteers, the Early Childhood Prevention Puppets bring an important message into schools: "It's What's Inside that Counts."[21]

Developing support groups

We sorely need support groups in secondary prevention efforts for students who struggle with eating, weight and body image issues, or who deprive themselves of food. That way, problems can perhaps be resolved early, before becoming severe.

Consciousness-raising support groups can be empowering in healing body shame and body dissatisfaction, say Carla Rice and Vanessa Russell, women's studies specialists at the Ontario Institute for Studies in Education in Toronto. In their teenage focus groups, the girls felt relief when they found the courage to share sexual harassment experiences and realized they were not alone.

As they connected the shame they felt about their bodies to incidents of violence or harassment, the girls grew outraged. Each had endured her humiliation in secret, ashamed because she feared she either deserved the hurtful comments or had provoked them. As they shared their experiences, the girls grew more affirming with each other, and became a force to be reckoned with. Their shame and self-loathing turned to anger as they realized most other girls had the same experiences. This transition from "I deserve to be violated," to "I have been violated," to "I do not deserve and will not tolerate violation," can be a key to empowerment, Rice and Russell suggest.

In organizing support groups for women and girls with eating issues, it is important to recognize that without the guiding hand of a professional, risks of perpetuating distorted thinking about eating, exercise and women's bodies exist.

Eating disorders screening

The annual National Eating Disorders Screening Program has remarkable success in getting help for the kind of individuals who are often reluctant to seek treatment. During a recent Eating Disorders

Awareness and Prevention Week, 35,897 people were screened at over a thousand sites around the nation. Attendees first take the screening test and attend information sessions, then those who meet the criteria are given referrals for further evaluation.

In 1998, a follow-up showed that over one-third of those screened tested positive, having a score indicating symptoms consistent with an eating disorder. Ninety percent of these were not in treatment, but half followed through and saw a clinician, and over three-fourths who did continued for further treatment. Interestingly, one-third of those screened said they improved just from going through the screening process, and 82 percent felt it had been helpful in some way, including helping friends and family.[22]

Eating disorder screening is an ongoing program that could be conducted much more widely, in all communities and schools. Less serious cases of disturbed eating could be assessed at the same time and targeted for secondary prevention.Moving ahead with eating disorder prevention, EDAP is training teams from around the country for Eating Disorder Awareness and Prevention Week, a February event in all 50 states and Canada. Every year these teams strengthen their awareness and preventive activities in local communities, highlighted by workshops, seminars, theater events, art and puppet shows and media promotions. Many continue activities throughout the year.

In Montana, these teams coordinate activities throughout the state in a program called *Pathways to Health: Preventing Eating Disorders*. They work through schools, community, and health care institutions in a systematic attempt to change the circumstances that promote, sustain, and intensify eating and weight problems.[23]

Obesity prevention programs

The first priorities in school-based obesity prevention programs are usually modifying school lunches, and making sure all students take physical education, and that PE does its job. More controversial are the next steps — from emphasizing the risks of overweight and screening kids, to putting them on weight loss plans.

But as with eating disorder prevention, the wrong kind of intervention is worse than the condition, warns Ellyn Satter. She advises that any programs for overweight children need to enhance psycho-social effects and ensure that no child is stigmatized. Don't rate progress by numbers on a scale, or how much weight kids lose, says Linda Omichinski, whose HUGS program, *Teens & Diets: No Weigh*, helps empower teens.[24]

Ongoing evaluations are important and need to measure, not just weight, but attitudes and behavior related to body image, dysfunctional eating, level of nourishment, weight loss practices, size prejudice, and medical risks. Increases in any adverse effects should be grounds for changing to another program proven safe and effective.

An awareness is needed by all who work with these programs that an emphasis on the risks of overweight can quickly escalate for vulnerable children into promoting thin mania, disturbed eating and social discrimination.

Teachers understand this. When the federal agency charged with implementing the Obesity Education Initiative in schools convened a major school conference in 1992, it likely expected an endorsement of plans to target large children for treatment.[25] But it was soon clear that educators were asking for a new approach. They warned policy makers not to just follow traditional thinking, but to provide sound information. They bluntly expressed concern that national messages on obesity can further stigmatize high-risk children and lead to worse problems. And they criticized changes that conference experts were recommending — to focus more on restricting diet than increasing physical activity.

The teachers recommended targeting all youth, not singling out those at high risk for special efforts. "Focus on how to make them healthier, as opposed to thinner, especially because making them thinner often does not make them healthy."

What teachers were asking for back in 1992 were preventive programs based on diet-free living and health at any size. They still are. Programs with this new approach empower and strengthen all youngsters.

CHAPTER 13

Healthy choices

■

Healthy lifestyle choices nourish the mind, body and spirit. They include nutritious eating, active living, and having a positive attitude toward life. It's important to teach children how to make healthy choices to prevent the weight and eating problems that dampen the spirits of so many kids today.

So how do we create an atmosphere that makes healthy choices for youngsters easy and fun, and show them it's the natural way to live? It involves families, teachers, schools, health professionals and communities.

"Feeling good about yourself starts by accepting who you are and how you look," the Canadian Vitality program reminds us. "Think positive thoughts. Laugh a lot. Spend some time with people who have a positive attitude — the type who look at the cup as being half full, not half empty. Positive vibes are contagious. Enjoy eating well and being active. Feel good about yourself. Have fun with family and friends, and you'll feel on top of the world!"[1]

Children need to make the connection between health and pleasure. We can help by emphasizing the positive, enjoyable aspects of a healthy lifestyle, and de-emphasizing weight. Helping them to feel good about their bodies gives them more freedom to choose a healthy lifestyle. Healthy bodies come in all shapes and sizes. Some store body fat more easily than others, or mature earlier or later. That's okay. Some stay small or lean. And that's okay, too. Every body is a good body, whether large or small. Each youngster is special, and we need to help them accept, respect and celebrate our differences.

We can help kids appreciate their strengths, abilities and uniqueness, to take pride in themselves and their accomplishments. We can help them find useful roles so they feel needed and important at home and in the community. We can teach them ways to relax and to cope with stress.

When kids feel good about themselves they'll be more likely to feel positive about making healthy changes in their lives.

Nutritious eating

Healthy food choices help youth grow, develop, do well in school, and feel at their best.Nutritious eating feeds the body and the spirit.

Balance, variety and moderation are the guiding principles. Balance occurs in eating enough of all five food groups: bread and grains, fruits, vegetables, meat and milk. The Food Guide Pyramid, a U.S. Department of Agriculture guide for consumers that is updated every five years, helps us visualize this balance. Eating a variety of foods from each group — especially a variety of fruits and vegetables — ensures that we get the more than 50 essential nutrients for growth, energy and health.

Eating moderately avoids the extremes — eating too much or too little. It reminds us not to overeat on high-fat or high-sugar foods, nor to deny them if we really want them. Kids who enjoy a variety of satisfying foods, and are not denied what they really want, are less likely to feel the sense of deprivation that can lead to eating and weight problems. Eating well means we usually choose whole grains, leaner meats, and lower-fat dairy products, along fruits and vegetables of all kinds.

Nutrient-dense foods are those high in nutrients and low in calories, fat and added sugars. They are highly satisfying. Some, such as eggs, fish or lean meat, pack a lot of nutrition into small size. Others are bulky and filling, high in fiber — like apples, corn and beans. Along with breads and milk, kids need to fill up on these.

Then there are the calorie-dense foods from the tip of the pyramid: fats, sweets, soft drinks, alcohol. They contain a lot of calories but not many nutrients. It's easy to eat too much of these, especially when they substitute for nutrient-dense foods. It's better to eat them less often and in smaller quantities.

Many kinds of sugars and syrups, fats and oils, are added to foods in processing or preparation, especially snack and dessert foods. Candy, cake, ice cream and cookies are major sources of added sugars. But soft drinks now top them all as the number one source of added sugars. Drinking more milk and water, and less soda pop or fruitade will quickly improve the diets of many youth.

The 1995 Dietary Guidelines for Americans, which I prefer to the later edition, offers this advice for healthful eating:

- Eat a variety of foods
- Balance the food you eat with physical activity — maintain or improve your weight
- Choose a diet with plenty of grain products, vegetables and fruits
- Choose a diet low in fat, saturated fat, and cholesterol
- Choose a diet moderate in sugars
- Choose a diet moderate in salt and sodium

It's sound advice for today's teens.

Vitality tells us, "Eating well doesn't mean giving up the foods you love; it means choosing wisely from a variety of foods that you enjoy. Your overall pattern of eating can include foods high, moderate and low in fat. If you want to enjoy a higher-fat food, balance it with staying active and enjoying a wide variety of foods the rest of the day. Children acquire attitudes about food first and foremost at home. Positive attitudes develop when food preparation and mealtimes are pleasant and fun experiences. So take time to enjoy meals and snacks with your children."

Even young children can help in buying and preparing food. It teaches them to make healthy choices at home, school, with friends, on trips, and through life.

Improving deficiencies

Surveys find that mostAmerican teens are eating quite well of the bread and grains group, the pyramid's solid foundation. However, they need to eat more fruits and vegetables to even come close to the five-a-day recommended. These are important sources for vitamins, minerals, fiber and the protective phytochemicals.

Teenagers don't drink enough milk, falling far short of the recommended three daily servings of dairy products. Calcium is essential for healthy bones throughout life and especially during the critical bone-building teenage years. Girls who fail to drink enough milk, and are thin, or often dieting, may never develop the strong bones they need to protect them osteoporosis.

Meat and its alternates, beans and peanut butter, too, are being neglected. Three-fourths of teenage girls fail to get recommended amounts from this group. They lack the high quality protein needed for healthy growth, and nutritionists are finding that some people feel much better when they eat even more protein. They lack high-quality, absorbable heme iron and zinc. Even a small amount of heme iron from animal sources will improve the absorption of nonheme iron from plants, from the legumes, dry beans and peas, leafy greens, iron-enriched bread and cereals. Vitamin C also helps.

Eating at least small amounts of meat has many benefits. (Vitamin B_{12} is only available in animal foods.) Currently there is no basis for the urban myth that eating less lean meat will improve health. Instead, it can cause severe problems. The Bogalusa Heart studies in Louisiana found that children who eat more meat are less likely to have nutrient deficiencies than children who eat little or no meat. Youngsters who have stopped eating meat, poultry, fish and eggs can benefit greatly from restoring these foods to their diets. They'll feel better and their immune system will be strengthened.

Teenage girls who fear meat produces fat, can be assured that it does not, if they make low-fat choices. Research suggests that protein, even in excess, is not stored as fat. And studies show that meals with meat satisfy longer. A Swedish study finds that people who ate a meat casserole at lunch, consumed fewer calories later in the day than when they ate a vegetable casserole.

At the same time, concerned parents need to keep in mind the basic principle that children are responsible for deciding what and how much they will eat. Parents need to respect these decisions, while guiding children toward healthy choices by having a variety of good-tasting foods available. A science-based vegetarian cookbook by a registered dietitian can be helpful if they don't — or won't — eat meat.

When parents choose vegetarian diets for their children, it's important to remember that the more restrictive vegan diets are not recommended for growing kids. It is possible to plan a diet entirely of plant foods that supplies most nutrient needs, but such a diet is so bulky that experts say it is unlikely a young child would eat enough calories, so growth may be stunted.[2]

While cutting down on fat is usually advisable when diets are high-fat, it should be remembered that babies have and need a high-fat diet until at least age two, because of their tremendous growth needs. These needs continue throughout childhood, so the transition to low-fat should be gradual. Canada advises a gradual transition that extends through the entire growth period until adult height is reached, before the low-fat diet of adulthood is recommended.

In the U.S., low-fat diets are being advised earlier, but this is controversial. Robert Olson, MD, PhD, professor of pediatrics at the University of South Florida, warns, "The recommendation to modify the diets of children is without merit."[3] A diet too low in fat may be risky at any age.

Fat is not a four-letter word. It's an essential nutrient that helps cells use vitamins and minerals more effectively. Fat is also protective. One of the most potent natural anticarcinogens ever identified is conjugated linolic acid (CLA), found almost exclusively in animal fat. Cutting out animal foods can deprive children of any cancer preventive benefits they may get from CLA.[4]

The Dietary Guidelines advise cutting dietary fat to 30 percent of total calories. Many nutritionists consider 30 to 35 percent reasonable, especially for children. Reducing fat to these levels is easily done if we bring less fat into the house, add less fat in cooking, and use less table fat.

Many kids do eat a lot of fat, and when they also overeat, this can contribute to excessive fat gain. However, surveys show that most

Food Guide Pyramid

A guide to daily food choices[1]

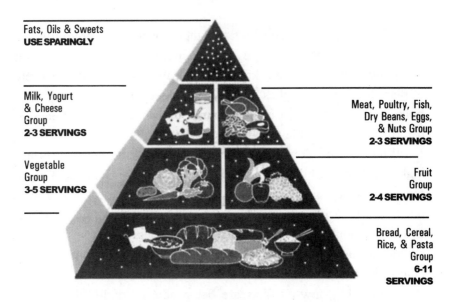

Fats, Oils & Sweets
USE SPARINGLY

Milk, Yogurt
& Cheese
Group
2-3 SERVINGS

Meat, Poultry, Fish,
Dry Beans, Eggs,
& Nuts Group
2-3 SERVINGS

Vegetable
Group
3-5 SERVINGS

Fruit
Group
2-4 SERVINGS

Bread, Cereal,
Rice, & Pasta
Group
**6-11
SERVINGS**

Use the USDA Food Guide Pyramid to help you eat better every day. Start at the pyramid base with plenty of grains, breads, cereals, rice and pasta: six to 11 servings depending on activity, size, growth, and individual preference. At the second level add vegetables and fruits — at least five a day. Moving up, add two to three servings of milk (three or more for older children and teens) and two to three servings from the meat group. Go easy on the fats, sweets and soft drinks at the tip of the pyramid, foods that provide calories but not much else.

Eating well focuses on balance, moderation and variety. Balanced food choices come from all five food groups. Eating moderately means eating enough for good nourishment, but not past the point of satiety, and choosing foods that balance out as moderately low in fat and sugars. Eating in variety from each food group ensures you'll get the many nutrients you need for health, energy and growth.[1]

DIETARY GUIDELINES FOR AMERICANS/AFRAID TO EAT 2001

What counts as one serving?
Food Guide Pyramid

Bread and grains group
- 1 slice of bread
- 1 ounce of ready-to-eat cereal
- 1/2 cup of cooked cereal, rice, or pasta

Vegetable group
- 1 cup of raw leafy vegetables
- 1/2 cup of cooked or
  chopped raw vegetables
- 3/4 cup vegetable juice

Fruit group
- 1 medium apple, banana, orange
- 1/2 cup of chopped, cooked or canned fruit
- 3/4 cup of fruit juice

Milk group
- 1 cup of milk or yogurt
- 1 1/2 ounces of natural cheese
- 2 ounces of processed cheese

Meat group (meat, poultry, fish, eggs, dry beans, nuts)
- 2-3 ounces of cooked lean meat, poultry or fish
  Equal to 1 ounce of meat, poultry or fish is:
  - 1/2 cup cooked dry beans
  - 1 egg
  - 2 tablespoons peanut butter
  - 1/3 cup nut

In using the pyramid, remember that serving sizes are a general guide. Small children will eat smaller servings; children in a growth spurt, larger teens and older boys may require more and larger servings. Even individuals of the same size differ in the amounts of food they choose and which satisfy their needs. Children should be encouraged to trust their bodies and respond to their natural signals of hunger, appetite and satiety.

DIETARY GUIDELINES FOR AMERICANS/AFRAID TO EAT 2001

have cut down on the fat they eat.

Most children do not eat too much, and apparently the number of calories they eat have not increased even though many kids are getting heavier. Recommended intakes are 2,000 calories increasing to 3,000 calories for boys between age seven and 18, and 2,000 to 2,200 calories for girls this age.[5] Girls on average are eating fewer calories than this, while boys are eating slightly more.

A recent USDA report concludes that energy intakes are already so low for some obese children that further restrictions could jeopardize their health. Therefore the positive message, "Be more active," is recommended, rather than the negative message, "Eat less food."[6]

Children mature at different rates, and their growth spurts may be unpredictable, so flexibility in feeding and trusting their natural responses is advised.

Parents who want to give children supplements should choose a simple multivitamin with levels at or below the Recommended Dietary Allowance, and from a company for which ingredients are regulated and reported fully on the label. Large amounts can be harmful. Supplements may help to meet special nutritional needs but are usually not needed and cannot substitute for healthy food choices.

Good foods, bad foods

When learning to make food choices, kids should be taught that there are no good foods or bad foods. All foods can fit in a healthy eating plan.

The idea that some foods are healthy and others unhealthy suggests that some foods can be used like medicine and others are toxic and disease producing. This is false and unscientific, although this notion is often promoted in the press, and even by health professionals who fail to understand nutrition.

While a balanced diet will usually be moderately low in fat and sugars, there's nothing wrong with occasionally eating high-fat, high-sugar foods in an overall nutritious diet.

People often refer to snack foods as junk foods, but it's better to say, *There are no junk foods, but there are junk diets.* It's not one or two tip-of-the-pyramid foods that matter, but having too much of them in the day's eating and omitting essential foods that counts.

It's all about you

In making a shift toward healthy lifestyles, it's helpful to move gradually into new patterns. A national group that advocates this through the new approach of enjoying food, taste and physical activity is the Dietary Guidelines Alliance, a coalition of health organizations, producers and government agencies. The Alliance campaign uses the theme "It's all about you." Key messages are:

- **Be realistic:** Make small changes over time in what you eat and the level of activity you do. After all, small steps work better than giant leaps.
- **Be adventurous:** Expand your tastes to enjoy a variety of foods. Try a new fruit or vegetable. Dig into a different grain.
- **Be flexible:** Go ahead and balance what you eat and the physical activity you do over several days. No need to worry about just one day or one meal.
- **Be sensible:** Enjoy all foods, just don't overdo it. Slow down. Have one helping and enjoy every bite.
- **Be active:** Walk the dog, don't just watch the dog walk. Set your goal at 30 minutes, most days. In 10-minute increments, it's easy. Take a walk. Try a fun new activity. You'll feel good and have more energy, too![7]

How parents can help

In their brochure *A Parent's Guide to Children's Weight*, Carol Hans and Diane Nelson of the Iowa State University Extension Service caution that children grow at different rates and may have very different body structures from their own brothers and sisters.[8]

They offer these suggestions for parents in helping kids make healthy food choices:

1. Be enthusiastic about eating a variety of foods. Help children learn what foods are in the different food groups and why it's important to eat some of each group daily.
2. Introduce new foods gradually. Offer the child a small portion but do not force the child to eat it. Tasting will come more

readily as the food becomes more familiar.

3. Serve realistic portions. The appropriate serving size depends on the child's age and size. One possible guideline is to offer one tablespoon of meat, fruit and vegetable per year of age up to age five. Physical activity and growth spurts also influence appetite. Plan meals to include some lower calorie food items that can be offered for second helpings.

4. Buy fewer high-calorie, low-nutrient foods. Encourage children to think of such foods as occasional treats, not regular fare. Involve children in planning, shopping, and label-reading.

Help kids choose active living

Living actively is widely accepted as a new, broader way of thinking about fitness than "exercise." Active living is concerned with long-term quality of life and total well-being. It's not focused on numbers, athletic training, or changing body size and shape.

Life is more fun when we live actively. It's the natural way for children and teens to live. It's a pleasurable part of a balanced life.

Vitality explains, "Being active means enjoying physical activity and finding fun ways to be active every day of the year — at home, at work, within your community. Whether it's bowling, mowing the lawn or playing hopscotch with the kids, an active lifestyle pays off. Make fitness a family activity: go ice-skating at the local rink, take an after-dinner walk together. Plan an active living vacation — a weekend hike, a cross-country ski holiday, a canoeing getaway."

Young children are the most active and physically fit of all — they're active because they want to be, not because it's good for them. On average, they spend an hour or two each day in moderate and vigorous physical activity.

We need to strengthen and extend the joy of activity that young children know, and help them carry it right through teen years and into adulthood. We need to find ways to halt the slide of less and less activity as kids grow older, especially for girls. Their activity falls off sharply after puberty.

It helps to emphasize the pleasure of being active, alone and with friends. After all, it's just for fun that 12-year-olds play softball

all afternoon in a vacant lot. It's for the joy and exhilaration of it that skiers and hikers challenge a mountain. It's for the social and rhythmic pleasure that young people dance for hours on a Saturday night.

In the active living approach, everyone can succeed, explains Gail Johnston, a health and fitness consultant in Walnut Creek, Calif. It's not necessary to count target heart rates, calories burned, or work up to training levels. Nor is it necessary to lose weight to achieve the benefits of fitness.[9]

In fact, focusing on weight loss can backfire and take the fun out of activity. So can focusing too much on excelling and winning, although children enjoy challenges and competitions if not outmatched.

Parents will want to keep tabs on their kids, their teams and coaches, to make sure they're having fun when playing hard. Of course, there'll be times of disappointment, anger or frustration, but it's important to keep this in perspective and create a sense of moderation in sports and active recreation. This keeps the activity fresh, fun and a learning experience. It keeps enthusiasm high. Sometimes it may be better to cut back on sports or change activities to avoid stress or burnout.

Help children be physically active

Children and adolescents benefit from physical activity in many ways. They need at least 60 minutes of physical activity daily. Here are ways parents can help:

- **Set a good example.** Arrange active family events in which everyone takes part. Join your children in physical activities.

- **Encourage your children to be physically active** at home, at school, and with friends by jumping rope, playing tag, riding a bike.

- **Limit television watching,** computer games, and other inactive forms of play by alternating with periods of physical activity.[2]

Dietary Guidelines for Americans 2000/ Afraid to Eat 2001

Benefits of exercise

Being physically active improves health in all sorts of ways. It lowers blood pressure. It improves cholesterol levels, increases good HDL cholesterol, reduces heart rate and lowers the risk of cardiovascular disease. It improves blood glucose levels and reduces risk of diabetes. It increases longevity.

The effect of exercise on bone density is particularly important during adolescence, because this is the time in life when bone mass builds rapidly. Think of bones as muscles. If they are actively used or stressed, they grow stronger. Tennis players, for instance, have much thicker and stronger bones in the tennis arm, the arm used more often, than in the non-tennis arm. Weight training, too, has a powerful effect on strengthening bones.

Being active may even make kids smarter. Brain research suggests that exercising the large muscles during adolescence helps increase nerve connections for higher brain development. This supports studies that show students involved in sports do better in academics. They are also less likely to drop out of school, take drugs or get pregnant while in school.

As important as are the physical benefits, mental, emotional and social benefits figure greatly in healthy activity, too. Being active gives a boost to self-esteem and mental outlook. It lowers stress and anxiety, lifts the mood, and is especially beneficial for youngsters who are anxious or depressed. It relieves tension and helps put problems in perspective. Best of all, it enhances the quality of life.

The good news is that youngsters don't have to reach competitive heights to achieve major benefits from physical activity. They need to be assured of this, and to have coaches and teachers who believe it. They can improve the quality of their lives by living actively in moderate ways. Regular, moderate activity:

- Improves self-image
- Boosts self-confidence
- More energy and zest for life
- Better looks
- Reduces stress and tension
- Less anxiety and depression

- Refreshes, relaxes
- Increases resistance to fatigue
- Improves sleep
- Increases lean body mass and reduces body fat
- Keeps weight stable, helps prevent overweight, may promote weight loss
- Increases strength and endurance
- Increases productivity at work
- Keeps heart and lungs working efficiently
- Lowers blood pressure and hypertension risk
- Helps prevent heart disease and diabetes
- Improves cholesterol levels, increases good HDL cholesterol
- Reduces heart rate
- Improves blood glucose levels; improves diabetic symptoms
- Reduces risk or symptoms related to some types of cancers
- Improves muscle function and joint problems
- Increases longevity
- Builds bone, slows bone loss, helps prevent osteoporosis
- Improves strength and function of elderly
- Provides social benefits: an easy way to meet and enjoy new friends; brings family and friends closer through shared activity

How much is enough?

Children differ in they type and amount of physical activity they enjoy. Some love it and will keep active throughout the day; others prefer less active pursuits. Parents can do much to help children enjoy activity by taking time for active family fun, and joining them in walking, biking or hiking.

The dietary guidelines suggest that children should be active at least an hour and adults 30 minutes on most days (five days a week or more). This can be broken up into several sessions.

Healthy People 2010 has set these goals for children and teens.

- Engage in moderate activity for 30 minutes five or more days a week
- Engage in vigorous activity for 20 minutes three or more days

a week

- Attend daily physical education classes.
- Keep physically active during at least 50 percent of PE class (or more than 20 minutes)
- Spend no more than two hours and perhaps less each day watching TV[10]

Healthy People 2010 recommends that children age 5 to 15 walk to school if it is less than a mile, and bike if less than two miles. Biking or walking other trips of these distances is also advised. Naturally, safety is an important consideration, and younger children will need to be accompanied. Some communities are working to establish safe school route zones, Walk your Child to School programs, and the Walking School Bus, in which adults walk the routes to school, picking up children as they go.

Schools are advised to require daily physical education for all students. Currently only 17 percent of middle and junior high schools and only 2 percent of high schools require this. Sixty percent of high school students are enrolled in PE classes. Only about one quarter attend classes daily, a decline from 42 percent during the first half of the 1990s. Yet overall, the outlook has improved greatly in the last decade. Schools are doing a better job in keeping more youngsters active in PE classes and after-school sports.

Sports enhance self-respect

A recent study by Melpomene Institute and *Shape* magazine of girls age 11 to 17 found girls who are physically active are more likely to have high body image, positive sense of self-satisfaction, higher perceived competence, and to like most things about themselves.

Being in athletics enhanced their self respect, and this was increased when they combined sports with other after-school activities. The researchers found that in all cases, girls who were in several after-school activities including athletics were more likely to have a higher sense of self than girls involved only in nonphysical activities or no activities. Girls in six or more after-school activities that included athletics were the most likely to feel good about themselves.

The authors suggest that after-school activities offer girls a way to define themselves in terms other than appearance. They allow girls to develop their interests, express commitment, and work with a group toward a common goal — all pursuits unrelated to appearance. The interest and encouragement of parents in these activities also had a big impact on the girls' self-esteem.[11]

Regular activity is important in preventing excessive weight gain for both children and adults, in keeping weight stable, and in maintaining long-term weight loss. However, kids and their parents and coaches should avoid a weight loss focus in activity. The purpose should not be to burn as many calories as possible or lose weight. This can be self-defeating and lead to discouragement and dropping out; often weight is not lost, but rather muscle gained. Keeping track of all the dials and numbers on fitness equipment, which supposedly add up to calories burned and pounds lost, is futile, too. This is not really the way it works.

The role of exercise in weight loss has often been exaggerated, bringing much disappointment and discouragement, warns Chester Zelasko, PhD, director of the Human Performance Laboratory at Buffalo State College in Buffalo, N.Y. People differ widely in the effect that activity has on their weight.[12]

Instead of focusing on losing weight, he says all people should exercise for the right reasons: "For the health of it! To improve the cardiovascular system; to improve the strength, endurance and flexibility of the muscular system; to effect positive changes on other body systems such as skeletal, digestive and immune systems; for other manifestations of improved health such as lower serum lipids and lower blood pressure."

Inspire the less fit

Most physically underdeveloped youth can become fit if they are motivated. It's time to focus more effort on identifying and helping these kids. The President's Council says this is "the most urgent task facing physical education and other youth activity programs."

The Council urges testing for fitness, as schools test for reading and math, and remedial programs for students who don't meet standards. A special class is recommended, or if this is impractical, a separate exercise program for part of the session or the entire class participating in activities needed by the underdeveloped.

Most of these kids can achieve appropriate levels of physical fitness, say experts. Teachers and parents need to understand the importance of fitness for each child in healthy growth, academic performance and prevention of weight problems.[13]

Parents help by understanding the importance of physical activity in their children's growth, performance and health, and by getting involved in their chosen sports and activities. Parents can also help by limiting screen time — television, videos, computer games and Internet browsing.

While school sports are important, it's clear that playing in sports doesn't automatically carry over into adulthood. Young athletes have just as great a chance of becoming middle-aged couch potatoes as their non-athletic buddies. In fact, a recent study conducted by Sallis at San Diego State University showed the only difference in activity between former high school athletes and nonathletes is that former athletes watch more televised sports.

Encouraging girls

The roadblocks that still keep many girls from being active in sports need to be removed. Making more facilities available for girls and encouraging girls to use them for pleasure and health will help. This focuses attention on ability and fitness, not appearance.

Research shows that for teenage girls who continue in sports, their primary motivator is having fun. Other motivators are gaining approval and respect, making their parents proud, feeling good about doing well, making friends and keeping in shape.[14]

Women's sports are still underrepresented in the media, even though this is changing. It is important for girls to have plenty of positive female role models, and to see healthy female athletes of all sizes in the media, not just thin ones. It will also help if journalists report on women athletes by emphasizing their ability, strength and skill, not exploiting femininity or appearance.

Activity programs

In planning an individualized activity or training program, Zelasko offers these recommendations for parents and health professionals:

- **Emphasize consistency first.** Since the goal is to maintain a lifetime of increased physical activity, it is most important to develop the exercise habit. Therefore, develop an easy, minimal workout and a consistent pattern of activity before moving to any in-depth, progressive fitness program.
- **Encourage duration, intensity and frequency.** Consistency is most important, but these factors are also important in building fitness and improving health as the program progresses.
- **Intermittent exercise is okay.** If the individual cannot sustain 10 or 20 minutes at one level, it is okay to break the sessions into segments. Alternating low or moderate intensity work is interval training, often used by athletes to increase strength and endurance.
- **Be a good example.** Parents who want their children to gain the benefits of lifetime physical activity are most helpful by modelling what lifetime activity means.
- **Respect the large youngster.** Everyone deserves respect no matter what his or her body weight. Nurturing is important. Maybe the child will lose weight or grow into the weight. Maybe not. But they can be healthier by exercising regularly and should be reassured of these benefits.
- **Understand physical and emotional needs.** For kids who have been inactive, it takes time to gain confidence in moving the body. They may need to overcome shyness about using their body. As they become more successful, they enjoy activity more, and are more likely to continue. When choosing a fitness facility, it is important to find one where trainers respect the emotional and physical needs of the child.

It also helps for parents to get involved with their youngsters in developing community opportunities for sports activities, safe biking and hiking trails, swimming pools, basketball and tennis courts, and local events and games.

CHAPTER 14

Changing to a child-friendly culture

■

In a culture that attacks people for being different sizes, we must accept some of the responsibility for allowing the messages. And we must make changes.

If we want our children to grow up in families that love and talk to each other, we can work toward that goal. If we want our children to grow up with solid, positive self respect and body images, we can work to encourage them. If we want girls to grow up free from sexual harassment, then we can stop it.

If we want the media to reflect to us images of healthy people in a range of sizes, then we can work toward that. If we want our children, who are afraid to eat, to grow up eating normally and making healthy lifestyle choices, then we can support these choices.

Taking back our culture

Changing culture is a monumental task, but it is possible. Strong forces and powerful commercial interests have molded today's society, and change won't be easy, nor will it happen overnight. But each of us can make a difference, starting now.

Changing our society into one that values healthy living and diverse sizes means enlisting professionals and the public.

There are numerous signs that people are ready for a change. Everywhere I find audiences enthusiastic about the health at any size philosophy, whether they are health professionals, teachers, or parents. People are hungry for messages of body acceptance, self-trust, normalized eating, freedom from dieting, balance, and getting on with life. The media is also receptive and interested.

The mood of the public is swinging toward a yearning for stronger family values, for safer and more nurturing communities. Leaders everywhere are taking up the cause of strengthening the family and lessening the impact of commercial culture's destructive elements.

Worldwide, there is backlash against fashion's excesses in portraying malnutrition as glamorous. When Omega decided to pull its ads from British *Vogue* in protest against skeletal models Trish Goff and Annie Morton showing underwear and sportswear, the public and media overwhelmingly supported the Swiss watchmaker. "It was irresponsible for a leading magazine, which should be setting an example, to select models of anorexic proportions," said Giles Rees, British Omega marketing manager.

Following a damning British Medical Association report that blamed the media's obsession with thin women as the main reason eating disorders have reached record levels, the British government convened a 2000 Body Image Summit. The meeting brought together medical experts, editors, media producers and designers. Medical concerns were raised about the thinness of catwalk models, actresses and singers such as Victoria Beckham (Posh Spice), Courtney Cox and Calista Flockhart, role models for many young women. The fashion world agreed they'd prefer self-regulation in trying to use "models who varied in shape and size" rather than federal monitoring.[1]

In Argentina the Senate passed a bill, June 2000, requiring clothing manufacturers to make clothes that fit women of all sizes, amid reports that one in 10 Argentine girls suffers from an eating disorder, and complaints that stores stock apparel only for thin women. "Every day the situation gets worse and more young people are affected by bulimia and anorexia," charged Leopoldo Moreau, the bill's sponsor.[2]

"The time is here to take all that energy and passion and together work through the process of actually starting a revolution, a health at any size revolution!" challenges Canadian dietitian Linda Omichinski.

We are at the point where the 100th monkey has jumped the

island, as in the story of how wisdom spreads. One monkey tells another and that monkey tells another and another, until they create such momentum that the 100th monkey and then many more jump from island to island, rapidly spreading the message.

With the magic of the Internet, island barriers are disappearing, and the health at any size revolution can quickly spread globally.

Female diversity in role models

In making changes, it's critical the media reflect the rich diversity of women in our society, depicting women as real people with diverse talents, deserving of respect. Girls need to see happy, popular, competent females in a wide range of sizes, ages, ethnicities, and even attractiveness, so girls who are not the most beautiful in class will be encouraged to feel good about themselves and their future.

We want our daughters to grow up as strong, capable, generous, loving women. So how do we shift their main role models to this, from today's thin, weak, sexually vulnerable, self-absorbed celebrities?

How do we combat beauty standards so narrow that women in the media all seem to look alike — hollow-cheeked, passive, focused on their appearance, vulnerable and extremely thin? As decorative or sexual objects to be admired, used, discarded? It's a stereotype that sets 9-year-olds dieting and teaches adolescent girls that their developing bodies will never be good enough. It compels young girls to live as if they are being constantly watched, desired, judged.

As women move into decision-making positions in the media, I have hoped this would change. It hasn't happened yet, despite the many advances made by women. Instead, female leaders have seemed all too willing to perpetuate the same stereotypes.

But I believe women are ready to turn this around and are in a position to do it. Those who are executives, producers, editors, reporters, models and actresses will make this needed shift, first in their own lives, then with powerful effect through their work. They will stop portraying women as objects and playthings, and liberate young women from conflicts over this role and its false images.

Leadership may also come from the women's movement, which can find a new cause in defending young girls and women from the excesses of the cult of thinness.

I've been encouraged by the public's enthusiastic response to women's athletic achievements, and to the few female entertainers who don't fit the stereotype, such as Camryn Manheim, Rosie O'Donnell, Roseanne, and Oprah Winfrey. I applaud women politicians like Janet Reno who, when she appears on television, doesn't look as if she's spent the last four hours in the beauty shop, but working at her desk like millions of women across the country. Yet why are these images so rare? How can we multiply them?

With pressure from subscribers and public criticism, the producers of girls' teen magazines can come to change their focus from today's tiresome replay of lookism and return to their missions. Once these magazines supported girls in improving their lives, but most now seem aimed only at delivering them to advertisers; they are little more than expensive catalogs. They will either include more stories on sports, careers, hobbies, and normal young women doing interesting things, or disappear — if readers will stop buying and tell the world why.

Fashion magazines may be even more damaging, and perhaps as in Britain, the threat of government regulation may bring changes.

Two or three visionary editors can turn this around. When a few leading magazines begin to depict girls and women of all sizes and ages in both editorial and advertising copy, rapid change is bound to follow. Can you imagine how stunned other editors, television producers, and Hollywood itself would be to discover the beauty, charm and unique talents of real women in all their diversity?

The new freedom of exchange on the Internet offers opportunities never before possible. It gives consumers unprecedented power in zeroing in on unscrupulous advertising and spreading the word to bring about change. An Internet campaign against an advertiser who exploits young people will have powerful effect — the threat may be enough. Unfortunately, we've already seen that not always will this be well-informed. But on balance, I believe it can work successfully against harmful elements in society.

Already the Internet is helping people break through barriers. After all, on the Net communication counts and appearance doesn't matter.

Boycott offensive advertisers

Taking on destructive media messages — in television, movies, books, magazines, newspapers, advertising, billboards, music — can be effective. Responsible journalists and media are powerful allies.

Multinational companies advertising throughout the world have seized unprecedented power in creating body dissatisfaction, negatively impacting cultures everywhere. But we need not accept their dominance. After all, they are pleading for our money, and that's a position of weakness, not strength. We can refuse to play their game.

We can reverse the adulation of malnourished female bodies. Will you refuse to buy any product that exploits body dissatisfaction in its advertising? Will you share your outrage with others? Will you refuse to watch television shows or movies that stereotype women — or if you do, contact producers, stations and advertisers about your dissatisfaction? If you are in the media or a media decision-maker, will you refuse to promote the thin stereotype? If so, you're part of the solution. Congratulations!

Regardless of difficulty, cultural changes *can* be made. In *Reviving Ophelia*, Mary Pipher calls on her readers to help girls fight cultural pressures, encourage their emotional toughness and self-protection, strengthen and guide them.

"Most important, we can change our culture. We can work together to build a culture that is less complicated and more nurturing, less violent and sexualized and more growth-producing. Our daughters deserve a society in which all their gifts can be developed and appreciated."

Pipher warns of the harm in today's portrayal of women in the media, as expensive toys, the ultimate recreation, "half-clad and half-witted, often awaiting rescue by quick-thinking, fully clothed men."[3]

Men and women concerned with these issues can work together to change the focus of responsible media and advertising, and to deflate the poisonous influence of its irresponsible fringe. The idealization of malnourished female bodies is continuing and worsening, not lessening, as rumored, so responsive action is sorely needed. A boycott can be extremely effective.

Letters, phone calls, faxes, email and Internet campaigns are effective in combatting these destructive images. Targeting offensive advertisers is important, but the medium that runs the ads should not be let off easy either. Magazines, newspapers and stations are responsible for ads they feed their audience. Editors keep a wary eye on marketing and routinely slant articles and shows to please their advertisers, often to the detriment of the public, as in smoking ads. They can be pressured, instead, to edit to reader demand.

On a more impulsive note, vigilantes are striking at offensive displays on billboards and buses by scrawling graffiti over thin women's bodies. "I'm So Hungry," lamented the caption on one gaunt model. "Please Give Me a Cheeseburger," another pleaded.

Parents and consumer groups can be vigilant in making strong complaints. I'd like to see an outpouring of organized support for positive portrayals, along with meaningful protests of the offensive. On their website, the Eating Disorder Awareness and Prevention group makes this easy. You can add your name to well-written letters of protest and support, report exploitive advertisers, and glean ideas to move ahead with other campaigns.

EDAP's Media Advocacy Campaign brought an end to four negative national advertising campaigns in a short time. Avia Sportswear no longer features an ad proclaiming, "Although fitness trainers gave advice, the mirror was her dedicated coach," and offered to involve EDAP in the early planning stages of future marketing programs.

Nicole Shoes apologized for claiming, "The pair you wear to your cooking class will also look fabulous at your weight loss seminar." A spokesman wrote, "We admit a mistake was made . . . and will follow the guidelines and principles you have outlined in your pamphlet for future advertising endeavours."[4]

It is my hope that readers of this book will be inspired to initiate changes aimed at respecting size diversity, and the diversity of women. You can't do everything, but if you are concerned with these issues, you can choose one or two ideas to work on personally or professionally. I believe each of us *can* make a difference, all alone. Together we can create a miracle.

"Never doubt that a handful of committed individuals can truly change the world," anthropologist Margaret Mead reminds us.

Inoculate with education, strong families

Our children do not have to be pawns in this game. They can be taught media literacy at home and school to protect their self concepts from narrow media stereotypes. Even young children can understand the advertisers' self-interest in creating body dissatisfaction to sell products. They can learn that extreme images do not represent real young people who have real lives and interesting futures.

Demonstrating the ease with which photos are computerized today makes media images even less believable. Both boys and girls need to learn a skepticism for advertising and the manipulative language that suggests a man's or woman's body and face always needs fixing — it's never quite good enough.

They can learn how media images constrain not just their body shape, but their behavior. Gail Huon, a psychologist at the University of South Wales in Sydney, Australia, says girls must be taught to critically review the media images, articles and advertising not only for female thinness, but also for passiveness and submissiveness. They need to examine how women are portrayed in advertising as "property," and as waiting, receptive, ready to contribute to someone else's life.[5]

We can pay more attention to the concerns diverse ethnic groups have for their children. An awareness is also needed for the problems encountered by immigrant teens — the loss and loneliness from missing out on shared experiences with peers; difficulty from their efforts to adapt and cope; feelings of rejection and helplessness in a new culture; confusion in terms of role expectations, values and identity.

Strong families that provide support for individuality and healthy development are the most powerful force in minimizing these effects. Perhaps the most resiliant factor for ethnic minority youth is identification with family and community. The bonding and sharing of values for families of people of color can provide strength and resources against the ravages of ethnic and gender discrimination. In this they need the support of the wider culture.[6]

Protecting youth from abuse

Eating disorders and other disturbed eating patterns may begin as ways of coping with the trauma, violence, sexual abuse, physical abuse, harassment, bullying or stigmatization that is so pervasive in our culture, and even glamorized in the media. Communities, schools and families can work together to protect our boys and girls from these violations of the self, which often impact body image, eating and weight in harmful ways.

Youth who are singled out for special torment by their peers, or stigmatized because of their size, appearance, disability, sexual orientation, or ethnicity deserve protection by the adults in their lives.

The National Education Association has declared itself against size prejudice in the schools. This largest teacher organization in the country pledged in 1994 to "support efforts to foster an improved teaching and learning environment for colleagues and students who have special needs due to physical size."[7]

Most teachers I speak with seem eager to support a policy of zero tolerance for size bias in the schools. They agree it's time to implement this policy.

Sexual harassment

Sexual harassment is one of the ways in which young girls' pleasure about their developing bodies is destroyed, experts say. It can alienate them from self, cause them to hate their bodies as a separate part of themselves, and oppress them with an overwhelming sense of shame.

Sexual harassment is seldom discussed, so victims bear their shame in secret. Boys, showing off for their peers, may not understand the harm they inflict with teasing or taunting remarks. Girls, too, are often the harrassers and oppressors. In combatting this, consciousness-raising groups are enlightening and empowering. They provide tools for young people to fight the weapons of oppression, share stories of resistance and empowerment, instill a sense of pride in their bodies and themselves, creating a force to be reckoned with.

Can you imagine girls, their parents and teachers taking power across the country in disallowing size bias or sexual harassment? I can, and it would make a big difference.

Consider this scenario: Instead of silently and individually absorbing abuse from disparaging remarks in the school hallway, a group of girls decides to view it as an opportunity to document what's going on. They pull out notebooks and write it all down — date, time, who said or did what. With this documentation over a period of several weeks, they present their case to school officials, teachers, counselors, parents, clergy and other adults willing to listen. Following through with effective action will confirm they are not powerless. Even getting together to discuss action can help to dispel the shame they might otherwise feel.

Both boys and girls can be taught to recognize sexual harassment and know its consequences. They need to know what is not acceptable, to strengthen their resistance and increase support when it is breached — so boys don't go on to become the men whose firms are sued for sexual harassment and they can't understand why. It has been said there are no rules in sexual behavior — until they are broken. This is true for young men as well as young women. When rules are broken, it's as if the offenders should have known all along what was acceptable, and they feel betrayed because they didn't know.

Somehow boys as well as girls need to learn acceptable limits. Teaching skills such as negotiation, communication, anger management, problem solving and coping strategies will help. Educating both boys and girls in how to be loving and gentle can help curb violence and harassment.

Prevention efforts will also address the cultural structures that promote sexual exploitation and the manipulation of children's and women's bodies. Charles Dinn, publisher of *Pageantry* magazine, estimates that 100,000 children under the age of 12 perform in U.S. beauty pageants every year. Is it helpful that our society still dotes on beauty contests for little girls and young teens, displaying their young bodies, even nearly bared in swimsuit competitions?

Preventing sexual abuse

As a responsible society, ours needs to be doing more to protect young people and women from sexual violations. Concerned adults must find ways to stop these abuses which cause so much shame and disruption. Currently the responsibility for prevention has been put on children and parents. But it's not enough to teach potential victims to protect themselves. The spotlight needs to be turned on perpetrators.

"Young men need to be socialized in such a way that rape is as unthinkable to them as cannibalism," says Pipher. Potential abusers need to clearly understand the impact of sexual crime. Being convicted can mean, besides serving prison time as the least popular of prisoners, having one's whereabouts and criminal background publicized by police, perhaps for life.

Some experts advise airing public service messages that emphasize adult responsibility, like these:

- Sexual molestation of children is a crime.
- A child is unable to give consent.
- Sexual molestation of children involves an abuse of power and trust based on coercion and intimidation.
- Sexual molestation is damaging to children.
- Preventing sexual abuse is the exclusive responsibility of adults.

This type of education may not fit easily into a society such as ours which flaunts sexuality and the availability of sex, but has many taboos about discussing sexuality and abusive sexual incidents. Yet it is imperative that ways be found to do this.

Abuse may occur where least expected. Piran and colleagues in Toronto advise informing first-time parents of the high incidence of sexual abuse within the family or by close relatives, the tendency to deny abuse, and how to build a protective environment for their children. They warn of incest, and recommend that new parents be targeted for intervention, informed about appropriate and inappropriate touching, and how to detect in oneself or one's mate an inclination toward inappropriate touching, and what to do about it. Discussing healthy sexuality with children in a positive context may provide opportunities to identify abnormal and destructive sexual situations they may have experienced.

In *Reviving Ophelia*, Pipher says the incidence of rape is increasing because of our culture's increasingly destructive messages about sexuality. "Sex is currently associated with violence, power, domination and status." She points out that rape hurts everyone, not just its victims. It keeps all women in a state of fear about men. Men are fearful for their women friends and aware that women are afraid of them. But mostly rape damages young women. Pipher quotes statistics that show 41 percent of rape victims expect to be raped again, 30 percent contemplate suicide, 31 percent go into therapy, and 82 percent say their lives are permanently changed.

We need to acknowledge the high rates of sexual abuse of women and children, boys as well as girls. Perhaps then more and more victims will break their silence, reveal their stories, and refuse to protect those who have abused them.

Above all, we need to respect and appreciate each other as human beings.

Stop fearmongering

Reducing our culture's confusion and fears over health and food issues would help children and their families eat normally again.

Elizabeth Whelan, president of the American Council on Science and Health, calls on scientists, policy makers, the media and consumers to stop the fearmongering and "food terrorism" in the press, and implement changes such as the following:[8]

- Emphasize that our food supply is safe. Keep reassuring the public of the truth: America's food supply is one of the safest and healthiest the world has ever known. The rarity of adverse incidents proves, rather than disputes, this fact.
- Return to mainstream science that defends reason and rationality. Many scientists don't want to get involved; yet they must explain science in terms that clarify relative risks and nonrisks.
- Emphasize healthy nutrition messages and insist on balance. Restore acceptance of the basic principle that health depends on the total diet, not on a few special components. Convey the message that all foods can fit in a healthy diet.
- Diffuse the power of "health terrorists" to grab headlines, whether ill-informed consumer groups, journalists on a mission, talk show hosts seeking higher ratings, radical animal rights groups, or scientists shoring up grant funding — spokesmen from the "Chicken Little School of Environmental Hyperbole."

- Expose the corruption of "politically correct science" that takes a stand against industry, technology, and free enterprise. This trendy ideology makes environmentalism and consumerism the new religion, and distorts reality by ignoring science, reason and rationality. Whelan says it has infused the press with false notions that health is at exaggerated risk from additives, preservatives and substances used to increase food production.

Whelan also calls for reducing the influence of the tobacco industry in its role of diverting attention from real health risks. She points out that when over 1,300 Americans die prematurely every day from tobacco use, and some 300 die of the affects of alcohol every day, it is almost ludicrous that nonrisks get the major headlines.

Federal policy impacts culture

National policy greatly influences how the media reports health issues, and how the public and health community respond. It sets the stage for what happens throughout the country. Unfortunately, national leaders in the United States are continuing to exaggerate the risks of obesity, based on selective research, to ignore the risks of eating disorders and related problems, and discount health professionals and consumer groups who disagree.

Canada is again showing leadership in bringing together a national consensus to develop a population health approach. This is dedicated to helping health professionals and policy makers use the most solid information available in making decisions, and to make sure that these decisions reflect the values and principles of Canadians.

We need to require that federal health officials and the National Institutes of Health take a more responsible role in this country. They have spent a quarter of a century and billions of tax dollars on the failed quest to make fat people thin. Certainly it is time to begin research on how to make them healthier, independent of weight.

Why does our culture ignore the deaths and damaging of so many children and young women from weight loss efforts and eating disorders? Why is there no public outcry about the nutrient deficiencies and malnutrition that haunt young girls — and increasingly, young boys — today?

Official recognition of eating disorders is, I believe, the key to bringing about needed change in federal policy. In the U.S. we have about 16 million girls between the ages of 13 and 20, according to the last census. If 10 percent of these girls have clinical eating disorders, and one-fourth are severely undernourished, what are the numbers here? Are they enough to gain a polititian's attention?

When eating disorders and related problems get the attention they need, policy makers will be forced to change their approach to obesity, so as not to exacerbate eating problems. A health-centered approach is the most logical when one looks at the big picture.

These policy changes are needed now:

- Include eating disorders prevention, awareness, and treatment in Healthy People 2010, the Women's Health Initiative, and obesity prevention programs. Related issues — dysfunctional eating, the undernutrition of teenage girls, hazardous weight loss, size prejudice and body image concerns — will follow naturally as part of this.
- Direct the National Center for Health Statistics to gather data on eating disorder prevalence, death and morbidity — a responsibility it has long neglected.
- Choose an independent panel to appoint federal obesity advisory groups. Set a firm policy to limit advisors with vested interests and include consumers of size, those most affected.
- Replace the NIH Guidelines definition of overweight (body mass index of 25) with a more realistic one. A metabolic fitness definition that depends on actual risk factors, not weight, is preferable. If BMI is part of the definition, set it at a higher level, adjusting for age and ethnicity.
- End the fiction that weight loss treatments are effective. Stop spending tax money on industry-serving reports like the NIH Guidelines on treating obesity. Stop promoting health insurance coverage of useless weight loss treatments.
- Require that five-year safety, effectiveness, and health outcome data be provided on all weight loss treatments *before* they are used or marketed to the public.
- Require weight loss programs to publish outcomes in ways that

are verifiable. Require they track changes in eating behavior, any complications, short- and long-term weight loss, and fat loss relative to loss of lean body mass.

- Regulate the weight loss industry in the same ways other health-related industries are regulated.
- Establish federal reporting of deaths and injuries related to weight loss efforts.

These problems are not simple, but unnecessary barriers are adding to the difficulty of solving them. Eating disorder prevention is stalled because of resistance at federal levels. Some leaders fear that addressing eating issues will set back anti-obesity efforts. Others dismiss eating problems as women's issues that affect only a few.

The answer may be new leadership. We especially need knowledgeable, visionary female leadership at the forefront. Already there is some progress. For the first time ever in July 1997, a congressional briefing focused on the problems of eating disorders.[9]

"Eating disorders is a women's issue that demands national attention. I believe that it's our responsibility to educate at the federal level," said Rep. Nita Lowey, of New York, one of the sponsors of the briefing. "What's amazing to me is that there is really no federal effort to educate the public."

Lowey and Rep. Louise Slaughter, New York, asked Congress to provide funding for research on prevention and treatment of eating disorders, to hold a concensus conference to examine the issues, and to launch an awareness and public education campaign.

The time has come to move forward. Visionary women and men working in federal policy and professional associations can take leadership now to make needed changes. The public can demand it. If we work together, it will happen. By taking action now, we can change our culture in positive ways. We can have an impact on what happens in Washington and in the pages of popular magazines.

CHAPTER 15

Call to action

■

It's time to move forward with vision. This is an urgent challenge for America and for the world community. We need to deal with the current weight and eating crisis in healthy ways — ways that don't repeat the mistakes of the past.

The new philosophy of Health at Any Size recognizes the interconnectedness of the six major problems: dysfunctional or disordered eating, undernutrition of teenage girls, hazardous weight loss, eating disorders, overweight and size prejudice. It promotes healthy growth and development of the whole person in mind, body and spirit, and it includes people of all sizes.

The process of furthering this vision needs to involve experts and lay people, teachers and parents, health care providers and community leaders — people of insight and integrity, with an understanding of the needs and concerns of children, women and minorities.[1]

How can we reach a shared vision and effectively communicate that vision? How can we promote wellness and wholeness in positive ways for children of all sizes? How can we help children understand that their bodies are good bodies? That their size is okay?

Encouraging health at any size challenges us to make changes in these five areas: attitude, lifestyle, prevention, health care, and knowledge.

1. Attitude shift

The health-centered approach advocates a shift in attitudes toward:

- Wider awareness and concern for weight and eating issues, for their interrelatedness, their importance to health and well-being.
- Greater appreciation for healthy lifestyles and balanced living (apart from size) to help children feel good about making healthy changes in their lives. Appreciation of the pleasurable aspects and benefits of a healthy lifestyle.
- Less concern for appearance and more on worth of the individual: on character, responsibility, talent, achievement, and relationships with family and community. Convey to girls and women who may be fixated on appearance that when well-nourished, they can live richer, fuller, more interesting lives.
- Acceptance of a wider range of sizes; more tolerance of differences, respect, appreciation of diversity, and recognition that beauty comes in all shapes and sizes. Rejection of extreme thinness (or any size or shape) as the ideal body type.
- Stronger sense of outrage and refusal to allow violations of persons — harassment, stigmatization, bullying, and mental, physical or sexual abuse.
- Increased determination to reduce the impact of negative media, and support for responsible media as an instrument for positive change.

2. Healthy lifestyles

The new approach promotes healthy lifestyles which embrace:

- Pleasurable, normal eating and a moderate, varied, balanced nutrition, moderately low in fat, avoiding extremes.
- Active living by improving physical education programs in schools and motivating youth to continue being active through life. Encourage active living through national public health programs.
- Promoting the attainment and maintenance for growing children of weights genetically appropriate for them, and stable weights for adults. Stop dieting; stop ineffective, unsafe weight loss.
- Managing stress levels. Promote effective ways to reduce and manage stress. Enhance self-respect, self-acceptance, feelings

of being needed, and positive relations with family, friends, community. Focus on balance, moderation and contentment in life. Avoid extremes.

- Reducing violence, sexual abuse, harassment and stigmatization, particularly against children and young women. Find effective ways to protect girls from aggressive men. Provide counseling accessibility and support for victims. Increase law enforcement and incarceration to separate abusers from potential victims.

- Promoting environments that support being active, eating well, reducing stress and appreciating size diversity through schools, health care providers, the community, media and home. Communities can do much to encourage active living: develop safe, well-lighted playgrounds, parks, swimming pools, skating rinks, and trails for walking, bicycling and cross-country skiing; open school gyms to the public, provide recreation centers, and organize community fitness events.

3. Prevention focus

The health-centered approach to prevention will:

- Promote prevention at three levels: primary (reducing eating and weight problems for all youngsters); secondary (identify and help high-risk youth or those with early stage problems, while avoiding stigmatization); tertiary (effectively treating youth with eating disorders or weight problems).

- Integrate prevention approaches. The prevention of obesity cannot be separated from the prevention of eating disorders and related problems. While trying to improve one area, do no harm in others.

- Continue to develop, test, evaluate and fine-tune preventive programs used in schools, community and health care. Recognize the risks in prematurely adopting preventive programs, without proof of safety and effectiveness.

- Move forward with tested programs. Integrate a needs assessment and measurable goals and objectives. Work with an active advisory council. Sustained, comprehensive efforts that encompass school, community and families will be most effective.

- Expand the National Eating Disorders Screening Program to more schools and communities. Follow up with participants needing or requesting help.
- Promote Eating Disorders Awareness and Prevention Week in February. Support and expand the work of EDAP-trained co-ordinators and teams.
- Develop consciousness-raising and support groups.
- Teach body image, growth and puberty changes in curricula from elementary through junior high.
- Teach media literacy at all levels, from elementary school through college classes in marketing, psychology, health and nutrition. Promote ability to question, evaluate, understand and respond.
- Enlist the media in promoting positive images, portraying strong, talented, intelligent women of diverse sizes, ages and ethnicity.
- Promote responsible reporting of health news, keeping risks in perspective, avoiding sensationalizing. Expose "health terrorists" and unsound politically correct views.

4. Health care

A health promoting shift in policy and health care services will:

- Ensure that health professionals consistently promote healthy lifestyles for children of all sizes, that they avoid weight cycling programs and ineffective weight loss for youthful patients.
- Reduce size prejudice in health care. Educate health care providers of the need for acceptance of patients of every size, and help them overcome size biases, so that large children feel assured of sensitive, respectful treatment.
- Identify and treat dysfunctional or disordered eating at early stages, when it is more easily treatable. Identify and treat under-nutrition among girls.
- Improve access to qualified services for high-risk populations.
- Call a moratorium on weight loss treatment — especially diets, drugs and surgery — until there is reasonable proof of long-term (five year) safety and effectiveness. It's time to up the ante and also insist on evidence of long-term health improvement (or at least the absence of harm), and optimal fat versus lean loss.

- Regulate obesity treatment. Require full disclosure and account-ability, reporting of weight loss and fat loss results, adverse effects, morbidity and mortality. Require adequate safety and effectiveness studies before going ahead with treatment, using five-year data as called for in American Heart Association guide-lines.[2]
- Add eating disorders, undernutrition and hazardous weight loss to the nutrition priorities in updates of Healthy People 2010 and other initiatives, establishing baselines and measurable targets.
- Develop a sound policy for use of weight loss drugs. The potential for abuse now and in the future is high. Require cred-ible studies demonstrating long-term safety and effectiveness, not one-year studies, as today. Begin dialogue on ethical use of drugs: When more effective drugs become available should they be prescribed widely for children? Should they be available without prescription?[3]

5. Knowledge expansion

In meeting challenges for research and information, the comprehensive health-centered approach, will:

- Ensure that nutrition and dietetic schools develop effective be-havior-change courses in weight and eating issues, preventive programs and support groups to deal with the high rates of eating disorders and related problems now rampant among col-lege students, including in their own departments. Solve the problem of sending out young professionals in the health sci-ences who have serious eating issues of their own.
- Provide medical school training and continuing education on eating and weight issues, eating disorders, and the risks and prevalence of undernutrition among children and young women.
- Encourage medical schools to require basic studies in eating disorders, obesity and nutrition. At the same time, encourage young doctors to rely on nutritionists and dietitians with special training in these areas, and to refer patients to specialists.
- Consolidate eating and weight studies into one academic de-partment within a specific field such as nutrition or health, de-

veloping graduate programs to train specialists. This will move the field ahead more rapidly. Bringing these now-fragmented specialties together into one field of study will mean the information is researched, analyzed and used in more comprehensive ways, and that the power of vested interests is lessened.

- Communicate and disseminate science-based information in more comprehensive, health-promoting ways to both health providers and consumers.

- Encourage women researchers to take more leadership positions, report at conferences, and publish in scientific literature. This will move forward more quickly issues related to women's health care and concerns, including eating disorders and related problems.

- Raise ethical standards. Require full disclosure of funding and commercial relationships at scientific conferences, on journal editorial boards and in public policy, to reduce the influence of vested interests, particularly by the weight loss industry. (Research and federal policy on obesity are uniquely vulnerable to vested interests.) Expose manipulative research reporting, in the public's best interest, and drop the fiction that current obesity treatments are safe and effective.

- Increase research study of the six major eating and weight problems (dysfunctional or disordered eating, undernutrition of teenage girls, hazardous weight loss, eating disorders, overweight, size prejudice), their etiology, causes, treatment and prevention. Extend study on normal eating; body regulation of weight, hunger, appetite and satiety; the physical and mental effects of starvation and semistarvation; the nature of the "thrifty gene" and how it impacts populations undergoing cultural change.

If we pull together to accomplish these goals, we can create a better world where children grow healthy and happy at their natural sizes and are no longer afraid to eat.

APPENDIX

Body Mass Index for Selected Weight and Stature

Stature m (in)

Weight kg (lb)	1.24 (49)	1.27 (50)	1.30 (51)	1.32 (52)	1.35 (53)	1.37 (54)	1.40 (55)	1.42 (56)	1.45 (57)	1.47 (58)	1.50 (59)	1.52 (60)	1.55 (61)	1.57 (62)	1.60 (63)	1.63 (64)	1.65 (65)	1.68 (66)	1.70 (67)	1.73 (68)	1.75 (69)	1.78 (70)	1.80 (71)	1.83 (72)	1.85 (73)	1.88 (74)	1.90 (75)	1.93 (76)
20 (45)	13	13	12	12	11	11	10	10	10	9	9	9	8															
23 (50)	15	14	13	13	12	12	12	11	11	10	10	10	9	9	9	9	8											
25 (55)	16	15	15	14	14	13	13	12	12	12	11	11	10	10	10	9	9	9										
27 (60)	18	17	16	16	15	15	14	13	13	13	12	12	11	11	11	10	10	10	9	9								
29 (65)	19	18	17	17	16	16	15	15	14	14	13	13	12	12	12	11	11	10	10	10	10							
32 (70)	21	20	19	18	17	17	16	16	15	15	14	14	13	13	12	12	12	11	11	11	10	10						
34 (75)	22	21	20	20	19	18	17	17	16	16	15	15	14	14	13	13	12	12	12	11	11	11	10					
36 (80)	24	22	21	21	20	19	19	18	17	17	16	16	15	15	14	14	13	13	13	12	12	11	11	11				
39 (85)	25	24	23	22	21	21	20	19	18	18	17	17	16	16	15	15	14	14	13	13	13	12	12	12	11			
41 (90)	27	25	24	23	22	22	21	20	19	19	18	18	17	17	16	15	15	14	14	14	13	13	12	12	12			
43 (95)	28	27	25	25	24	23	22	22	21	20	20	19	18	18	17	17	16	16	15	15	14	14	14	13	13	13	12	
45 (100)	29	28	27	26	25	24	24	23	22	21	21	20	19	19	18	17	17	16	16	15	15	14	14	14	13	13	13	12
48 (105)	31	30	28	27	26	25	24	24	23	22	21	21	20	19	19	18	17	17	16	16	16	15	15	14	14	13	13	13
50 (110)	32	31	30	29	27	27	25	25	24	23	22	22	21	20	19	19	18	18	17	17	16	16	15	15	15	14	14	13
52 (115)	34	32	31	30	29	28	27	26	25	24	23	23	22	21	20	20	19	18	18	17	17	16	16	15	15	15	14	14
54 (120)	35	34	32	31	30	29	28	27	26	25	24	24	23	22	21	20	20	19	19	18	18	17	17	16	16	15	15	15
57 (125)	37	35	34	33	31	30	29	28	27	26	25	25	24	23	22	21	21	20	20	19	19	18	17	17	17	16	16	15
59 (130)	38	37	35	34	32	31	30	29	28	27	26	26	25	24	23	22	22	21	20	20	19	19	18	18	17	17	16	16
61 (135)	40	38	36	35	34	33	31	30	29	28	27	27	25	25	24	23	22	22	21	20	20	19	19	18	18	17	17	16
64 (140)	41	39	38	36	35	34	32	31	30	29	28	27	27	26	25	24	23	23	22	22	21	20	20	19	19	18	18	17
66 (145)	43	41	39	38	36	35	34	33	31	30	29	28	27	27	26	25	24	23	23	22	21	21	20	20	19	19	18	18
68 (150)	44	42	40	39	37	36	35	34	32	31	30	29	28	28	27	26	25	24	24	23	22	21	21	20	20	19	19	18
70 (155)	46	44	42	40	39	37	36	35	33	33	31	30	29	29	27	26	26	25	24	23	23	22	22	21	21	20	19	19
73 (160)	47	45	43	42	40	39	37	36	35	34	32	31	30	29	28	27	27	26	25	24	24	23	22	22	21	21	20	19
77 (170)	50	48	46	44	42	41	39	38	37	36	34	33	32	31	30	29	28	27	27	26	25	24	24	23	23	22	21	21
79 (175)		49	47	46	44	42	40	39	38	37	35	34	33	32	31	30	29	28	27	27	26	25	24	24	23	22	22	21
82 (180)		51	48	47	45	44	42	40	39	38	36	35	34	33	32	31	30	29	28	27	27	26	25	24	24	23	23	22
84 (185)			50	48	46	45	43	42	40	39	37	36	35	34	32	31	30	29	28	27	27	26	25	25	24	23	23	22
86 (190)			51	49	47	46	44	43	41	40	38	37	36	35	34	32	32	31	30	29	28	27	27	26	25	24	24	23
88 (195)				51	49	47	45	44	42	41	39	38	37	36	35	33	33	31	31	30	29	28	27	26	26	25	25	24
91 (200)					50	48	46	45	43	42	40	39	38	37	35	34	33	32	31	30	30	29	28	27	27	26	25	24
93 (205)					51	50	47	46	44	43	41	40	39	38	36	35	34	33	32	31	30	29	29	28	27	26	26	25
95 (210)						51	49	47	45	44	42	41	40	39	37	36	35	34	33	32	31	30	29	28	28	27	26	26
98 (215)							50	48	46	45	43	42	41	40	38	37	36	35	34	33	32	31	30	29	28	28	27	26
100 (220)							51	50	47	46	44	43	42	40	39	38	37	35	35	33	33	32	31	30	29	28	28	27
102 (225)								51	49	47	45	44	42	41	40	38	37	36	35	34	33	32	32	30	30	29	28	27
104 (230)									50	48	46	45	43	42	41	39	38	37	36	35	34	33	32	31	30	30	29	28
107 (235)									51	49	47	46	44	43	42	40	39	38	37	36	35	34	33	32	31	30	30	29
109 (240)										50	48	47	45	44	43	41	40	39	38	36	36	34	34	33	32	31	30	29
111 (245)											49	48	46	45	43	42	41	39	38	37	36	35	34	33	32	31	31	30
113 (250)											50	49	47	46	44	43	42	40	39	38	37	36	35	34	33	32	31	30
116 (255)												50	48	47	45	44	42	41	40	39	38	37	36	35	34	33	32	31
118 (260)												51	49	48	46	44	43	42	41	39	38	37	36	35	34	33	33	32
120 (265)													50	49	47	45	44	43	42	40	39	38	37	36	35	34	33	32
122 (270)													51	50	48	46	45	43	42	41	40	39	38	37	36	35	34	33
125 (275)														51	49	47	46	44	43	42	41	39	38	37	36	35	35	33
127 (280)															50	48	47	45	44	42	41	40	39	38	37	36	35	34
129 (285)															50	49	47	46	45	43	42	41	40	39	38	37	36	35
132 (290)																50	48	47	46	44	43	42	41	39	38	37	36	35
134 (295)																50	49	47	46	45	44	42	41	40	39	38	37	36
136 (300)																	50	48	47	45	44	43	42	41	40	39	38	37

© 1995 American Medical Association

Median daily intake — male

Percent of Recommended Dietary Allowances (RDAs)

Nutrient	12-15 years			16-19 years			20-59 years			≥60 years		
	NHW	NHB	MA	NHW	NHB	MA	NHW	NHB	MA	NHW	NHB	MA
Food energy	102	92	84	106	89	82	90	84	82	81	67	72
Protein	184	160	187	173	163	156	149	140	152	117	103	113
Vitamin A	85	55	70	77	55	67	78	53	62	91	55	61
Vitamin E	68*	74	67	93	92	77	90	75	80	70	51	59
Vitamin C	194	204	180	112	188	137	140	153	148	138	108	125
Thiamin	146	122	134	148	120	109	119	108	109	135	102	120
Riboflavin	169	120	147	148	120	118	129	102	116	139	108	119
Niacin	140	115	120	135	122	96	140	131	120	146	112	108
Vitamin B_6	110	92	95	104	93	83	100	89	98	89	65	67
Folate	203	133	169	140	106	132	146	114	144	141	100	122
Vitamin B_{12}	242	188	212	258	248	244	248	210	225	210	165	164
Calcium	90	60	85	103	76	79	113	74	103	90	62	82
Phosphorus	118	97	114	141	126	122	188	155	196	152	121	148
Magnesium	103	85	97	78	68	70	95	74	96	83	58	74
Iron	128	110	119	146	119	114	161	139	152	140	102	127
Zinc	77	59	70	90	82	80*	87	75	84	72	57	55
Copper	81	76	79	93	87	84	100	82	97	81	59	79
Sodium	154	137	134	194	179	134	161	151	143	128	98	118

NHW-nonHispanic white   NHB-nonHispanic black   MA-Mexican American

Shaded values indicate median intakes that are below recommended amounts, (for sodium, above) for boys and men. Considered to be current public health issues are the intakes of food energy (calories), calcium, iron and zinc. Potential public health issues for which further study is needed are the intakes of vitamin A, vitamin C, vitamin B_6 and folate. Values represent percentage of Recommended Dietary Allowances (RDAs); for food energy, values represent percentage of the Recommended Energy Intake (NRC, 1989a). An asterisk (*) indicates a statistic that is potentially unreliable. Third Report on Nutrition Monitoring in the U.S. Vol 1, p135. 1995. USDA, HHS, NHANES III, 1988-1991. *For intake of girls and women, see Chapter 9.*

National eating disorders screening program

Age ____   Sex ___   Height _____

Current weight _____   Highest weight _____   Lowest adult weight _____

EATING ATTITUDES TEST (EAT-26)

Please check a response for each	Always	Usually	Often	Sometimes	Rarely	Never
1. Am terrified about being overweight.	☐	☐	☐	☐	☐	☐
2. Avoid eating when I am hungry.	☐	☐	☐	☐	☐	☐
3. Find myself preoccupied with food.	☐	☐	☐	☐	☐	☐
4. Have gone on eating binges where I feel that I may be able to stop.	☐	☐	☐	☐	☐	☐
5. Cut my food into small pieces.	☐	☐	☐	☐	☐	☐
6. Aware of the calorie content of foods that I eat.	☐	☐	☐	☐	☐	☐
7. Particularly avoid food with a high carbohydrate content; i.e. bread, rice, potatoes, etc.	☐	☐	☐	☐	☐	☐
8. Feel that others would prefer if I ate more.	☐	☐	☐	☐	☐	☐
9. Vomit after I have eaten.	☐	☐	☐	☐	☐	☐
10. Feel extremely guilty after eating.	☐	☐	☐	☐	☐	☐
11. Am preoccupied with a desire to be thinner.	☐	☐	☐	☐	☐	☐
12. Think about burning up calories when I exercise.	☐	☐	☐	☐	☐	☐
13. Other people think that I am too thin.	☐	☐	☐	☐	☐	☐
14. Am preoccupied with the thought of having fat on my body.	☐	☐	☐	☐	☐	☐
15. Take longer than others to eat my meals.	☐	☐	☐	☐	☐	☐
16. Avoid foods with sugar in them.	☐	☐	☐	☐	☐	☐
17. Eat diet foods.	☐	☐	☐	☐	☐	☐
18. Feel that food controls my life.	☐	☐	☐	☐	☐	☐
19. Display self-control around food.	☐	☐	☐	☐	☐	☐
20. Feel that others pressure me to eat.	☐	☐	☐	☐	☐	☐
21. Give too much time and thought to food.	☐	☐	☐	☐	☐	☐
22. Feel uncomfortable after eating sweets.	☐	☐	☐	☐	☐	☐
23. Engage in dieting behavior.	☐	☐	☐	☐	☐	☐
24. Like my stomach to be empty.	☐	☐	☐	☐	☐	☐
25. Have the impulse to vomit after meals.	☐	☐	☐	☐	☐	☐
26. Enjoy trying new rich foods.	☐	☐	☐	☐	☐	☐
TOTAL EAT SCORE	__	__	__	__	__	__

Copyright David M. Garner and Paul E. Garfinkel, 1979. David M. Garner et al., 1982.

BEHAVIORAL SCREENING QUESTIONS

1. Have you gone on eating binges where you feel that you may be able to stop? (Eating much more than most people would eat under the same circumstances)

   NO   YES How many times in the last 6 months? _____

2. Have you ever made yourself sick (vomited) to control your weight or shape?

   NO   YES How many times in the last 6 months? _____

3. Have you ever used laxatives, diet pills or diuretics (water pills) to control your weight or shape?

   NO   YES How many times in the last 6 months? _____

4. Have you ever ben treated for an eating disorder?

   NO   YES When? _____

5. Have you recently thought of or attempted suicide?

   NO   YES When? _____

The five criteria for referring particpants for a follow-up evaluation are:

1. a score of more than 20 on the EAT-26;
2. a "yes" to any one of the behavioral screening questions;
3. a body mass index (BMI) below 18 *(see BMI chart, page **)*;
4. a respondent who feels that he or she has significant eating or weight concerns and therefore specifically requests a referral; or
5. the clinician, based on interview, believes that there is reason for referral.

Scoring instructions for EAT-26

Responses for items 1-25:
   always - 3; usually - 2; often - 1; sometimes, rarely, never - 0

Responses for item 26:
   always, usually, often - 0; sometimes - 1; rarely - 2; never - 3

Add to find the total EAT score.

Source: Garner DM, and Garfinkel PE. The Eating Attitudes Test: An index of the symptoms of anorexia nervosa. Copyright David M. Garner and Paul E. Garfinkel, 1979. *Psychological Medicine* 1979:9:273-279. David M. Garner et al., 1982.

Vegetarian self-test

Origin of vegetarian choice

1. I ate a variety of protein products as a child, but have gradually narrowed my protein choices to a few "acceptable" items.　　T　　F

2. I avoid animal-based foods as much as possible, but find that I get cravings that turn into binges.　　T　　F

3. I feel superior to others when I eat differently than them.　　T　　F

4. I eat nut butters, avocados, seeds, and fats on a regular basis.　　T　　F

5. Sometimes I think I would like to eat a piece of meat, but I am afraid to.　　T　　F

6. I feel less guilty about myself when I eat a vegetarian diet.　　T　　F

7. I can eat meatless products that look, taste, and smell exactly like meat without discomfort.　　T　　F

8. I am willing to eat 1/3 more volume of food and add a serving of fat to my meal plan to insure that my diet has the necessary amount of fat, calories, and protein.　　T　　F

9. I feel that people who eat less meat are more "perfect" or "acceptable" than people who eat meat.　　T　　F

10. Eating meat makes me feel uncomfortable.　　T　　F

Score 1 point for each *true* answer on numbers 4, 7 and 8; score 1 point for each *false* answer on numbers 1, 2, 3, 5, 6, 9 and 10. A score of 0 indicates a high probability that the vegetarian choice is disordered in its origin, and a score of 10 indicates a low probability of disordered motivation. In-between scores indicate the degree of disordered thoughts contributing to the vegetarian decision.

Reprinted with permission. Copyright 1996, Monika M. Woolsey, MS, RD, A Better Way Health Consulting, Glendale, Arizona. /WOMEN AFRAID TO EAT 2000

How to help a friend with eating and body image issues

- Make a plan to approach the person in a private place when there is no immediate stress and time to talk.

- Present in a caring but straightforward way what you have observed and what your concerns are. Tell him or her that you are worried and want to help. (Friends who are too angry with the person to talk supportively should not be a part of this discussion.)

- Give the person time to talk and encourage them to verbalize feelings. Ask clarifying questions. Listen carefully; accept in a non-judgmental manner.

- Do not argue about whether there is or is not a problem — power struggles are not helpful. Perhaps you can say, "I hear what you are saying and I hope you are right that this is not a problem. But I am still very worried about what I have seen and heard, and that is not going to go away."

- Provide information about resources for treatment. Offer to go with the person and wait while they have their first appointment with a counselor, physician, or nutritionist. Ask them to consider going for one appointment before they make a decision about ongoing treatment.

- If you are concerned that the eating disorder is severe or life-threatening, enlist the help of a doctor, therapist, counseling center, relative, friend, or roommate of the person before you intervene. Present a united and supportive front with others.

- If the person denies the problem, becomes angry, or refuses treatment, understand this is often part of the illness. Besides, they have a right to refuse treatment (unless their life is in danger). You may feel helpless, angry, and frustrated with them. You might say, "I know you can refuse to go for help, but that will not stop me from worrying about you or caring about you. I may bring this up again to you later, and maybe we can talk more about it then." Follow through on that — and on any other promise you make.

- Do not try to be a hero or a rescuer; you will probably be resented. If you do the best you can to help on several occasions and the person does not accept it, stop. Remind yourself you have done all it is reasonable to do. Eating disorders are stubborn problems, and treatment is most effective when the person is truly ready for it. You may have planted a seed that helps them get ready.

- Eating disorders are usually not emergency situations. But, if the person is suicidal or otherwise in serious danger, *get professional help immediately.*

Marcia Herrin and Heidi Fishman, Dartmouth College Health. Copyright 1996, EDAP.

LETTER OF PROTEST TO RED ROBIN
Englewood, Colo.

We at EDAP (Eating Disorders Awareness & Prevention) are writing to protest Red Robin's current gift certificate advertising campaign, specifically the "Co-worker who thinks you've lost weight" ad. Please discontinue this harmful advertising campaign immediately.

EDAP is very concerned about the impact of various media messages on the body image and eating habits of women and young girls. We feel that it is our responsibility as health professionals (psychologists, physicians, dietitians, counselors, nurses, health educators, etc.), as people recovering from eating disorders, and as parents, to unite in an effort to promote healthy self-esteem and body image in our community.

While your advertisement may be designed to be humorous, the underlying message — that it is more important to be thin than to be smart or funny — is not humorous at all, because it is a message that is taken to heart by too many people in our country. Some of these people (five to ten million American women and one million American men) even develop life-threatening eating disorders in their drive for thinness as a result of media messages like yours. For these people, being thin truly is their most sought-after goal. This desire to lose weight at any cost often results in kidney failure, sterility and even death.

Research has shown that the pervasive presence of thinner and thinner body ideals is associated with an increased prevalence of body dissatisfaction and eating disorders. While we certainly don't mean to accuse your advertisement of being the sole cause of eating disorders, the message in the advertisement contributes to the weight-conscious context within which eating disorders, widespread negative body image, and unnecessary calorie-restrictive dieting occur.

I would like very much to speak with you further about the concerns that EDAP and the undersigned have about this issue. A number of corporations have recently enjoyed positive publicity as a result of reshaping their advertising campaigns and we would like nothing more than to see Red Robin celebrated as a company brave enough to take a stand. Please call me at (206) 382-3587 as soon as possible.

To join EDAP's Media Advocacy Campaign, become a Media Watchdog, or to add your name to letters expressing concerns and praise for current media advertisements, contact EDAP (Eating Disorders Awareness and Prevention, Inc.) 1-800-931-2237, or sign on at their website www.edap.org

A doctor's weight loss education
by Allen King, MD

For the past 20 years I have seen over 5,000 obese patients for weight reduction and weight-related diseases. The results of my attempts to improve their disease state by weight loss were, at best, short-lived. Initially, I thought obesity was caused by lack of knowledge. I gave patients an outline of the caloric content of foods. In a follow-up period of four weeks to four months, the average patient lost eight ounces. Half gained weight!

I next tried behavior modification and recruited a dietitian to provide a more individualized diet. In a three month follow up, the average patient lost only five pounds.

With the popular movement to liquid diets and their initial great success, I then tried a rigidly controlled program. Over 500 patients were placed on 500 to 1000 calorie diets with behavior modification. The average patient lost 50 pounds in six months. I felt we had finally succeeded. A three year follow up, however, uncovered an average 60 pound regain.

Certainly, I thought, what was needed was more control. Gastric surgeries were unacceptable due to the mortality and morbidity rate. Anorexic medications were of limited use. My two patients who elected jaw wiring lost weight initially, then regained. The Garren Gastric bubble seemed the ideal solution — a plastic balloon inflated in the stomach. Weight loss did occur, but only in patients who developed ulcers and bowel obstructions.

I then became disillusioned and found myself avoiding discussing diet approaches with patients. Each method was followed by failure, and worse, guilt on the patient's part for "failing."

[Then] my dietitian colleague, Dana Armstrong, brought to my attention the pioneering [nondiet approaches]. Open and frank conversations with patients confirmed many of the points advocated in this approach. With patient feedback and the gentle support of my colleagues, I have changed from the diet doctor-control model to allowing self acceptance, and removing the masks for both patient and doctor.

I now realize it is not the doctor's role to control the patient. Responsibility for change is with the patient. . . . Change takes time and progress is variable. I now tell patients it takes five years to change. Patients who are able to change benefit greatly from their increased self knowledge and self acceptance.

Reprinted from *Healthy Weight Journal* 1993;7:104. Allen King, MD, uses a nondiet approach in treating diabetic patients with Dana Armstrong, RD, in private practice in Salinas, Calif.

Working with teenagers
How to deliver the health at any size message

Teens & Diets: No Weigh
by Linda Omichinski, RD

The importance of breaking the diet cycle at an early age can't be overemphasized. As health professionals we can take some new directions and responsibility to change the cultural message.

What legacy are we passing on to the next generation? Are we a society of dieters unhappy with the way we look because media messages tell us we should be slim? Food preoccupation and dieting has become an obsession for too many. The right to enjoy food and accept the inherent satisfaction and sustainment that comes from nourishing your body seems to have been stolen away.

The good news is that healthy, nondieting is a valid lifestyle choice that comes with a freeing set of parameters and characteristics far surpassing the restrictions of a diet lifestyle. There is no better time for establishing a new way of living than the teen years.

Part of working with teens involves letting go of the control and enabling them to make the decisions. Comments like, "That's a very interesting point of view. Could you tell me more about that?" lets teens express their own perspective.

Empowerment techniques are ideally suited for teen development.

It's critical to have an open attitude about the seeming negatives in this age group so that true learning can take place. Personal qualities of openness, caring and a good sense of humor aid educators of any age group and particularly for teens.

Build a relationship based on trust; share personal stories and some background so they can identify with you. Treat teens as adults, with the acceptance that will enable feeling good, relaxing and opening up to occur. Emphasize that no question is stupid. Use lots of humor.

We recommend four prongs to reach the public with a nondieting health message for teens: through schools, teen grapevines, parental concern, and the medical and health professional community.

Reprinted with permission from the HUGS teen facilitator package *Teens & Diets: No Weigh,* by Linda Omichinski, Copyright 1995. HUGS International Inc., Box 102A, RR#3, Portage la Prairie, Manitoba, R1N 3A3, Canada (1-800-565-4847) www.hugs.com

Child-centered resources
Based on the health at any size approach

Books, videos, information, materials

Secrets of feeding a healthy family, by Ellyn Satter. E. Satter Associates, 4226 Mandan Crescent, Madison, WI 53711 (800-808-7976) www.ellynsatter.com **Child of Mine — Feeding with love and good sense,** by Ellyn Satter. **How to get your Kid to Eat — But not too much,** by Ellyn Satter. Bull Publishing, Box 208, Palo Alto, CA 94302 (415-322-2855; 800-676-2855).

EDAP (Eating Disorders Awareness and Prevention). Information, resources, how to help a friend, what parents can do, puppet show. 603 Stewart St., #803, Seattle, WA 98101 (206-382-3587, 800-931-2237) www.edap.org

National Eating Disorder Information Centre (Canada). College Wing 1-211, 200 Elizabeth St., Toronto ON M5G 2C4, Canada (416-340-4156) www.nedic.on.ca

Vitality Leader's Kit. Canadian health centered materials that focus on a fundamental shift to health at any size, and prevention of weight and eating problems. Health Services and Promotion, Health and Welfare Canada, 4th Floor, Jeanne Mance Bldg., Ottawa, Ontario, Canada K1A 1B4 (613-957-8331; fax 613-941-2399).

Children and Weight. University of California Cooperative Extension Resources. **If My Child is Too Fat, What should I do about it?** Booklet for parents. **Children and Weight: What's a parent to do?** and **Food Choices for Good Health.** Low-literacy booklets for parents. **Am I Fat? Helping Young Children Accept Differences in Body Size,** age 10 and under. ANR Publications, University of California, 6701 San Pablo Ave., Oakland, CA 94608 (800-994-8849), website: http://danrcs.ucdavis.edu

Childhood and Adolescent Obesity in America: What's a Parent To Do? by Betty Holmes. University of Wyoming Cooperative Extension publication #B-1066. (307-766-2115) www.uwyo.edu/ag/ces/PUBS/b1066.pdf

A New Look at Adolescent Girls: Strengths and Stresses. American Psychological Association, 750 1st st., NE, Washington DC 20002 (202-336-6031) bfreeman@apa.org

Gurze Books. Catalog, specializes in eating disorder books. Gurze Books, PO Box 2238, Carlsbad, CA 92018 (800-756-7533) www.gurze.com

All Kids are Our Kids, by Peter Benson. Search Institute, 40 developmental assets kids need. What communities must do to raise healthy, successful, caring kids. San Francisco: Jossey-Bass Publ.

Body Talk. 28 minute video on body acceptance. Teen girls and boys on how they accept themselves and reject pressures to be thin. New video will focus on grades 4-6. Body Positive, Connie Sobczak, Exec. Director, 2417 Prospect St., #A, Berkeley, CA 94704 (510-841-9389).

Good News for Big Kids. National Association to Advance Fat Acceptance. Pamphlet. NAAFA, PO Box 188620, Sacramento, CA 95818 (1-800-442-1214; 916-558-6880; fax 916-558-6881).

Size Wise, by Judy Sullivan. Resources of all kinds for persons of size, some youth materials. Avon Books, 1350 Ave. of Americas, New York, NY 10019.

Council on Size & Weight Discrimination, PO Box 305, Mt. Marion NY 12456 (914-679-1209) www.cswd.org

Amplestuff. Catalog, large sizes, equipment. PO Box 116, Bearsville, NY 12409 (914-679-3316) amplestuff@aol.com www.amplestuff.com

Largely Positive, Carol Johnson, PO Box 17223, Glendale WI 53217, (414-299-9295) positive@execpc.com

National Association to Advance Fat Acceptance (NAAFA) , PO Box 188620, Sacramento CA 95818 (916-558-6880; 800-442-1214) www.naafa.org

Dads and Daughters. Networking, resources, promotions. DADs, PO Box 3458, Duluth, MN 55803 (fax: 218-728-1997) www.dadsanddaughters.org

AABA. American Anorexia/Bulima Association, www.aabainc.org

ANAD. Association of Anorexia Nervosa and Associated Disorders, PO Box 7, Highland Park, IL 60035 (847-831-3438) www.members.aol.com/anad20/ index.html

ANRED. Anorexia Nervosa and Related Disorders. PO Box 5102, Eugene OR 97405 (503-344-1144).

NEDO. National Eating Disorders Organization. 6655 S. Yale Ave., Tulsa, OK 74136, www.laureate.com

Breaking Size Prejudice. Promotes respect and size acceptance; 20-minute video developed by youth, includes skits, teacher's packet, activities, grade 6-9.

DietBreakers, Mary Evans Young, Church Cottage - Barford St. Michael, Banbury Oxon, England 0X15 OUA (0869-37070)

Largesse, the Network for Size Esteem www.eskimo.com/~largesse

Melpomene Institute for Women's Health Research, 1010 University Avenue, St. Paul NM 55104 (612-642-1951) www.melpomene.org

Are You Too Fat, Ginny? by Karin Jasper. For young girls, challenges myths about fatness and dieting in adolescents and offers the healthy alternative of self-acceptance. Introduction for parents and teachers. New York: Is Five Press.

Belinda's Bouquet, by Leslea Newman. Small book for all ages. When Belinda is teased about her weight, a flower garden shows her the beauty of diversity. Boston: Alyson Publications.

Blubber, by Judy Blume (about a girl); **Jelly Belly,** by Robert Kimmel Smith (about a boy). New York: Bantam Doubleday Dell books for young readers.

How did this happen? A practical guide to understanding eating disorders. Coaches, teachers, parents. Institute for Research and Education HealthSystem Minnesota, 1999.

Eating Disorders and Men, by Ira M. Sacker. www.eatingdis.com/men.htm

Making Weight: Healing Men's Conflicts with Food, Weight, Shape & Appearance, by Arnold Andersen, Leigh Cohn, Thomas Holbrook. Issues for boys and men. Gurze Books (800-756-7533) www.gurze.com

Mirror-Mirror. Eating disorders information. www.mirror-mirror.org

Your Dieting Daughter: Is she dying for attention? by Carolyn Costin, 1997, Brunner/Mazel Publ., NY.

Like Mother, Like Daughter: How (girls and) women are influenced by their mother's relationship with food and how to break the pattern. Debra Waterhouse. New York: Hyperion Publications.

Creating Health Behavior Change: How to Develop Community-wide Programs for Youth, by Cheryl L. Perry. Book gives a 10-step process in developing effective health behavior programs for children and teens, $32.95. Minneapolis: University of Minnesota Sage Publications. www.sagepub.com

Building Blocks for Children's Body Image, by Marius Griffin. From the Body Image Task Force, PO Box 360196, Melbourne, FL 32936-0196. http://home.earthlink.net/~dawn_atkins/children.htm

The Girl's Guide to Life, by Catherine Dee. New York: Little, Brown and Co.

Food Fight: A Guide to eating disorders for preteens and their parents, by Janet Bode, New York: Aladdin Paperbacks.

All Shapes and Sizes: Promoting fitness and Self-Esteem in Your Overweight Child, Teresa Pitman and Miriam Kaufman. Toronto: Harper Collins.

Little Girls in Pretty Boxes: The Making and Breaking of Elite Gymnasts and Figure Skaters, Joan Ryan. New York: Warner Books.

When Girls Feel Fat: Helping Girls Through Adolescence, Sandra Susan Friedman. Harper Collins.

Preventing Childhood Eating Problems: A Practical, Positive Approach to Raising Children Free of Food and Weight Conflicts, Jane Hirschmann and Lela Zaphiropoulos. Available from Gurze Books.

National Women's Health Information Center. Information for school nurses, counselors, teachers, coaches, administrators. (800-994-8662) www.4woman.gov

Kids Packet. Women's Sports Foundation, Eisenhower Park, East Meadow, NY, 11554 (800-227-3988).

National Association for Girls & Women in Sport, American Alliance for Health, Physical Education, Recreation and Dance. 1900 Association Dr., Reston, VA 22091 (800-213-7193), mborysowicz@aahperd.org

Take Charge of Your Health: A Teenager's Guide to Better Health. WIN (Weight-control Information Network. 1 WIN Way, Bethesda, MD 20892 (toll free 877-946-4627) www.niddk.nih.gov/health/nutrit/nutrit.htm

Magazines, publications

New Moon: Magazine for girls and their dreams. PO Box 3587, Duluth, MN 55803 (218-728-5507) www.cp.duluth.mn.us/

Girls' Life. 4517 Harford Rd., Baltimore MD 21214 (410-254-9200)

Teen Voices: The magazine by, for and about teenage and young adult

women. Age 15 up. Women Express, PO Box 6009, Jfk Post Office, Boston, MA 02114 www.1USA1.com/womenexp

Healthy Weight Journal. Reports research, news and commentary on eating and weight. Editorial office: 402 S 14th Street, Hettinger, ND 58639 (701-567-2646) www.healthyweight.net. Subscriptions: Decker Periodicals (800-568-7281) www.bcdecker.com

After the Diet Newsletter. A Better Way Health Consulting. PO Box 11985, Glendale, AZ 85318-1985 (623-486-0737) www.afterthediet.com

Radiance. Magazine for large women; some special youth issues, materials. PO Box 30246, Oakland CA 94604 (510-482-0680) www.radiancemagazine.com

BBW (Big Beautiful Woman). Some youth materials. 4045 Sunset Lane, #4, Shingle Springs, CA 95682 (1-877-BBW-STYLE) www.bbwmagazine.com

Programs, curricula, training

EDAP (Eating Disorders Awareness and Prevention) Programs. Healthy Body Image — Teaching Kids to Eat and Love Their Bodies Too, by Kathy Kater (grades 4-6). **A 5-Day Lesson Plan on Eating Disorders,** by Michael Levine and Laura Hill (grades 7-12). **GO GIRLS!** (Giving Our Girls Inspiration & Resources for Lasting Self-Esteem) 12-week media program. Sponsors Eating Disorder Awareness Week, training workshops, resources, information, activist programs, puppet show. 603 Stewart St., #803, Seattle, WA 98101 (800-931-2237) www.edap.org

Children and Weight: What health professionals can do about it. In-service training kit for health professionals, 5 lesson plans, activities, overheads, handouts, videotape. ANR Publications, University of California, 6701 San Pablo Ave., Oakland, CA 94608 (800-994-8849). website: http://danrcs.ucdavis.edu

Feeding with Love and Good Sense, by Ellyn Satter. Training workshops, resources, videos, baby through preschooler. **Feeding with Love and Good Sense Training Manual,** 103 pages, reproducible teaching materials. **Ellyn Satter's Vision workshops for leaders.** Ellyn Satter Associates, 4226 Mandan Crescent, Madison, WI 53711 (800-808-7976) www.ellynsatter.com

Teens & Diets — No Weigh: Building the road to healthier living, by Linda Omichinski. Prevention programs, leader training. **Home Study Course: Weight Management for Teens.** HUGS International, Box 102A, RR3, Portage la Prairie, Manitoba, Canada R1N 3A3 (204-428-3432; 800-565-4847) www.hugs.com

Girls in the 90s. Sandra Susan Friedman. Eating disorders preventive program for pre- and early-adolescent girls. Open-ended groups, 10-12 weeks. Salal Books, Box 309, 101-1184 Denman St., Vancouver, BC, Canada V6G 2M9 (604-689-8399).

Kid's Project, Packet of size acceptance materials. Kids Come in all Sizes workshops. Council on Size & Weight Discrimination, Miriam Berg, P.O. Box 305, Mt. Marion, NY 12456 (914-679-1209; fax 914-679-1206).

National Eating Disorders Screening Program. Schools, community screening. One Washington St Ste 304, Wellesley Hills MA 02481 (781-239-0071) info@nmisp.org www.nmisp.org

Girl Power! National public education campaign, Department Health and Human Services, for girls age 9-14. www.health.org/gpower/index.htm

This is Your Life! Food Play. Video, theater show, teachers' activity guidebook for health education that includes nutrition, fitness, body image, media literacy. FoodPlay, 221 Pine St., Northampton, MA 01062 (800-FOODPLAY), www.foodplay.com

It's All About You: Make healthy choices that fit your lifestyle so you can do the things you want to do. 28-minute video, Leaders guide, handouts, masters, owners manual. Dietary Guidelines Alliance, 233 N Michigan Ave., #1400, Chicago, IL 60601.

Celebrate Healthy Eating. Nutrition education packet for preschool children. From Penn State Nutrition Center, Dannon Institute, and Scholastic Early Childhood Today. Teacher guide, activities, posters, two parent newsletters, colorbook. Call (914-332-1092) or email dannon.institute@dannon.com

Pyramid Explorer: Nutrition Adventures CD-ROM, grades 5-9; Pyramid Plus: Guide to Food Choices for Better Health, for teens and young adults. Oregon Dairy Council. www.oregondairycouncil.org

Kids Module — Parents and Children Sharing Food Tasks, by Rita Mitchell. Leaders guide, videotape, handouts for parents. $60 each packet. Rita Mitchell, 209 Morgan Hall, U of California, Berkeley, CA 94720 (510-642-3080).

SPARK Active Recreation. For leaders of youth ages 5-14. Also four books for school PE programs K through 6. Sports, Play, and Active Recreation for Kids. www.foundation.sdsu.edu/projects/spark/index.html

Girls on the Run. International, PO Box 268, Huntersville, NC 28070 (800-901-9968; 704-948-7016) www.girlsontherun.com

Media literacy

Slim Hopes, by Jean Kilbourne. Video on how female bodies are depicted in advertising. Online from www.healthyweight.net

Media Mayhem: more than make believe; kids look at movies, television, music and video games, NEWIST/CESA, Green Bay, Wisc.

Kids Talk TV: Inside out. Office of Communication, United Church of Christ, Cleveland, Ohio.

Media Watch. Information, newsletter. Grade 7 up. PO Box 618, Santa Cruz, CA 95061-0618 (408-423-6355)

Living in the Image Culture: An introductory primer for media literacy education, by Francis Davis. AdSmarts: A media literacy curriculum. Center for Media and Values, Los Angeles, CA.

Center for Media Literacy (1-800-226-9494) www.medialit.org

WEBSITES

Health and Wellness
HUGS International .... www.hugs.com
Healthy Weight Network .... www.healthyweight.net
WIN Wyoming .... http://uwacadweb.uwyo.edu/winwyoming
National Women's Health Information Center www.4women.gov
Women's Health Initiative .... www.nhlbi.nih.gov/nhlbi/whil
Federal Juvenile Justice/Delinquency Prevention .... www.parentingresources.ncjrs.org
Ellyn Satter Associates .... www.ellynsatter.com
Office of Minority Health Resource Center .... www.omhrc.gov
Weight Information Network (WIN) .... www.niddk.nih.gov/health/nutrit/win.htm
    (information may not be size accepting)

Nutrition
USDA Food and Nutrition Information Center .... www.nal.usda.gov/fnic
National Network for Childcare Nutrition .... www.exnet.iastate.edu
American School Food Service Assoc. .... www.asfsa.org/childnutrition
Food Play .... www.foodplay.com
Oregon Dairy Council .... www.oregondairycouncil.org

Physical activity, sports
SPARK (Sports, play)...........www.foundation.sdsu.edu/projects/spark/index.html
Walk our children to school program .... www.walktoschool-usa.org
President's Council on Physical Fitness Sports .... www.indiana.edu/~preschal
Girls on the Run .... www.girlsontherun.com
National Association for Girls & Women in Sport ... www.aahperd.org
Melpomene Institute for Women's Health Research.. www.melpomene.org

Body Image, self-esteem
Body Wise www.4woman.gov/BodyImage/bodywise
Dads and Daughters .... www.dadsanddaughters.org
GO GIRLS! .... www.edap.org/gogirls.html
Girl Power! .... www.health.org/gpower
Self acceptance...................http://home.earthlink.net/~dawn_atkins/children.htm

Media Literacy
Media Education Foundation .... www.igc.org/mef
Center for Media Literacy .... www.medialit.org
Slim Hopes .... www.mediaed.org
PBS .... www.pbs.org/mix/imgguide.html

Eating disorders
EDAP (Eating Disorders Awareness and Prevention)...www.edap.org
National Eating Disorder Information Centre .... www.nedic.on.ca
National Eating Disorders Screening Program .... www.nmisp.org

Massachusetts Eating Disorders Assoc. .... www.medainc.org/parents.htm
ANRED .... www.anred.com
ANAD www.members.aol.com/anad20/index.html
AABA .... www.aabainc.org
NEDO .... www.laureate.com
Gurze Books .... www.gurze.com
Mirror Mirror .... www.mirror-mirror.org
Something Fishy .... http://somethingfishy.org
Eating Disorders and Men .... www.eatingdis.com/men.htm

Size acceptance
National Association to Advance Fat Acceptance .... www.naafa.org
Council on Size & Weight Discrimination .... www.cswd.org
Largesse, the Network for Size Esteem .... www.eskimo.com/~largesse
Amplestuff (catalog of resources) .... www.amplestuff.com
Size Wise .... www.SizeWise.com
Radiance Magazine .... www.radiancemagazine.com
BBW (Big Beautiful Woman) .... www.bbwmagazine.com

Magazines
New Moon (teen magazine) .... www.cp.duluth.mn.us/
Healthy Weight Journal .... www.healthyweight.net.
Healthy Weight Journal (subscriptions) .... www.bcdecker.com
After the Diet Newsletter .... www.afterthediet.com

Quackery and fraud
National Council Against Health Fraud .... www.ncahf.org
Quackwatch .... www.quackwatch.com

Many of the above link to other useful websites.

EVENTS

Healthy Weight Week, 3rd full week in January; celebrates healthy lifestyle habits; provides an antidote to January dieting. **Rid the World of Fat Diets and Gimmicks Day,** on Tuesday of Healthy Weight Week; exposes fraud and quackery in weight loss industry; annual Slim Chance Awards given for the "worst" weight loss products of the year. **Women's Healthy Weight Day,** on Thursday of Healthy Weight Week; celebrates size diversity in women; Women's Healthy Weight Awards given for businesses that portray size diversity in women.

Eating Disorder Awareness and Prevention Week. February, U.S. and Canada. Special events and eating disorder screening.

Fearless Friday. Friday of Eating Disorder Awareness and Prevention Week. A day to reject dieting and restriction of food.

No Diet Day. May 6. International day to reject dieting and restriction of food.

References

Chapter 1

1. Berg F. Harmful weight loss practices widespread among adolescents. *HWJ/Obesity & Health* 1992;6:4:69-72.
2. Wolf N. Hunger. 1994. In *Feminist perspectives on eating disorders*, eds. P Fallon, M Katzman, and S Wooley. New York: Guilford Press.
3. *P.L.E.A.S.E. Newsl.* Spring-Summer 1996;2.
4. Fern Gale Estrow, email communication. 3/8/00.
5. *Third report on nutrition monitoring in the US*, Vol 1-2, Dec 1995. Life Sciences Research Office, US Health/Human Serv, US Dept of Agriculture. Natl Ctr for Health Statistics, NHANES III. Advance Data Nov 14, 1994.
6. *Third report on nutrition, see Ch1:5.*
7. *Youth Risk Behavior Surveillance — US*, 1995. MMWR, CDC, US Public Health Serv. Sep 27, 1996:45:SS-4. JAMA 1991;266:2811-12.
8. *Youth Risk Behavior, 1995, see Ch1:7.*
9. *Vitality Leader's Kit, 1994.* Health Services/Promotion, Health and Welfare Canada. Ottawa, Ontario, Canada K1A 1B4 (613-957-8331).
10. *JAMA* 1996;276:1907-1915.
    Berg F. Task Force advises against diet drugs. *Healthy Weight Journal* 1997;11:2:27.
11. *NIH-NHLBI Clinical Guidelines on Identification, Evaluation, and Treatment of Overweight and Obesity.* National Institutes of Health, National Heart, Lung, and Blood Institute. Preprint June 1998. Bethesda, MD.
12. *Choosing a safe and successful weight-loss program,* WIN, NIDDK.
13. *Weighing the Options.* 1995, Natl Academy Press, Wash., DC.
14. Berg F. Review: Weighing the Options. *Healthy Weight J* 1995;9:3:57-58.
15. NIH Technology Assessment Conference: *Methods for Voluntary weight loss and control.* 1992. Office Medical Research, Bethesda, MD 20892.

Chapter 2

1. Pipher M. *Reviving Ophelia.* 1994. Ballantine Books, Random House, NY.
2. Kennedy E, Goldberg J. What are American children eating? Implications for public policy. *Nutr Rev* 1995;53:111-126.
3. Stevens J, et al. Attitudes and behaviors in Russian adolescents. *Obesity Res.* 1997;5:227-236.
4. Hesse-Biber S. *Am I Thin Enough Yet?* 1997. New York: Oxford U. Press.
5. Levine P. President's message. *Eating Disorders Awareness and Prevention Newsletter.* Spring 1995:1-3.
6. Barker M. Girls on the Run: Coping with the crisis of cultural pressure. *Healthy Weight J* 1998;12:89-91.
7. *Newsweek.* Feb 1, 1993, 64-65.
   Berg F. Gaunt idols. *HWJ/Obesity & Health* 1993;7:2:23.
8. Fallon P, M Katzman, S Wooley, edits. *Feminist perspectives on eating disorders.* 1994. Guilford Press, NY.
   Health Risks of Weight Loss, 1995;89. Healthy Weight J, Hettinger, ND.
9. *Eating Disorders* 1993;1:1:52-61.
   Berg F. Television ads promote dieting. *HWJ/Obesity & Health* 1993;7:6:106.
10. Kilbourne J. *Still killing us softly: Advertising and obsession with thinness.* Fallon, *see Ch2:8.*
11. Wolf N. *The beauty myth: how images of beauty are used against women,* 1991. Morrow, NY.
12. Rubinstein S. Is Miss America an undernourished role model? *JAMA* 2000;283:1569.
13. *I J Eating Disorders* 1992; 11:1:85-89.
14. Berg F. Thin mania turns up pressure. *HWJ/Obesity & Health* 1992;6:5:83.
15. Berg F. *Health Risks of Weight Loss,* 1995;90. Healthy Weight J, ND.
16. Morgan L. Why are girls obsessed with their weight? *Seventeen* Nov. 1989;118-119, 145, 150, 154.
17. Kalodner C. Media influences on male and female non-eating-disordered college students. *Eat Dis* 1997;5:47-57.
18. Communication, Jessica Setnick, MS, RD. 3/2/00.
19. Reported from New Scientist by *American Anorexia/Bulimia Assoc Newsletter* Spring 1994;8.
    Berg, *see Ch2:15:92.*
20. Oswalt R, Davis J. *Societal influences on thinner body size in children.* Proceedings Eastern Psychological Assoc. Philadelphia, Apr 1990.
21. Eating Disorder Awareness Week Kit:

Celebrating our natural sizes. 1996, National Eating Disorder Information Centre, Toronto.

22. *Eating Disorders* 1993;1:2:109-114.
    Berg F. False media messages. *HWJ/Obesity & Health* 1994;8:1:5.

23. Nutr Forum Sep/Oct 1989, from *Pediatrics* 1989 83:393-397.
    Berg F. Weight Terror. *HWJ/Obesity & Health* 1990;4:1:1.

24. Morgan, *see Ch2:16.*

25. Pope H, Olivardia R, Gruber A, et al. Evolving ideals of male body image as seen through action toys. *Int J Eat Disord* 1999;26:65-72.

26. Grange D, J Tibbs, J Selibowitz. Eating attitudes, body shape, and self-disclosure in adolescent girls and boys. *Eating Dis* 1995:3:3:253-264.

27. Crisp A. Anorexia nervosa in a young male. In *Treating Eating Disorders*, J Werne, edit. Jossey-Bass Inc, San Francisco. 1996:6.

28. Smolak L, M Levine. Toward an empirical basis for primary prevention of eating problems with elementary school children. *Eat Disorders* 1994;2:4:293-307.

29. Gustafson-Larson, AM, RD Terry. Weight-related behaviors and concerns of fourth-grade children. *J of the Am Dietetic Assoc* 1992:818-822.

30. 30. *Food Nutr News* 1993;65:1:4.
    Berg, *see Ch2:15.*

31. Nichter M, S Park, M Nichter, *Body image and weight concerns among African American and white adolescent females.* Anthropology, U of Arizona, Tucson, AZ.
    Berg F. Beauty ideas are fluid. *Healthy Weight Journal* 1995;9:2:26.
    Berg, *see Ch2:15:123.*

32. Rothblum E. *I'll die for the revolution but don't ask me not to diet.* 1994;53-76.
    Fallon, *see Ch2:8.*
    Berg, *see Ch2:15:91.*

33. Berg F. Girls and dolls. *Healthy Weight Journal* 1997;11:1:6.

34. Meletiche. *NAAFA News* Sep/Oct 1991:5.
    Meletiche L. Barbie: Symbol of oppression. *HWJ/Obesity & Health* 1993;7:5:96.

35. Gerhart A. More young women choose surgical perfection. *Washington Post* 6/23/99.

36. Tolman D, E Debold. Conflicts of body and image, 301-317. In Fallon, *see Ch2:8.*

37. Sexual harassment. *USA Today.* 7/23/96.

38. Larkin J, C Rice and V Russell. Slipping through the cracks: sexual harassment, eating problems, and embodiment. *Eat Disorders* 1996;4:1:5-26.

39. Levine P. The Last Word. *Eat Disorders* 1995;3:1:92-95.

Chapter 3

1. Niven C, D Carroll. *The Health psychology of women.* Harwood Academic Publ., Chur, Switzerland. 1993:115.

2. Berg F. Kids fear being fat early. *HWJ/Obesity & Health* 1993;7:3:46-47.
   J Am Diet Assoc 1992;92;92:7:851-53.

3. Hartung L. Disordered eating patterns in the the college environment. *J Am Diet Assoc* 1997;97:9:SupplA-60.

4. *Clin Psych Rev* 1991;11:729-780
   Berg F. Nondiet movement gains strength. *HWJ/Obesity & Health* 1992;6:5:85-90.

5. Satter, Ellyn. *How to Get Your Kid to Eat . . . But Not Too Much*, 1987; also Satter, *Child of Mine*, 1983. Bull Publishing, Palo Alto, CA.

6. Smolak, *see Ch2:28.*

7. Reiff, D, KK Lampson Reiff, *Eating Disorders: Nutrition Therapy in Recovery Process*, 1992, p162. Aspen, Gaithersburg, MD.

8. Eating disorder awareness, *see Ch2:21.*

9. Young M Evans. *Diet Breaking: Having it all without having to diet.* Hodder and Soughton, London. 1995:41-42, 56-57.

10. Estes L, M Crago, C Shisslak. Eating disorders prevention. *The Renfrew Perspective,* 1996;2:1:3-5.
    Fallon, *see Ch2:8.*
    Berg, *see Ch3:2.*

11. Smolak, *see Ch2:28.*

12. Fallon, *see Ch2:8.*

13. *Restaurants USA* 1994;14:18-21.
    Berg, F. Customers want bigger meals *Healthy Weight Journal* 1995;9:2:26.

14. Rolls B, Engell D, Birch L. Serving portion size influences 5-year-old but not 3-year-old children's food intakes. *J Am Diet Assoc* 2000;100:232-234.

15. Taste, Health, and the Social Meal. Special issue. *Journal of Gastronomy.* Winter/Spring 1993. Berg F. Review of special issue, J Gastronomy. *Healthy Weight J* 1994;8:3:59.
16. Birch LL, Development of eating behavior among children. *Pediatrics, Suppl.,* 1998, pp 539-549.
17. Peck P. Baby fat cute, but contributes to adult heart disease. *WebMD Medical News* 3/3/00 (San Diego).
18. Stice E, Agras WS, Hammer LD. Risk factors for emergence of childhood eating disturbances. *Int J Eat Disord 1999;25:375-387.*
19. *HUGS Club News,* Jan. 1997, p6.
20. Berg F. Weight-loss programs for children and adolescents. *HWJ/Obesity & Health* 1989;3:10:78. *Nutrition News* 1988;51:2:5-7.
21. Fabrey W. Big News. *Radiance.* Fall 1995.
22. Pollitt E. Does breakfast make a difference in school? *J Am Diet Assoc* 1995;95:10:1134-1139.
23. Satter, Ellyn. *Secrets of feeding a healthy family.* 1999. Madison, Wis: Kelcy Press
24. Davis KS. *Resetting the American table.* National Pork Producers. Presentation at Family and Consumer Science Annual Meeting, Atlanta 1998.
25. Reinhardt M. American Foodways. *SNE Communicator,* Fall 1997.

Chapter 4
1. *Youth Risk Behavior, 1995, see Ch1:7.*
2. Third report nutrition, *see Ch1:5.*
3. USHHS, *Healthy People 2010,* Conf Edition. Wash., DC: Jan 2000.
4. Institute of Medicine. *Dietary Reference Intakes for Calcium, Phosphorus, Magnesium.* Wash., DC: National Academy Press, 1997.
5. Kretchmer N, J Beard, S Carlson. The role of nutrition in the development of normal cognition. *Am J Clin Nutr* 1996;63:997S-1001S.
6. Kenyon G. Dieting may harm girls' IQ. Reuters Health (London) 8/1/00.
7. Duyff RL. 1996. *The American Dietetic Association's Complete Food and Nutrition Guide.* Minneapolis, MN: Chronimed Publ.
8. Keys, Ancel et al. *The Biology of Human Starvation.* 1950. U of Minnesota Press, Minneapolis, MN.
9. Turnbull, Colin. *The Mountain People.* 1972, Simon and Schuster, NY.
10. Reiff, *see Ch3:7.* Reiff D. Personal communication. 1996.

Chapter 5
1. Kassirer JP, Angell M. Losing weight — an ill-fated New Year's resolution. *N Engl J Med* 1998;338:52-54.
2. Berg F. The weight loss industry. Regulation is needed. *HWJ/Obesity & Health* 1990;4:6:41-46.
3. NIH Technology Conf., *see Ch1:15. Annals Int Med* 1993;119:688-770.
4. Fraser, Laura. 1994. *Losing it: America's obsession with weight and the industry that feeds on it.* New York: Penguin/Dutton.
5. NIH Guidelines, *see Ch1:11*
6. Coulston AM. Obesity as an epidemic: facing the challenge. *J Am Diet Assoc* 1998;98:10(S2):16-22.
7. Dieting and purging behavior in black and white high school students. *J Am Diet Assoc* 1992;92:3:306-312. Adolescents dieting. *JAMA* 1991;266: 2811-2812. Berg F. Harmful weight loss practices widespread among adolescents. *HWJ/ Obesity & Health* 1992;6:4:69-72.
8. *JADA, JAMA,* Berg, *see Ch5:7.*
9. *JADA, JAMA,* Berg, *see Ch5:7.*
10. Marchessault G. Weight perceptions and practices in American Indian youth. *Healthy Weight J* 1999;13:71-73, 79.
11. *JADA, JAMA,* Berg, *see Ch5:7.*
12. Garner D, L Rosen. Eating disorders among athletes. *J Applied Sport Sci Research* 1991;5:2:17.
13. Berg F. The case against PPA. *HWJ/ Obesity & Health* 1991;5:1:9-12.
14. *JADA, JAMA,* Berg, *see Ch5:7.*
15. Berg F. 1997 Slim Chance Awards. *Healthy Weight J,* 1997;11:1:7.
16. Berg F. *Weight Loss Quackery and Fads,* 1995:16. Healthy Weight J., Hettinger, ND.
17. FDA to Consumers: "Good luck with dietary supplements." *NCRHI Newsletter* 2000;23:1.
18. *FDA Consumer,* May 1995;3.
19. Berg F. Bee pollen "cures" truckers. *HWJ/Obesity & Health* 1991;5:2:30.
20. Rosencrans K. Diet pills suspected in

deaths. *Healthy Weight J,* 1994;8:4:68.

21. Berg, *Quackery, see Ch5:16.*
22. *JADA, JAMA,* Berg, *see Ch5:7.*
23. *Youth Risk Behavior,* 1995, *see Ch1:7.*
24. Baker D and A, R Sansone. Overview of eating disorders. 1994. NEDO. Berg, *see Ch2:15.*
25. Mehler P, K Weiner. Frequently asked medical questions about eating disorder patients. *Eating Disorders,* 1994;2:1:22-30.
26. Kaplan A, P Garfinkel. *Medical issues and the Eating Disorders.* 1993. Brunner/Mazel, New York.
27. *JADA, JAMA,* Berg, *see Ch5:7.*
28. *JADA, JAMA,* Berg, *see Ch5:7.*
29. Kaplan, *see Ch5:26:101-122.*
30. *HP 2010, see Ch4:3.*
31. *NEJM* 1995;333:1165-1170/1214-1216. Berg F. Smoking cessation impacts weight. *Healthy Weight J,* 1996;10:2:27-28.
32. *Healthy People 2000.* 1990:140, 147. USDHHS, PHS.
33. Williamson D, R Anda, G Giovino, T Byers, CDC, J Madans, Kleinman. Weight gain caused by cessation of smoking. Natl Ctr for Health Statistics. 1993;324:739-745. Berg F. Smokers who quit gain to average. *HWJ/Obesity & Health* 1991;5:6:92.
34. Berg, *Quackery,see Ch5:16.*
35. Berg, *Quackery, see Ch5:16.* See also Questionable features, each issue; Slim Chance Awards, each January, *Healthy Weight J.*
36. *Obesity Research* 1993;1:1:51-56. Berg F. Linking gallstones with weight loss. *HWJ/Obesity & Health* 1993;7:3:45.
37. *Options, see Ch1:13.*
38. *NIH Guidelines, see Ch1:11.*
39. FDA News Release, Sept. 15, 1997. Berg F. Redux, fen-phen withdrawn from market. *Healthy Weight J* 1997;11:6:105.
40. Levitsky D. Diet drugs gain popularity. *Healthy Weight J* 1997;11:1:8-12. Ernsberger P. Adverse reactions to dexfenfluramine. *Healthy Weight J* 1997;11:1:13-14, 16.
41. FDA discussion paper, 11/24/97; AP Washington, 11/25/97. FDA committee backs another anti-

obesity drug. AP, Bethesda, MD, 5/25/97.
42. FDA, *see Ch5:41a.*
43. FDA, *see Ch5:41b.*
44. Mayer K. *Real Women don't Diet.* 1993:149.
45. Hall L. *Full Lives: Women who have freed themselves from food & weight obsession.* 1993:96-97. Gurze Books, Carlsbad, CA.
46. Rand C, A MacGregor. Adolescents having obesity surgery. *Southern Med J* 1994;87:12:1208-1213.
47. Bloomers T, Exec Mgr Am Society for Bariatric Surgery, interview 1994;5.
48. *Guidance for Treatment of Adult Obesity,* 1996. Shape Up America! and American Obesity Assoc.
49. Droze K. Considering Liposuction? *eDiets.com online news* 2/3/00.
50. *Food & Nutr News* Nov/Dec 1989;61:5 Berg F. Summer weight loss camps: Not a quick fix for overweight teens. *HWJ/Obesity & Health* 1990;4:3:29.
51. AP Feb 27, 1991.
52. Wisconsin Interscholastic Athletic Association, 41 Park Ridge Drive, PO Box 267, Stevens Point, WI 54481; 715-344-8580.
53. Steen S, S McKinney. Nutrition assessment of college wrestlers. *Phys Sportsmed* 1986;14:100-116. Berg F. Weight cycling; crash dieting drops metabolism for wrestlers. *HWJ/Obesity & Health* 1989;3:2:1-4. Berg, *see Ch2:15:52.*
54. Hyperthermia and dehydration-related deaths in three collegiate wrestlers. CDC, *MMWR* 2/20, 1998;47:105-108. Wrestling training deaths, AP 12/20/97.
55. Garner, *see Ch5:12.*
56. NIH Conf, *see Ch1:15.*
57. Allison DB, Zannolli R, Faith MS, et al. Weight loss increases and fat loss decrease all-cause mortality rate. *I J Obesity* 1999;23:603-611.

Chapter 6
1. Alexander-Mott L, DB Lumsden. *Understanding Eating Disorders.* Taylor & Francis, Washington, DC 1994:290.
2. Personal communication with Doris Smeltzer, Napa, Calif., Jan-Feb 2000, www.andreasvoice.org.

3. Alexander-Mott, see Ch6:1.
4. Reiff, see Ch3:7.
5. Efron S. Eating disorders in Asia. Los Angeles Times. Oct. 21, 1997.
6. Hoek H. 1995. Distribution of eating disorders. In Eating Disorders and Obesity, K Brownell and C Fairburn. p207-211. NY: Guilford Press.
7. Levine M. Prevalence of eating disorders. EDAP. Feb 1, 1996.
   Also, National Association Anorexia Nervosa and Associated Disorders.
8. Scand J Med Sci Sports 1999;9:304. Eating disorders and personality among active women. Eating Disorders Rev 1999;10:7.
9. Marx R. Questions & Answers. Eat Disorders 2000;8:77-79.
10. Pawluck D, Gorey K. Secular trends in incidence of anorexia nervosa. Int J Eating Disorders 1998;23:347-352.
11. Lucas AR, Crowson CS, et al. The ups and downs of anorexia nervosa. Int J Eat Disord 1999;397-405.
12. Pawluck, see Ch6:10.
13. Eating disorders awareness see Ch2:21.
14. Levine, Michael. Personal communication, August 2000.
15. Gordon RA. Eating disorders: Anatomy of a social epidemic (2nd ed.) 2000. New York: Blackwell.
16. HP 2010, see Ch4:3.
17. Garner D. Effects of starvation on behavior: Implications for dieting, disordered eating, and eating disorders, Healthy Weight J 1998;12:5:68-72.
18. Bruch H. 1973. Eating disorders: Obesity, anorexia nervosa and the person within. New York: Basic Books.
19. Reiff, see Ch3:7.
20. Kaplan, see Ch5:26.
21. Lowinger K, Griffiths RA, Beumont PJV, et al. Fluid restriction in anorexia nervosa. Int J Eat Disord 1999;26;392-396.
22. Stice, see Ch3:18.
23. Fallon, see Ch2:8.
24. Fallon, see Ch2:8.
25. Goodman E. Eating disorders: Columbine for girls. Boston Globe 5/28/99.
26. Berg F. Eating disorders — physical and mental effects. Healthy Weight J 1995;9:2:27-30.
27. Wilson, GT. The controversy over dieting. Guilford Press, NY 1995:87-92.
28. Position of American Dietetic Association: Nutrition intervention in treatment of anorexia nervosa, bulimia nervosa, binge eating. ADA, Chicago.
29. Reiff, see Ch3:7:162.
30. Allis Tim, et al. Weight and See. People 1/31/94; p 50-58.
31. Krasnow M. My Life as a Male Anorexic. 1996. Haworth Press, N.Y.
32. Berning J, S Steen. Sports Nutr for the 90s. 1991:156-158. Aspen, Gaithesburg, MD.
33. Diagnostic criteria eating disorders. Diagnostic and Statistical Manual, Fourth Edition, 1994. American Psychiatric Association, Washington, DC.
34. Position ADA, see Ch6:28
35. Are (Were) You like me? The Healthy Weigh 1995;1:1:3.
36. Reiff, see Ch3:7:162.
37. Costin C. The eating disorder handbook. Los Angeles, CA: RGA Publishing Group, 1997;28-44.
38. Berg F. Eating disorders affect mind and body. Healthy Weight J 1995; 9:2: 27-30.
39. Berg F. Competitive bodybuilding. Healthy Weight J 1996;10:3:47-48.
40. Wooley S. Recognition of Sexual Abuse: Progress and Backlash. Schwartz M, L Cohn, editors. Sexual abuse and eating disorders. 1996. Brunner/Mazel, New York.
41. Brewerton T. Sexual and physical assault are risk factors for bulimia nervosa. NEDO Newsl 1994;7:4:1-5.
42. Schwartz M, L Cohn, eds. Sexual abuse and eating disorders. 1996. Brunner/Mazel,NY.
43. Levenkron S, One man's experience treating a woman's disorder. Renfrew Perspective 1995;1:2:1-15.
44. Kaplan, see Ch5:26.

Chapter 7
1. Davis D. Radiance, Fall 1987, p29-31.
2. Nutrition News 1988;51:2:5-7.
   Berg, see Ch3:20.
3. Eating and Its Disorders, edit Albert J. Stunkard and Eliot Stellar, 1984, Raven Press, NY. p 175.
4. Dietz W and Scrimshaw N. Potential advantages and disadvantages of human obesity. Social Aspects and Beach Publ. Luxembourg.
5. Parade Magazine 11/4/1990.
6. Brownell K, Fairburn C, Edits. Eating

Disorders and Obesity. 1995. Guilford Press, N.Y. p 417-421.

7. Stunkard A, Wadden T. Psychopathology and obesity. *Human Obesity*, Eds. Wurtman T, J. NY Academy of Sci 1987:57.

8. Report on Size Discrimination, NEA, Adopted Oct. 7, 1994. NEA, 1201 16th St. NW, Washington, DC 20036-3290 (202-822-7700)

9. Johnson C A, *Self-Esteem Comes in All Sizes.* 1995:8-10, Doubleday, N.Y.

10. Erdman, C K. *Nothing to Lose: A Guide to Sane Living in a Larger Body.* 1995. HarperCollins, N.Y.

11. Mayer, *see Ch5:44.*

12. Brownell, *see Ch7:6.*

13. Hall, *see Ch5:45.*

14. *Fort Lauderdale Sun-Sentinel* 8/27/96. *Canada Wyde*, Fall 1996:6. AP Ft. Lauderdale, March 23, 1997.

15. Goodman C. *The Invisible Woman: Confronting Weight Prejudice in America.* 1995:ix-xi. Gurze Books, Carlsbad, Calif.

16. Summer, N. Teaching kids about size awareness. *Healthy Weight J* 1996;10:5: 95-96.

Chapter 8

1. Kumanyika S. *Epidemiologic Reviews* 1987;9:31-50.

2. Troiano R, K Flegal, et al. Overweight prevalence and trends for children and adolescents. *Arch Pediatr Adolesc Med* 1995;149:1085-1091.

3. Center for Chronic Disease Prevention and Health Promotion. CDC Growth Charts, 2000. www.cdc.gov/nccdphp/dnpa/bmi/bmi-for-age.htm

4. *Obesity Res* 1996;4:1S:68S. Berg F. Heaviest children log increases. *Healthy Weight J* 1997;11:1:6.

5. HP 2010, *see Ch4:3.*

6. Shear C, D Freedman, et al. The Bogalusa Heart Study. *Am J Public Health* 1988;78:75-77.

7. Morrison J, et al. Mothers in black and white households: the NHLBI growth and health study. *An J Pub Health* 1994;84:1761-1767. Obarzanek E, G Schreiber, et al. Energy intake and physical activity in relation to indexes of body fat. National Heart, Lung, and Blood Institute.

8. Ogden C, et al. Prevalence of over-weight among preschool children, 1971-1994. *Pediatrics* 1997; 99:4:1.

9. Pediatric Nutrition Surveillance System (PedNSS), Division of Nutrition, Centers for Disease Control, Atlanta. Berg F. High rates of childhood obesity in assistance programs. *HWJ/Obesity & Health* 1992;6:2:26-27, 34.

10. Berg F. Prevalences of obesity rises for minorities. *HWJ/Obesity & Health* 1993;7:4:72.

11. Fontvieille, A M and E Ravussin. Metabolic Rate and body composition Indian and Caucasian children. *Critical Rev in Food Sci and Nutr* 1993;33(4/5):363-368.

12. Becque MD, K Hattori, et. al. *Em J Phys Anthro* 71;423-249. Berg F. *Health Risks of Obesity.* 1993. Healthy Weight J, Hettinger, ND.

13. Bouchard C, F Johnston. *Fat distribution during growth and later health outcomes.* 1988. Alan Liss, NY. Berg F. Ethnic differences in fat patterning. *HWJ/International Obesity Newsletter* 1988;2:12:5.

14. Peck EB, Ulrich HD. *Children and Weight: A changing perspective.* U of Calif. Berkeley.

15. Heitmann BL, Erikson H, Ellsinger BM, et al. Mortality associated with body fat, fat-free mass and body mass index among 60-year-old Swedish men. *I J Obesity* 2000;24:33-37.

16. Kline G. Analyzing BMI: Can it measure individual risk? *Healthy Weight J* 2001;15 in press.

17. Federal Update: BMI poor indicator of body fat in individual kids. *J Am Diet Assoc* 2000;100:628.

18. Lohman T, S Gonig, et al. Concept of chemical immaturity in body composition estiamtes. *Am J Hum Biol* 1989;1:201-204.

19. CDC growth charts, *see Ch8:3.*

20. NIH-NHLBI Guidelines, *see Ch1:11.*

21. Faith MS, Pietrobelli A, Nunez C, et al. Evidence for independent genetic influences on fat mass and body mass index in a pediatric twin sample. *Pediatrics* 1999;104:918-924.

22. Mayer J. Genetic factors in human obesity. *Ann NY Acad Sci* 1965;131:412-421. Mayer 1965, PubEd wkshop report, p27.

23. Kumanyika, *see Ch8:1.*

Wendorf M, I Goldfine, *Diabetes* 1991;40:161-165.

Berg F. Thrifty gene may set stage for obesity in blacks. *HWJ/Obesity & Health* 1991:5:1:6-7.

Berg F. Former big game hunters succumb to diabetes, *HWJ/Obesity & Health* 1991;5:6:98.

Berg F. Thrifty gene threatens the good life. *Healthy Weight J* 1995;9:4:64.

24. Bouchard C, L Perusse, et al. Inheritance of the amount and distribution of human body fat. *Int J Obesity* 1988;12:205-215

Berg F. NAASO highlights. *HWJ/Obesity & Health* 1992:6:1:5.

25. Obarzanek, *see Ch8:7.*

26. Williamson D. US adolescents are inactive, at risk for health problems. UNC-CH News Service 9/14/99. *Pediatrics* Sept. 1999.

27. Kotani K, Nishida M, et al. Two decades of medical exams in Japanese obese children. *Int J Obes* 1997;21: 912-921.

28. Obarzanek, *see Ch8:7.*

29. Prentice A. Manipulation of dietary fat or calorie density? *Healthy Weight J* 1998;12:6:87-88.

30. Willett W. Is dietary fat a major determinant of body fat? *Am J Clin Nutr* 1998;67(Suppl):556-562S.

31. *Nutr Review* 50:9:267-270.

32. World Health Organization. Obesity: Preventing and managing the global epidemic. Report of WHO Consultation, Geneva, June 3-5, 1997.

33. Klesges Robert, *J Applied Behavior Analysis* Winter 1983.

Berg F. Urging children to eat more. *HWJ/International Obesity Newsl* Jan 1987:1:1-2.

34. Johnson S, L Birch. Parents' and children's adiposity and eating style. *Pediatrics* 1994;94:653-661.

35. Stice E, Cameron RP, et al. Naturalistic weight-reduction efforts predict growth in weight and onset of obesity among female adolescents. *J Consult Clin Psych* 1999;67:967-974.

36. *JADA* 1991 Sp191:9:A-81.

Berg F. Family communication. *HWJ/ Obesity & Health* 1992:6:2:24.

Berg F. Infants and young children, family tendencies hold strong influence. *HWJ/Obesity & Health* 1989;3: 12:89, 91-92.

37. WHO, *see Ch8:32.*

38. Williamson DF. Smoking cessation and severity of weight gain in a national cohort. *NEJM* 1991;324;739-745.

39. WHO, *see Ch8:32.*

40. Filer L J. Summary of Workshop on Child and Adolescent Obesity, *University critical reviews in food science and nutrition* 1993:33:4/5:287-305.

41. Filer, *see Ch8:40.*

42. Mogan J. *Int J Nurs Stud* 1986;23:3: 255-264.

43. Crawford P, L Shapiro. How obesity develops: A new look at nature and nurture. *HWJ/Obesity & Health* 1991;5: 3:40-41.

Berg F. Fat cells: An increase in number or in size? *HWJ/Obesity & Health* 1988;2:8:1-2.

44. Giblin W P. *JADA* 1984;436-438.

45. *Epidemiologic Reviews* 1987;9:31-50.
Berg, Berg and Berg, *see Ch8:23.*

46. Frisch R, Edit. *Adipose Tissue and Reproduction.* 1990. Karger, Basel, Switzerland.

Berg F. High body fat brings early puberty. *HWJ/Obesity & Health* 1990;4: 10:73-76.

47. AP Chicago 4/8/97.

48. Astrup A, et al. Is obesity contagious? *Int J Obes* 1998;22:375-376.

49. *Critical Review Food Sci and Nutr* 1993;93(4/5);423-430.

50. NIH Strategy Development Workshop for Public Education on Weight and Obesity, National Heart, Lung and Blood Institute, 1992, p35.

51. Kotani, *see Ch8:27.*

52. Conference on the Prevention of Obesity. NIDDK, 1993:64. Abstracts:64.

53. NIH Strategy, *see Ch8:50:51.*

54. Tufts U Diet Nutr Ltr Jan 1993;1-2.
Berg F. Teen obesity increases heart risk. *HWJ/Obesity & Health* 1993; 7:2:31.

55. Smoak C, G Burke, et al. Relation of obesity to clustering of risk factors in children. *A J of Epidemiology* 1987; 125:3:364-372.

56. WHO, *see Ch8:32.*

57. Berg F. Obesity in children and teens. *HWJ/International Obesity Newsl* 1986;pilot:8:1-2.

Chapter 9
1. Kennedy, *see Ch2:2*.
2. Johnson R, Panely C, Wang MQ. Association between noon beverage consumption and diet quality. *J Child Nutr & Mngt* 1998;22:95-100.
3. USDA press release: what and where our children eat — 1994 nationwide survey results, 4/18/96, #0197.96.
4. Youth Risk Behavior Surveillance — 1997. CDC, USDHHS, *Morbidity and Mortality Weekly Report* 8/14/98.
5. USDA, *see Ch9:3*.
6. Johnson, *see Ch9:2*.
7. Center for Science in Public Interest, 10/21/98, website www.cspinet.org/sodapop/liquid_candy.htm
8. Johnson, *see Ch9:2*.
9. Eaton S B, M Konner. Paleoplithic. *NEJM* 1985;312:5:283-289.
10. Kennedy, *see Ch2:2*.
11. Nicklas T. Dietary studies of children: The Bogalusa Heart Study. *J Am Diet Assoc* 1995;95:1127-1133.
12. Gayle Alleman WSU extension alleman@coopext.caahe.wsu.edu.
13. Gugliotta G. Supplement marketers target kids. *Washington Post* 6/18/00.
14. Kennedy, *see Ch2:2*.
15. Nicklas, *see Ch9:11*.
16. 7th European Congress on Obesity, Barcelona, Spain. *I J Obesity* 1996; 20(4):53.
17. *Recommended Dietary Allowances*, Natl Research Center, 1989, p33. Washington, DC. National Academy Press.
18. Jarvis W. Why I am not a vegetarian. *Nutrition & Health Forum*, 1996;13: 6:57-64.
19. AMA Statement, Sept 29, 1992.
20. Woolsey M. The eating disordered vegetarian. *Healthy Weight J* 1997;11: 2:32-34.
21. Kennedy, *see Ch2:2*.
22. Whelan E. Smoking report. *Priorities* 1996;8:1:4-9.
23. AP Atlanta, Feb. 7, 1997.
24. HP 2010, *see Ch4:3*.
25. Johnson P. TV grabs biggest share of kids' time. *USA Today* 11/18/99.
26. Gordon-Larsen P, McMurray RG, Popkin BM. Adolescent physical activity, inactivity vary by ethnicity. *J Pediatr* 1999;135:301-306.
27. HP 2010, *see Ch4:3*.
28. Youth Risk, *see Ch1:7*.
29. Sallis, J F. Epidemiology of physical activity and fitness in children and adolescents, *Crit Rev in Food Sci and Nutr* 1993;33(4/5):403-408.
30. Iverson, et al, Public Health Reports, 1985;100(2):212.
31. HP 2010, *see Ch4:3*.
32. Iverson, *see Ch9:30*.
33. *Melpomene J* Fall 1993;14-18, 19-26. Berg F. Why teenage girls drop out of sports. *HWJ/Obesity & Health* 1994; 8:1:13.
34. Allen JE. Female athletes at risk. *Los Angeles Times* 6/17/00.)
35. *Melpomene, see Ch9:33*. Berg F. Picture books portray mostly males in sports. *HWJ/Obesity & Health* 1994;8:1:13.
36. Glass J Exercise benefits, risks and precautions for women. *Healthy Weight J* 1999;13:4:56.
37. Berg, *see Ch2:15:24-38*.
38. Loosli AR, and Ruud JS. Meatless diets in female athletes: A red flag. *The Physician and Sportsmedicine.* 1998;26:11:45-48, 55.
39. *Muscle & Fitness.* 1996:137-138, 221-222.
40. Dwyer E, D Silbiger, J Ryan. The red flags of over-training. *Shape* Apr 1996;122-123.

Chapter 10
1. Omichinski L. 1999, 1992. *You Count, Calories Don't; Teens and Diets: No Weigh.* Portage La Prairie, Manitoba: HUGS Internationl, (www.hugs.com).
2. Hawks SR, Gast JA. The ethics of promoting weight loss. *Healthy Weight J* 2000;14:25-26.
3. Campfield LA. 1997. Role of pharmacological agents in the treatment of obesity. In *Overweight and weight managment*, ed. S Dalton. p471-473. Gaithersberg, MD: Aspen Pub.
4. Satter, Satter, *see Ch3:5*.
5. Vitality, *see Ch1:9*.
6. Berg F. 2000. *Women Afraid to Eat*, p222-223. Hettinger, ND: Healthy Weight Network.
7. Ernsberger P, Koletsky RJ. Rationale for a wellness approach to obesity. *Healthy Weight J* 2000;14:20-24, 29.
8. Miller W. Health promotion strategies for obese patients. *Healthy Weight J* 1997:11:3:47-51.

9. Berg F, Marchessault G. Naming the Revolution. *Healthy Weight J* 2000:14:12, 14.
10. Search Institute, *Healthy communities, healthy youth.* Minneapolis, MN (www.search-institute.org)

Chapter 11

1. Search, *see Ch10:10.*
2. Vitality, *see Ch1:9.*
3. Satter, *see Ch3:5.*
4. Hans C, RD, and Nelson D. *A parent's guide to children's weight,* 1994. Iowa State Extension, Iowa State U, Ames.
5. Walsh K. Nutrition for busy families I. *Herald-Press* 3/8/97, Fessenden, ND.
6. Satter, *see Ch3:23.*
7. Child Nutrition and Health Campaign. *J Am Diet Assoc* October 1995.
8. Fortin S. Supporting adolescents with eating problems. *National Eating Disorder Information Centre Bulletin* 1995;10:2:1-4.
9. Robin Arthur L. *J Am Acadmy of Chi and Adol Psych* Dec 1999.
10. Johnson S, L Birch. Parents' adiposity and children's adiposity and eating style. *Pediatrics* 1994;94:653-660.
11. Crawford, *see Ch8:43.*
12. *I J Eat Disorders* 1986;5:335-346.
13. Satter E. Childhood obesity demands new approaches. *HWJ/Obesity & Health* 1991;5:3:42-43. 5.
    Satter E. Internal regulation and the evolution of normal growth as the basis for prevention of obesity in childhood. *J Am Diet Assoc.* In press. Diag/Stat Manual IIIR, 1988. Am Psych Assoc
14. Bruch, *see Ch6:18.*
15. Satter, Satter, Diag/Stat, *see Ch11:13.*
16. Ikeda J, et al. Two approaches to adolescent weight reduction. *J Nutr Educ* 1982;14:90.
17. Ikeda J. *Winning weight loss for teens.* 1989. Bull Publishing, Palo Alto, CA.
18. Ikeda J, Peck E. California takes action on children weight concerns. *HWJ/ Obesity & Health* 1991;5:3:39.
19. Ikeda J. *If My Child is Too Fat, What Should I do?* Nutrition Education, Cooperative Extension, Dept. Nutritional Sciences, U of Calif. Berkeley.
20. Johnson C. 1995. Reprinted with permission from materials compiled by Largely Positive, Inc. Glendale, Wisc.

21. Johnson, *see Ch7:9.*

Chapter 12

1. Allensworth D and Kolbe L. Comprehensive school health program. *J School Hlth* 1987 57;10:409-412.
2. Kolbe L. An essential strategy to improve the health and education of Americans. p55-80. In Cortese P, and Middleton K, eds. *The Comprehensive School Health Challenge,* Vol 1: Promoting health through education. 1994. ETR Assoc., Santa Cruz, CA.
3. Petersmarck K. Shaming heavy kids at school. *Healthy Weight J* 1999;13:45-46.
4. Website: www.olemiss.edu/depts/nfsmi/time.html
5. What time is lunch? *J Am Diet Assoc* 1996;96.
6. Summer, *see Ch7:16.*
7. Project SPARK, *Sports Play and Active Recreation for Kids,* National Heart, Lung and Blood Institute, March 1995. NIH Healthline, Bethesda, MD (301-496-1766).
8. Seebacher N. Student athletes' health at stake. *HealthSCOUT* 7/9/00.
9. Wisconsin, *see Ch5:52.*
10. Piran N. The Last Word: Prevention of eating disorders: The struggle to chart new territories. *Eating Dis* 1998;6:365-371.
11. Levine MP. 1999 Prevention of eating disorders, eating problems and negative body image. In *Controlling eating disorders with facts, advice and resources,* 2nd ed. R Lemberg. P64-72. Phoenix, AZ: Oryx Press.
12. Johnson, Linda. 1999. *Prevention: Does it really work?* p3-99. Dept. Public Instruction. Bismarck, ND.
13. Price RH, Cowen EL, Lorion RP, et al. edits *14 ounces of prevention: A casebook for practitioners.* Washington, DC: American Psychological Assoc.
14. Latzer Y, and Shatz S. Comprehensive community prevention of distrubed attitudes to weight control: A three-level intervention program. *Eating Disorders* 1999;7:3-31.
15. Levine MP, and Piran N. 1999. Approaches to health promotion in the prevention of the eating disorders. *Unpublished manuscript,* Kenyon College, Gambier, OH.

Piran N. Prevention: Can early lessons lead to delineation of an alternative model? *Eating Dis* 1995;3:28-36.

16. Piran N. Eating disorders: Trial of prevention in a high risk school setting. *J Primary Prevention* 1999;20:75-90.

Piran N. On prevention and trasnformation. *The Renfrew Perspective* 1996;2:1:8-9.

Levine, *see Ch12:15*.

17. Levine MP, Piran N, Stoddard C. Mission more probable: Media literacy, adtivism and advocacy as primary prevention. 1999. In *Preventing Eating Disorders, see below*.

Levine MP, Piran N. Prevention of Eating Disorders: Reflections, conclusions and future directions. 1999. In *Preventing Eating Disorders*, p3-25, eds. N Piran, MP Levine, and C Steiner-Adair. Philadelphia: Brunner/ Mazel.

18. Springer EA, Winzelberg AJ, Perkins R, et al. Effects of a body image curriculum for college students on improved body image. *Int J Eat Disord* 1999;26:13-20.

19. Smolak, *see Ch2:28*.

20. Levine, *see Ch2:5*.

21. Eating Disorders Awareness and Prevention (EDAP). (www.EDAP.org)

22. Garner DM, Reizes JM, Deutsch NL, et al. National Eating disorders Screening Program. Academy for Eating Disorders Annual Meeting, San Diego, 6/11-12/99.

23. Paul, Lynn. *Helping a friend with an eating disorder — What can you do?* Power Point presentation. Lynn Paul, MSU Extension, 101 Romney Hall, Bozeman, MT 59717 (406-994-5702; lpaul@montana.edu).

24. Omichinski L. *Teens & Diets: No Weigh.* HUGS International, Portage la Prairie, Manitoba, Canada.

25. NIH Strategy, *see Ch8:50:51*.

Chapter 13

1. Vitality, *see Ch1:9*.

2. Beck P. Vegetarian Diets. Aug 1990. NDSU Extension Service, Fargo, N.D.

3. Olson R. Folly of restricting fat in the diet of children. *Nutrition Today* 1995;30:6:234-245.

4. Reiner S. CLA: Does fat have a silver lining? *Priorities* 1996;3:4:42-47.

5. RDA, *see Ch9:17*.

6. Kennedy, *see Ch2:2*.

7. Reaching consumers with meaningful health messages: Putting the Dietary Guidelines into action. 1996. Dietary Guidelines Alliance.

8. Hans, *see Ch11:4*.

9. Johnston G. New vision for exercise. *HWJ/Obesity & Health* 1992;6:6:108.

10. HP 2010, *see Ch4:3*.

11. Jaffee L, P Wu. After-school activities and self-esteem in adolescent girls. *Melpomene J*, summer 1996;15:2:18-25; *Shape* Nov. 1995.

12. *J Am Diet Assoc* 1995;95:1414-1417. Berg F. Avoid weight loss focus. *Healthy Weight J* 1996;10:4:75.

13. The physically underdeveloped child, 1984: 0-438-699. USHHS, President's Council on Physical Fitness, Washington, DC.

14. *Melpomene,* Berg, *see Ch9:33*.

Chapter 14

1. Cartner-Morley J. The coat-hanger look is mainstream, but who's to blame? *The Guardian* 6/1/2000.

2. Lawmakers back real clothes sizes. Buenos Aires, *Reuters* 6/22/2000.

3. Pipher, *see Ch2:1*.

4. *EDAP Matters* Spring 1998:5.

5. Huon G. Health promotion and the prevention of dieting-induced disorders. *Eat Disorders* 1996;4:1:27-32.

6. *A new look at adolescent girls: Strengths and stresses*. 1999. Am Psychological Assoc., Wash., DC.

7. NEA, *see Ch7:8*.

8. Whelan, *see Ch9:22*.

9. Berg F. Congress asked to take eating disorders seriously. *Healthy Weight J* 1998;12:41-44.

Chapter 15

1. Berg, *see Ch2:15:122-132*.

2. Berg F. Connecticut law curbs diet claims. *Healthy Weight J* 1996;10:6:109. (Law: 1/10/96, SHB 5621;Pub Act 96-126.) Conn. Dept Consumer Protection, Hartford CT (203-566-4499).

3. *Am J Clin Nutr* 1994;60:153-156. Berg F. Is drug abuse the next miracle cure? *Healthy Weight J* 1994;8:5:84.

Chart references

Chapter 3
1. Berg F. Dysfunctional eating: A new concept. *Healthy Weight Journal* 1996;10:5:88-92.

Chapter 4
1. National Center for Health Statistics. Unpublished data, 1997. NHANES III, Phase 1, 1988-91.
2. NCHS, *see chart ref Ch4:1.*
3. NCHS, *see chart ref Ch4:1.*
4. *Third report nutrition, see Ch1:5.*

Chapter 5
1. JADA, JAMA, Berg, *see Ch5:7.*
2. *Youth Risk Behavior, 1995, see Ch1:7.*

Chapter 6
1. APA, *see Ch6:33.*
2. NEDO materials. National Eating Disorders Organization, 6655 S Yale Ave, Tulsa, OK 74136.

Chapter 8
1. Update: Prevalence of overweight among children, adolescents and adults — U.S., 1988-1994. MMWR March 7, 1997;46:9:199-202.
   Troiano, *see Ch8:2.*
2. Update, *see chart ref Ch8:1.*
3. Bouchard, Berg, *see Ch8:13.*
   Berg, *Health Risks Obesity, see Ch8:12.*
4. Klesges R. J Applied Behavior Analysis. Winter 1983.

Chapter 9
1. *Youth Risk Behavior, 1995, see Ch1:7.*
2. *Youth Risk Behavior, 1995, see Ch1:7.*
   Surgeon General's Report on Physical Activity and Health, NHIS-YRBS data, 1996, CDC, HHS, PHS.

Chapter 10
1. *Vitality, see Ch1:9.*

Chapter 11
1. Plain talk about adolescence. National Institute of Mental Health, USDHHS. Rockville, MD. See also: An Adolescent in Your Home, and Parent-Teenager Communication. Consumer Info. Center, Pueblo, CO 81009.

2. Wisconsin, *see Ch5:52.*
3. Levine M. 10 things parents can do to help prevent eating disorders. Menninger, EDAP.
4. 10 tips for Dads with Daughters. 1-888-824-DADS; www.dadsanddaughters.org.
5. Ikeda J. With permission, from *If My Child Is Too Fat, What Should I Do About It?* Booklet for parents. University of Calif.
6. Satter E. *Feeding with Love and Good Sense: Training Manual.* 1995. Ellyn Satter Associates, Madison, WI.

Chapter 12
1. 10 things coaches can do to help prevent eating disorders in their athletes. NEDO Newsl. EDAP. Eating disorders Awareness & Prevention.
2. Levine M. and Maine M. *Guide to the primary prevention of eating disorders,* brochure EDAP. 1993, 1999. Eating disorders Awareness & Prevention, www.edap.org.

Chapter 13
1. *Dietary Guidelines for Americans,* 1995. USDA, USDHHS.
2. *Dietary Guidelines for Americans,* 5th edition, 2000, USDA, USDHHS.

Index

Chart index

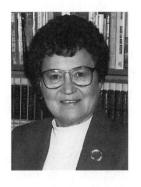 An internationally known authority on eating and weight, FRANCES M. BERG, M.S., LN, is a licensed nutritionist, family wellness specialist, and Adjunct Professor at the University of North Dakota School of Medicine. As the editor and founder of *Healthy Weight Journal,* Berg has reported eating and weight-related research for over 16 years to health professionals and educators worldwide.

The author of ten books and a weekly column, *Healthy Living,* published in more than 50 newspapers, she has presented at numerous national and international conferences, and been a guest on national television, including Oprah, Leeza and Inside Edition. Her master's degree in family social science and anthropology is from the University of Minnesota, and she holds a Family and Consumer Science degree from Montana State University.

Francie Berg serves as National Coordinator of the Task Force on Weight Loss Abuse, National Council Against Health Fraud, and on advisory boards working with prevention of childhood obesity, eating disorders, and quality health care for people of all sizes. She is a member of the Society for Nutrition Education (Chair of Weight Realities Division), the Academy for Eating Disorders, the North American Association for the Study of Obesity, the National Association to Advance Fat Acceptance, and the Society for the Study of Ingestive Behavior. She has four children and lives with her husband Bert, a veterinarian, in Hettinger, North Dakota.

A personal note

A question I'm often asked is: Why did you write this book? The easy answer is that I was growing more and more concerned as I read the appalling research on kids' eating problems, and as I watched that research personified in the gaunt, vacant-looking girls I was seeing everywhere at high school basketball games, hanging out in malls, in school hallways, wherever kids gather.

Someone has to do it, I kept thinking uneasily. Someone needs to tell parents and teachers what's happening, and why we can't do this to our kids. But no one did. And when I'd tell other writers in the field of my concerns, they'd say, it's you. But I didn't want to take a year out of my already busy life.

There were personal reasons, too. I'd experienced acute pain in the seasonal dieting of our two wrestling sons. Both were champion high school wrestlers in the lower weights, and every wrestling parent knows what that means: they cut weight, cut food and even cut water to "make weight" for each match.

Still, this isn't the complete answer. In Vancouver a Canadian dietitian told me, "We need to know where you're coming from, it will help us process our own feelings. We can accept others, but it's not easy to accept ourselves."

So yes, there's more. I can understand the desperation to lose weight, because I recall only too well how, as an overweight teenager, I lived through the miseries of gazing into the mirror wishing I could pull off a hunk here, and here, of watching my best resolutions dissolve into uncontrolled eating binges.

Then by a lucky accident I lost my excess weight. I was on my first job out of college, living alone, trying each new diet that came along. I'd begin the diet with enthusiasm and high hopes — and always lose weight. But as the excitement faded the pounds returned. The diets made no real changes in my life, except they kept me thinking about food and weight and hunger. I skipped meals and filled up on snack foods. I fasted and binged by turns.

The lucky accident came when I happened to acquire a roommate with amazingly simple and sensible eating habits. Unlike my other friends, Carol didn't diet. She didn't even talk about dieting. She didn't need to, I told myself — she was slender and athletic.

Carol insisted straight off that we eat three meals each day beginning with a good breakfast. She couldn't mean scrambled eggs, toast and cereal? She did. I was dismayed. Breakfast was the one meal I could and did skip with ease.

Reluctantly I gave in, sure I'd gain weight fast. (At the same time, I knew she was right. As a nutrition educator, I taught the value of balanced meals. I just didn't apply it to myself.)

Nonetheless, Carol won me over. At noon we fixed quick hot food, such as soup and toasted cheese sandwiches. Our evening meals were based solidly on meat, potatoes, vegetables, salad, bread and milk. I couldn't get Carol to understand that I'd certainly fatten up on such fare. She'd just look at me in mild surprise and say, "Well sure, we have to eat potatoes. We need to keep up our strength."

No more eating on the run, reading as I ate, rushing back to work, hunger unsatisfied. Carol insisted we sit at the table and enjoy the food. Meals became a relaxing and pleasant time.

A couple of months passed before I happened to step on a scale. What a surprise. The scale was wrong, I thought. How could I have shed 10 pounds without so much as a struggle? But it was no mistake. My clothes began fitting easier. Soon I bought them in a smaller size.

Surprisingly, I wasn't caught up in the fervor of losing weight as I had been in the past. I was busy, active and having fun. My stomach was satisfied and my days were filled. Food just wasn't very important in my life anymore. Even my precise weight wasn't important. The pounds slipped off rather slowly, but in a natural, painless and lasting way. That year I lost another 10 pounds and some months later another 10. My weight stabilized at about 125 pounds — the very point I'd struggled so long and hopelessly to reach. All those years of agonized dieting, frustration and despair had accomplished exactly nothing. It was only when I forgot about eating and turned my energy toward other areas of living that I shed my excess weight in a lasting way.

The weight stayed off naturally until my fourth baby was born. I tried a couple of diets, then decided to recreate that earlier experience: gradually change some bad habits and let the weight come off as it may. I returned to eating normally, dropped those "Mommy habits" I'd acquired — nibbling when fixing a meal, clearing up, unloading groceries, skipping meals because I "wasn't hungry." I began running a couple of miles a day, which I'd always loved, and which has been a continuing pleasure. This time I used a contract system and records to keep track of habit changes, and again over the course of a year the extra weight came off.

Then midlife came along, and with it 15 pounds or so. Research tells me this is normal. Nearly all women gain some weight (and it tends to settle around the middle). By this time I was reading sad studies about the bitter fights many women put up against this, even into their 70's or 80's, and I recalled my aunt at 86, 120 pounds, wondering how to rid herself of that tummy roll.

Should I double my activity, then? No. Sure, that could make a difference, but it's not worth it. I enjoy my life, just as it is. If this weight gain is normal, maybe there's a good reason. And there is — a little extra weight is protective against the fragile bones and osteoporosis that many women suffer at midlife, especially if they're thin or dieting. Research suggests it may be protective in other ways, too. So I'm happy to regard it as natural and protective — and a good time to buy some new clothes.

America is afraid to eat!

Learn how you can break free, live free and
help others attain health at any size —

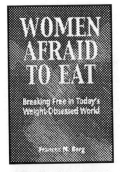

■ **Women Afraid to Eat: Breaking Free
in Today's Weight-Obsessed World**
A startling indictment on the obsession with thinness
and its devastating effect on women. Examines the crisis in eating, weight and body image, and gives clear
guidelines on how women can move ahead in healthy
ways. An innovative and thought-provoking book!

384 pages   19.95 softcover   0-918532-62-0
               27.95 hardcover   0-918532-63-9

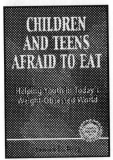

■ **Children and Teens Afraid to Eat: Helping
Youth in Today's Weight-Obsessed World**
At last, a book that challenges America's obsession
with weight and documents its tragic effect on children.
Helps parents, teachers and health professionals find
new ways to nurture youth and promote wellness and
wholeness for every child of every size!

352 pages   19.95 softcover   0-918532-55-8
               27.95 hardcover   0-918532-56-6

Both are award-winning books by Frances M. Berg. Visit our website for more information and valuable resources using the Health at Any Size approach.

www.healthyweight.net

✁ —

	Softcover	Hardcover
Women Afraid to Eat	___ $19.95	. . . . ___ $27.95
Children and Teens Afraid to Eat	___ $19.95	. . . . ___ $27.95

Shipping: $3.20 1st book, $1.50 ea. add'l book.   Subtotal   _____

(U.S. priority; Foreign surface)   Shipping   _____

We accept check, VISA or MasterCard.   TOTAL   _____

Name _____

Address _____

_____

_____

CALL, MAIL OR FAX TO: Healthy Weight Network, 402 S 14th St, Hettinger, ND 58639
Tel 701-567-2646•Fax 701-567-2602•hwj@healthyweight.net•www.healthyweight.net

REVIEWER ACCLAIM FOR

Women Afraid to Eat

"Highly recommended to all readers"

THE MOST COMPREHENSIVE AND SOCIALLY responsible guide to dealing with weight-obsession available to date. Its scope, intensity and integrity is simply unparalleled.

Berg systematically and eloquently argues that women need to know the risks associated with extreme dieting: "It's time to confess we don't know the answers . . . Time to get serious about solving weight problems instead of letting weak or unethical leaders, a relentless diet industry, doctors who dispense 'rainbow pills,' advertisers and the media lead us into even deeper trouble."

Highly recommended to all readers — from undergraduates and the general public to faculty and professionals.
— *CHOICE, American Library Association*

THIS BOOK SPEAKS THE PAINFUL TRUTH all women need to hear so that we can come home to our bodies.
— *Jeanine Cogan, PhD, Research Psychologist*
Washington, D.C.

A MUCH-NEEDED BOOK. . . . The author addresses the problems while providing direction in how to break free with a new approach that helps people and does not harm them. . . . Includes self-help tools, questionnaires, health-centered resources, websites, references, and an index.
— *Doody's Journal, Health Sciences Libraries*

A MUST READ for women . . . an amazing read for men!
— *Nancy King, MS, RD, Nutrition Therapist*
La Canada, Calif.

THE GURU OF THE NONDIETING MOVEMENT has struck again. Frances Berg scores a direct hit, plunging an arrow into the heart of the dieting industry. . . . (She) plunks the missing piece into the puzzle with a resounding "clink" — a federal policy that works too closely with the weight-loss industry.

Berg reiterates her theme that weight loss is disproportionately promoted as the means to improve health to the detriment of women. Well-written, thought-provoking . . . a reference as well as an inspiration . . . belongs on every dietitian's bookshelf.

— *Today's Dietitian*

PACKED WITH INSIGHT AND INFORMATION relevant to the plight of women today living in a weight-obsessed world. Berg exposes the unhealthy collusion between government, pharmaceutical companies, and scientific research in the multi-billion dollar a year diet industry.

— *Ventures, American Dietetic Association*

FRANCIE'S WORK IS CONSISTENTLY on the cutting edge. She asks questions that must be answered if we are to truly assist people in improving health.

— *Karin Kratina, MA, RD, PhD*
Eating Disorder Therapist, Cocoanut Creek, Fla.

"HEALTH AT ANY SIZE!" is this book's emphatic message to American women. Berg argues that the media and society cause women to obsess over the numbers on the scale and subsequently abuse their bodies and minds.

Recommended for libraries serving consumers, educators, health professionals.

— *Library Journal*

AN EXCEPTIONAL BOOK that can help high school students improve their health and well-being.

— *What's New Magazine*

A COMPREHENSIVE OVERVIEW of our major weight and eating problems, and a delightfully simple, integrated framework for working to resolve them. . . . All of this is packaged in a personal, easy-to-read style.

— *Gail Marchessault, RD, PhD (Cand.), Winnipeg, Canada*

EVERY PAGE IS PACKED with information, support and encouragement for women of all sizes. Bravo!

— *Pat Lyons, RN, MA, Co-Author, Great Shape*

AMERICAN WOMEN ARE CAUGHT UP in a body-image crisis, afraid they'll gain weight, afraid they will not lose down to their goal, afraid to fully nourish themselves. *Women Afraid to Eat* probes why this is happening at a time when women have more freedom than ever before. . . . How did it happen that a woman's value now is being judged by her degree of slimness, not her talent, insight or generosity?

All public libraries will want at least two copies, one for the reference desk and a second for the circulating collection.

— Public Library Quarterly

WOMEN AFRAID TO EAT is a refreshing antidote to our culture's preoccupation with weight. . . . Affirming, liberating, and a must-read for any woman who has ever obsessed over the size of her thighs.

— Sally E. Smith, Editor, BBW Magazine

A DANGEROUS EPIDEMIC is plaguing women desperate to lose weight: They've become too afraid to eat! In her startling new book *Women Afraid To Eat*, Berg warns that the all-too-common end result is damage to the body from dysfunctional eating and to the mind from distorted self-image.

— eDIETS.com

FRANCIE KNOWS THE RESEARCH and presents it in a way that the reader cannot but be profoundly changed for having listened to her arguments.

— Monika M. Woolsey, MS, RD, After the Diet Newsletter

SHOWS IN STARTLING DETAIL what the current warped norm for body shape is doing to women, how it harms them physically, emotionally, and socially. . . . *Women Afraid to Eat* is also a handbook for change at the personal and cultural level. It offers women positive feelings, reaffirming that they can be healthy and attractive at any size.

— Midwest Book Review

SHOULD BE REQUIRED READING for all students in medical, nursing or dietetics programs. Perhaps then they would not be so flippant in recommending weight loss.

— Joanne Ikeda, MA, RD, State Nutrition
Specialist, University of California Berkeley